D1446653

Diet, Nutrition, and Health

Diet, Nutrition, and Health

Edited by
K.K. Carroll, F.R.S.C.

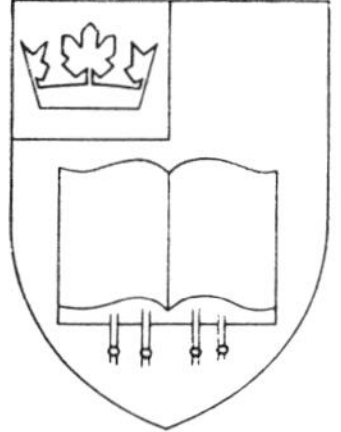

Published for the Royal Society of Canada by
McGill-Queen's University Press
Montreal & Kingston • London • Buffalo

ISBN 0-7735-0741-8 (paper)
ISBN 0-7735-0733-7 (cloth)
Legal deposit first quarter 1990
Bibliothèque nationale du Québec

Printed in Canada on acid-free paper

Canadian Cataloguing in Publication Data

Main entry under title:
Diet, nutrition, and health

"These papers were prepared for a symposium held at the University of Western Ontario, London, Ontario, Canada, 27 to 30 May, 1987, under the sponsorship of the Royal Society of Canada and the Food and Nutrition Board of the U.S. National Research Council – National Academy of Sciences."
Includes bibliographical references.
ISBN 0-7735-0733-7 (bound) –
ISBN 0-7735-0741-8 (pbk.).

1. Nutrition. 2. Diet in disease. 3. Nutritionally induced diseases. I. Carroll, K. K. (Kenneth Kitchener) II. Royal Society of Canada. III. National Research Council (U.S.). Food and Nutrition Board.

RA784.D43 1989 613.2 C89-090357-3

These papers were prepared for a symposium held at the University of Western Ontario, London, Ontario, Canada, 27 to 30 May 1987, under the sponsorship of the Royal Society of Canada and the Food and Nutrition Board of the U.S. National Research Council – National Academy of Sciences.

Contents

Foreword/K.K. Carroll
xi

Acknowledgments
xv

Contributors
xix

KEYNOTE ADDRESS

W.P.T. JAMES
Dietary Guidelines and the Development of a European Policy
3

DIET AND CARDIOVASCULAR DISEASE

RICHARD J. HAVEL
Dietary and Hereditary Factors in Coronary Heart Disease
19

SONJA L. CONNOR AND WILLIAM E. CONNOR
Coronary Heart Disease: Prevention and Treatment by Nutritional Change
33

J. ALICK LITTLE
Coronary Heart Disease Prevention Trials
73

PIRJO PIETINEN
A Public Health Program for Prevention of Cardiovascular Disease
85

DIET AND SELECTED HEALTH PROBLEMS

NORMAN M. KAPLAN
Diet and Hypertension
93

THOMAS M.S. WOLEVER AND DAVID J.A. JENKINS
Diet and Diabetes
103

DANIEL A.K. RONCARI
Individual Susceptibility to Obesity in Response to Dietary Factors
121

WILLIAM E. MITCH
Diet and Kidney Disease
130

DIET AND HEALTH MAINTENANCE

ERNST L. WYNDER, J. BARONE, AND JAMES R. HEBERT
The Role of Diet in the Maintenance of Health throughout Life
141

PHILIP J. GARRY AND ROBERT L. RHYNE
Nutritional Problems of the Elderly
155

HAROLD KALANT
Alcohol Use and Nutrition
176

ANTHONY B. HODSMAN
Diet in Relation to Osteoporosis
188

DIET AND CANCER

TAKASHI SUGIMURA, KEIJI WAKABAYASHI,
MINAKO NAGAO, AND HIROKO OHGAKI
Mutagens and Carcinogens Formed during Cooking
207

JOZEF V. JOOSSENS AND J. GEBOERS
Salt, Stomach Cancer, and Stroke
229

ANTHONY B. MILLER
Epidemiology of Breast and Colon Cancer
243

DAVID KRITCHEVSKY
Calories and Cancer
250

DIETARY GUIDELINES

C. WAYNE CALLAWAY
Development and Use of Dietary Guidelines for Whole Populations versus Populations at Risk
259

LEWIS E. LLOYD AND CLAIRE CRONIER
Dietary Guidelines: Implications for Agriculture
268

GILBERT A. LEVEILLE
Dietary Guidelines: Steps for the Food Industry
284

HEATHER NIELSEN
Dietary Guidelines: Steps for Dietitians/Public Health Nutritionists
287

JOAN DYE GUSSOW
Dietary Guidelines: Steps for Nutrition Educators
292

RICHARD B. GOLDBLOOM
Nutrition, Diet, and Health: The Physician's Role
298

JOYCE L. BEARE-ROGERS
Dietary Guidelines: Steps by Government Agencies
303

PUBLIC HEALTH AND MORTALITY

JOHN CAIRNS
The History of Mortality
309

Index
345

K.K. CARROLL

Foreword

Diet is a subject that interests everyone, and many people are concerned to know whether their diet is providing good nutrition. Much of the concern stems from evidence that diet has significant effects on health and on susceptibility to various chronic diseases, including heart disease and cancer. This has resulted in a great renaissance in the science of nutrition in recent years. The increased emphasis on research in nutrition has encompassed nearly every component of the diet, including the macronutrients (protein, carbohydrate and fat), the micronutrients (vitamins and minerals) and non-nutritive dietary components such as fibre.

These were some of the considerations that led to a proposal that the Royal Society of Canada sponsor a symposium on Diet, Nutrition and Health. It appeared that the topic was timely, and that the subject would be of interest to many segments of the population. It was also felt that a symposium on this topic would serve as a stimulus to further emphasis on nutrition research and teaching in Canada.

It seemed particularly appropriate that such a symposium be sponsored by the Royal Society, whose membership encompasses a wide range of disciplines including the arts, the humanities, and the physical, biological and social sciences. The Society was founded over one hundred years ago, in 1882, with the objective of promoting learning and research in the arts and sciences. One of its founding members was Sir William Osler, the greatest physician of his day.

In pursuing its objective, the Society arranges separate symposia, as well as those at annual meetings, for the presentation and discussion of national issues, on matters of interest to the membership and the public. Thus, when the proposal to sponsor a symposium on diet, nutrition and health was considered and approved by the committee on symposia, they indicated that they would prefer to hold it as a separate event rather than as part of an annual meeting. They also suggested that it be held at the University of Western Ontario, commenting that the Society had never sponsored a symposium in London, Ontario, and would welcome an opportunity to do so.

As the symposium was being planned, the Food and Nutrition Board of the U.S. National Research Council-National Academy of Sciences appointed a committee to conduct a three-year study on Diet and Health. Because of their interest in the subject, the Food and Nutrition Board agreed to co-sponsor the symposium on Diet, Nutrition and Health. This is particularly appropriate since Canada and the United States share mutual concerns over the role of diet in health and disease and since fellow scientists from the United States made an important contribution by their participation in the symposium.

This volume contains the proceedings of the symposium, which was held in Middlesex Theatre Auditorium at the University of Western Ontario on May 27th to 30th, 1987. The aim was to provide an overview of the role of diet in maintaining good health and minimizing the risk of chronic disease. The theme also included the development and implementation of dietary guidelines for this purpose, and the opening session on the evening of May 27th featured a keynote address on Development of Dietary Guidelines in Britain and Other European Countries.

The program for the next two days consisted of four sessions of four speakers each, dealing with various aspects of the role of diet in health and disease. The first session was devoted to cardiovascular disease, which is the major cause of death in Canada and for which there is a long history of dietary guidelines. Four diet-related health problems were selected for discussion in the second session: hypertension, diabetes, obesity, and kidney disease. The third session opened with a presentation on the role of diet in maintenance of health throughout life and continued with surveys of nutritional problems of the elderly, concerns over alcohol usage, and a discussion of osteoporosis. The fourth session dealt with diet and cancer, a developing field which has been the subject of much recent research.

The final half-day of the symposium featured two presentations on the development, use and implications of dietary guidelines. These were followed by a panel discussion of the implementation of dietary guidelines, including steps for the food industry, dietitians, public health nutritionists, nutrition educators, the medical profession, and government agencies.

Social events included a trip to the Shakespearian Theatre in the neighbouring city of Stratford, and a banquet in the Great Hall of the University of Western Ontario. The latter was followed by an after-dinner address on the History of Mortality, the text of which is included as part of the proceedings.

This permanent record of presentations given at the symposium contains information of interest to biomedical scientists (not necessarily experts in the field), nutritionists, dietitians and other professionals concerned with interpretation of research findings and their implementation for the general public. It can also be read for pleasure and profit by the educated lay person.

Acknowledgments

The encouragement and support of the Royal Society of Canada in the organization of this symposium are gratefully acknowledged. Dr. Keith Laidler, the Chairman of the Committee on Symposia, provided helpful advice and suggestions, and the Executive Secretary of the Society, Pierre Garneau, and members of his office staff assisted greatly by accepting responsibility for the financial arrangements, correspondence, printing of the program, registration and other administrative details. The new Executive Director, Michael Dence, the Editor of the Royal Society Publications, Dr. John M. Robson, and Philip Cercone of McGill-Queen's University Press, have been very helpful in the preparation of this volume. The then President of the Royal Society, Dr. Alexander McKay, graciously participated in the opening ceremonies of the symposium by giving an overview of the history and activities of the Royal Society of Canada.

I am particularly indebted to Dr. Sushma Palmer, the Executive Director of the Food and Nutrition Board, U.S. National Research Council-National Academy of Sciences, for her assistance in developing the program for the symposium, in preparing the statement of purpose, and in co-chairing the final session of the symposium. The Chairman of the Food and Nutrition Board, Dr. Kurt Isselbacher, was present at the opening ceremonies and gave a description of the organization and activities of the Food and Nutrition Board.

The National Institute of Nutrition of Canada supported the symposium by sponsoring Dr. Takashi Sugimura as the NIN lecturer. The former President of the Institute, Dr. Keith Murray, and the Council provided valuable advice during development of the symposium program, and the new President, Dr. Nancy Schwartz, participated in the opening session by providing a summary of the aims and activities of the Institute during the three years of its existence.

We are grateful to the University of Western Ontario for the use of its facilities and for the excellent cooperation provided by the staff in the physical arrangements for the symposium, including residence accommodation and food services. The President of the University, Dr. K. George Pedersen, attended the opening ceremony and welcomed participants to the symposium and to the University.

The symposium would not have been possible without the financial support provided by a number of different organizations whose contributions are greatly appreciated. I also wish to express my personal appreciation to the members of the symposium committee and to those who served as chairmen of symposium sessions and assisted in the work of editing this volume. These individuals and the organizations that provided financial support are listed below:

Financial Contributors

Agriculture Canada, Research Branch
Boehringer Mannheim Canada
Canadian Atherosclerosis Society
Canadian Life & Health Insurance Association Inc.
Canadian Meat Council
General Mills Canada Inc.
Health and Welfare Canada
Heart & Stroke Foundation of Ontario
Hoffmann-La Roche Ltd.
Medical Research Council of Canada
Mutual Life Insurance Co. of Canada
National Institute of Nutrition
Ontario Government Hospitality Fund
Ontario Ministry of Health
Parke-Davis Canada Inc.
University of Western Ontario

Symposium Committee

Ms. E.J. Brownridge, HBB & Associates, London, Ontario
Dr. S.E. Evers, Dept. of Health Studies, University of Waterloo, Waterloo, Ontario

Dr. P.M. Giovannetti, Dept. of Home Economics, Brescia College, University of Western Ontario
Dr. J.T. Hamilton, Assistant Dean of Medicine (Research), University of Western Ontario
Dr. J.A. Leith, Dept. of History, Queen's University, Kingston, Ontario (representing the Academy of Humanities and Social Sciences of the Royal Society of Canada)
Dr. G.J. Mogenson, Dean of Graduate Studies, University of Western Ontario
Dr. K. O'Hea, Dept. of Physiology, University of Western Ontario
Dr. R. Roth, Dept. of Zoology, University of Western Ontario
Dr. M.-A. Tremblay, Dept. of Anthropology, Université Laval, Québec City, Québec (representing l'Académie des Lettres et des Sciences humaines of the Royal Society of Canada)
Dr. B.M. Wolfe, Dept. of Medicine, University of Western Ontario
Chairman: Dr. K.K. Carroll, Dept. of Biochemistry, University of Western Ontario

Session Chairmen

Dr. G. Harvey Anderson, Dept. of Nutritional Sciences, University of Toronto
Dr. Aubie Angel, Clinical Sciences Division, University of Toronto
Dr. W. Robert Bruce, Ludwig Institute for Cancer Research, Toronto, Ontario
Dr. Kenneth K. Carroll, Dept. of Biochemistry, University of Western Ontario
Dr. Harold H. Draper, Dept. of Nutrition, University of Guelph
Dr. John Dupre, Dept. of Medicine, University of Western Ontario
Dr. M. Daria Haust, Dept. of Pathology, University of Western Ontario
Dr. Sushma Palmer, Food and Nutrition Board, U.S. National Research Council-National Academy of Sciences, Washington, D.C.
Dr. Bernard M. Wolfe, Dept. of Medicine, University of Western Ontario
Dr. Ernst Wynder, American Health Foundation, New York, N.Y.

Contributors

Ms J. Barone
American Health Foundation
320 East 43rd Street
New York, NY 10017

Dr. Joyce L. Beare-Rogers
Health Protection Branch
Health & Welfare Canada
Tunney's Pasture
Ottawa, Ontario K1A OL2

Dr. John Cairns
Department of Cancer Biology
Harvard School of Public Health
Boston, MA 02115

Dr C. Wayne Callaway
2112 F Street N.W.
Suite 703
Washington, DC 20037

Dr Kenneth K. Carroll
Department of Biochemistry
Room M316, Health Sciences Centre
University of Wesern Ontario
London, Ontario N6A 5C1

Dr Sonja L. Connor
Department of Medicine
Oregon Health Sciences University
Sam Jackson Park Road
Portland, OR 97201

Dr William E. Connor
Department of Medicine
Oregon Health Sciences University
Sam Jackson Park Road
Portland, OR 97201

Ms Claire Cronier
Food Research Centre
Research Branch
Agriculture Canada
Ottawa, Ontario K1A OC6

Dr Philip J. Garry
University of New Mexico
School of Medicine
Surge Building, Room 236
Clinical Nutrition Laboratory
2701 Frontier Place N.E.
Albuquerque, NM 87131

J. Geboers
Division of Epidemiology
School of Public Health
Sint-Rafael University Hospital
University of Leuven
Leuven, Belgium

Dr Richard B. Goldbloom
Isaac Walton Killam Hospital
5850 University Avenue
Halifax, Nova Scotia B3J 3G9

Dr Joan Dye Gussow
Department of Nutrition Education
Teachers College
Columbia University
P.O. Box 137
New York, NY 10027

Dr Richard J. Havel
Cardiovascular Research Institute
University of California
School of Medicine
San Francisco, CA 94143

Dr. James R. Hebert
Division of Preventive
and Behavioural Medicine
University of Massachusetts
Medical Center
55 Lake Avenue North
Worcester, MA 01655

Dr Anthony B. Hodsman
Department of Medicine
St Joseph's Hospital
268 Grosvenor Street
London, Ontario N6A 4V2

Dr W.P.T. James, Director
Rowett Reseach Institute
Greenburn Road
Bucksburn, Aberdeen
AB2 9SB UK

Dr David J.A. Jenkins
Department of Nutritional Sciences
University of Toronto
Toronto, Ontario M5S 1A8

Dr Jozef V. Joossens
Division of Epidemiology
School of Public Health
Sint-Rafael University Hospital
University of Leuven
Leuven, Belgium

Dr Harold Kalant
Addiction Research Foundation
33 Russell Street
Toronto, Ontario M5S 2S1

Dr Norman M. Kaplan
University of Texas
Health Sciences Center
5323 Harry Hines Boulevard
Dallas, TX 75235

Dr David Kritchevsky
Associate Director
The Wistar Institute
36th & Spruce Streets
Philadelphia, PA 19104

Dr Gilbert A. Leveille
Nabisco Brands Inc.
DeForest Avenue
East Hanover, NJ 07936

Dr J. Alick Little
Clinical Investigation Unit
St Michael's Hospital
Toronto, Ontario M5B 1W8

Dr Lewis E. Lloyd
Food Research Centre
Research Branch
Agriculture Canada
Ottawa, Ontario K1A 0C6

Dr Anthony B. Miller
NCIC Epidemiology Unit
McMurrich Building
University of Toronto
Toronto, Ontario M5S 1A1

Dr William E. Mitch
Department of Medicine
Emory University School of Medicine
1364 Clifton Road N.E.
Atlanta, GA 30322

Dr Minako Nagao
National Cancer Center
1-1, Tsukiji 5-chome, Chuo-ku
Tokyo 104, Japan

Mrs Heather Nielsen
Nutrition Programs Unit
Health Promotion Directorate
Health and Welfare Canada
Tunney's Pasture
Ottawa, Ontario K1A 1B4

Dr Hiroko Ohgaki
National Cancer Center
1-1, Tsukiji 5-chome, Chuo-ku
Tokyo 104, Japan

Dr Pirjo Pietinen
National Public Health Institute
Department of Epidemiology
Mannerheiminitie 166
Helsinki, Finland 00280

Dr Daniel A.K. Roncari
Sunnybrook Medical Centre
2075 Bayview Avenue
Toronto, Ontario M4N 3M5

Dr. Robert Rhyne
Department of Family, Community and Emergency Medicine
University of New Mexico School of Medicine
Albuquerque, NM 87131

Dr Takashi Sugimura, President
National Cancer Center
1-1, Tsukiji 5-chome, Chuo-ku
Tokyo 104, Japan

Dr Keiji Wakabayashi
National Cancer Center
1-1, Tsukiji 5-chome, Chuo-ku
Tokyo 104, Japan

Dr Thomas M.S. Wolever
Department of Nutritional Sciences
University of Toronto
Toronto, Ontario M5S 1A8

Dr Ernst L. Wynder, President
American Health Foundation
320 East 43rd Street
New York, NY 10017

Keynote Address

W.P.T. JAMES

Dietary Guidelines and the Development of a European Policy

Those of us engaged in medical and nutritional research all too often fail to understand the difference between the three entirely different processes involved in initiating a program of health promotion, that is medical/nutritional research, policy-making, and, finally, the practical implementation of policy by health promotion in its widest sense. Only too clear, however, is the need to produce coherent, simple documents that illustrate and explain the link between diet and disease. And non specialists need such tools if they are to understand and use the information efficiently. Such an undertaking would, of course, from a research scientist's point of view, need a major treatise.

Policy-making is an area in which few clinical scientists are skilled. In the analysis of the research base for policy-making, many experts contribute their own findings while critically assessing data in fields ranging from epidemiology through clinical studies, metabolic investigations, animal studies, and detailed cellular biochemistry. Indeed much of our training is geared to the unceasing drive to maintain a critical, even sceptical, view of new evidence. Yet in policy-making one must take a broad view, recognizing that proof of efficacy and validity of a particular community program will often be obtained only after the proposal of a policy change. Yet, as laboratory scientists, even though we might want to implement that specific program, it is best to be cautious in intervening if there seem to be risks from intervention, but bold in proposing change if the prevalence of a disease in the population is high and the probability of successful intervention reasonably good. Of course judging the balance of evidence is very difficult my assessment would be that those unwilling to sully themselves with such crude assessments are best left in their laboratories, there to nurture their critical faculties! Unfortunately, a widely acclaimed academic is often assumed, incorrectly, to be suitable for policy-making.

The third component requires translation of that policy into practical action. Such an activity requires a variety of processes and skills unfamiliar to many people in both the medical science or policy-making areas. For many years we in Europe have neglected this third component medical field. Indeed, within Europe, and particularly in Britain, the critical scientist so dominates, culturally, that any proposal for a health promotion campaign would be greeted with suspicion or scorn. Such an attitude, combined with a highly conservative medical establishment, only handicaps the process. In fact the various Royal Colleges of Physicians may soon find themselves drawn into maintaining traditional stances rather than fulfilling their role as leaders. The cautious nature of British policy-making will thus be further amplified, underlined by groups within the food industry who perceive that their livelihood may be threatened by changes in the population's eating patterns.

Developing a Food Policy in Britain: The Political Dimension

In Britain, the Department of Health issued guidelines in 1974 which called for a reduction in the population's dietary fat intake and particularly in the intake of saturated fatty acids. No specification for the degree of change was given nor advice on how to alter the national diet. The report was set in very cautious scientific terms. As a result no national policy or practical measures were developed; British preventive medicine drifted, with the U.K. becoming the European country noted for its neglect of health promotion and for its conservative stance on nutritionally related diseases.

The one bright spot was the Royal College of Physicians which, under its then President, Sir Douglas Black, set up working parties and produced reports on the prevention of coronary heart disease (1), on the role of dietary fibre in health and disease (2), and on the importance of obesity (3). These reports highlighted the public health significance of the national diet and the need to promote a different pattern of eating. The 1976 report on cardiovascular disease was produced in conjunction with the British Cardiac Society and was remarkable in many ways. It specified a goal for average national nutrient intakes for the first time in Britain, specified the extent to which the average diet of the population should change, and produced a coherent set of dietary guidelines for use by the medical profession and by the public. The report, however, had little impact, perhaps because neither the Royal College nor the British Cardiac Society had any mechanism for developing the next step, i.e., a health promotion program. Indeed, neither organization has much expertise in relating to journalists, still less in initiating a coherent national campaign. The report may, however, have stimulated the Department of Health to produce a booklet called *Eating for Health* (4) which included, surprisingly, a call for a reduction in sugar intake in an effort to control dental caries. This is the only report produced by the British government so far which includes a recommendation on sugar.

Most attempts to have sugar discussed as a specific or general health problem in Britain have provided an illustration of how any political decision relating to food can become a very contentious issue. In the case of sugar there are well recognized vested interests which have long been known to organize highly co-ordinated campaigns in public and private to ensure that sugar intake is maintained. Thus sceptical nutritional scientists have been nurtured through a series of well publicized conferences organized on a lavish scale and the individual scientist's research has been bolstered by commercially sponsored research grants. Only recently has the possible link between commercial research funding and the public stance of nutritionists been highlighted after a year of detailed analysis of public and other records. This link has now been published by a campaigning investigative journalist, Geoffrey Cannon (5), who is widely perceived as the scourge of a cosy network of academics, civil servants, and industry.

Despite the British tradition for settling matters of public interest in the privacy of government offices, it became apparent in the late 1970s that the British public had an extreme interest in diet and its relationship to health. This became clear when the British Broadcasting Corporation began a series of short nutrition and health education programs. The emphasis in these programs was, for the first time, on the role of diet in diseases of public health importance and was produced with a popular entertainer who used the author as an "expert." The response from the public, retailers, and food manufacturers was remarkable; complaints from the millers and retailers came thick and fast because they were unprepared to meet the new massive demand for foods with a lower fat, higher fibre content! They then started intense advertising for particular food products. However, some sectors of the food industry, the sugar sector for example, were alerted to the possible damage to their trade and began to prepare their defences.

In parallel with these developments attempts were being made to produce a coherent set of practical dietary guidelines for use by schools, health visitors, health educationalists, and the Health Education Council. To this end a National Advisory Committee on Nutrition Education (NACNE) had been formed by both the Health Education Council and the British Nutrition Foundation. This Foundation is wholly supported by the food industry but aims to act as an independent source of impartial information on food and nutrition as well as serving as a focus for nutritional scientists and doctors to interact with representatives of the food industry. The NACNE committee in 1980 invited two nutritional advisers (Mr Derek Miller and myself) onto the main committee to seek guidance on what constituted the current perceptions on nutrition and health. It soon became clear that the committee's professional groups had a perspective on nutrition which could only be described as very old fashioned; dominant was the idea that nutritional problems were only to be seen in a small minority of vulnerable groups in society, e.g. in pre-term babies, immigrants, and the elderly. Otherwise the only requirement was to teach children how to avoid protein and vitamin deficiencies.

However, once a totally different approach had been outlined to the committee relating diet to the problems of obesity, cardiovascular disease, bowel disorders, and dental health, it became clear that a new simple document for those involved in health and nutrition education was needed. To this end I was asked to organize a meeting to establish the new proposals while retaining the principle of relying on policy documents generated by authoritative bodies such as the Royal College of Physicians, WHO, and the government. As the need for practical, coherent, and quantified advice became evident, a set of nutritional goals were produced, essentially based on the WHO document for the prevention of coronary heart disease and on the Royal College Report on Obesity which I was drafting at the same time. It soon became apparent, however, that the officials representing the Department of Health and the British Nutrition Foundation (BNF) were very unhappy with what they perceived as new policy-making. The Department of Health resented the usurping of their power and the BNF was appalled by what they perceived as a radical program for changing fat and sugar consumption. The then Director

General of the BNF has since publicly confirmed that the constant criticism of the various drafts of the NACNE report and the attempts to delay and modify its impact and importance were part of a carefully co-ordinated campaign between some Department of Health officials and representatives of the food industry. Meanwhile, as author of the NACNE report (6), I was asked to extend, illustrate, and reference the report in response to pressure from the NACNE committee, which wished to make the report substantial, and as readable and understandable as possible for those lay people involved in health promotion. These changes, however, courted the criticism that the document was a policy statement rather than the helpful health education document which had been my aim.

By early 1983 the Department of Health was able to claim that the NACNE document could not be used and certainly not published because the Department had set up its own policy-making committee; all therefore seemed lost, with delays anticipated for at least another two to three years. However, the editor of *The Lancet*, Dr Ian Munro, was taking an interest, and Geoffrey Cannon, a highly effective journalist, had somehow gained access to all the drafts and correspondence which I had distributed to the Committee. There then ensued a public exposé of the conspiracy by officials within the Department of Health and the BNF to obstruct the publication of the document. A major quality Sunday newspaper broke the news as its front-page feature and questions to the Prime Minister followed in the House of Commons on the following Tuesday. Investigative journalists and those involved in food or in health immediately took interest. The Department and the BNF professed total innocence and a wish to see the report published, but it was only the publication of extracts in *The Lancet* which led to a frantic rush to see the document in print. Thus a short document, never originally intended for publication, was launched with publicity which could not have been bettered by the most brilliant of advertising agents.

There then followed a curious phase during which a variety of methods were used by government officials as well as by some sectors of the food industry to reduce the impact of the report by blurring its message, by casting doubt on the validity of its findings, or by questioning the competence of its promoters. Some of the criticisms were, of course, justified, as any scientist would agree when scrutinizing a simplified statement of current ideas on nutrition and health. Unfortunately for the officials concerned, there was intense public interest with an incessant demand by the media for information and guidance. Major establishment groups, e.g. the Church of England's Social Responsibility Committee, the main women's organizations, such as the Women's Institute, and teaching and trade union organizations all decided to promote the need for change. Central government continued to refuse to endorse the NACNE report, but it immediately became the basic document which community dietitians and health officials used to formulate their health promotion campaigns. Thus, four years later, over 85% of all health districts in Britain now have a diet and health policy which incorporates the NACNE guidelines, and a host of local initiatives are just beginning.

Given this intense public discussion and new evidence of remarkable dietary changes in a population that was considered by both industry and nutritional scientists to be highly conservative, the attitude to policy-making began to change. The Department of Health and the Ministry of Agriculture both formally accepted that their new expert (COMA) committee report (7) would become official government policy before it had even been finalized. This reflected the effects of a continuous barrage of questioning by Members of Parliament and by journalists and the increasingly aggressive role of the Coronary Prevention Group – a voluntary organization without commercial links and with a new Director, Ms Anne Dillon, who had considerable knowledge of and skill in parliamentary lobbying.

The COMA report was received in 1985 with acclaim for three principal reasons. First, it was written very carefully, in short, terse paragraphs, without citing any detailed evidence to justify its policy-making. In this way it avoided the usual British savaging by critics who were left simply having to specify their disagreement. More important, however, was the careful emphasis in the report on the fact that none of the experts (including the Chairman of the WHO committee, Professor Rose, and myself) considered the evidence for dietary change proven. Instead we were dealing cautiously with probabilities. This statement came as an enormous relief to those in nutrition and in industry because at last it was recognized that policy-making was an uncertain business; it also meant that critics could continue with their own sometimes quirky views until "proof" was obtained! The third reason for the report's acceptability was that it accorded with the medical profession's and the public's view of the importance of the individual. The NACNE document had taken the WHO approach of specifying targets for the average fat intakes of the population and advocated shifting the distribution of intakes in the population. This had the connotation of crude social engineering with general advice for everybody to eat less fat; this applied even to those who were already eating very little. More socially acceptable was the COMA report's call for all those eating more than 35% of their energy as fat to bring their intake below this value. This is philosophically much more acceptable, since it seems to deal with only those who need to change their diet. As a member of the COMA committee I readily accepted this because I surmised that the overall effect would be very similar, although I was unsure of how any individual could readily estimate his dietary fat content nor how many of the population would be affected.

These compromises seemed to be worthwhile because other recommendations in the COMA report on the fat labelling of foods and on changing agricultural practices to limit the fat content of carcasses immediately forced the Ministry of Agriculture to consider new measures despite its traditional role of simply endorsing the recommendations of a somewhat benighted British food and farming industry. So, by 1985, the opportunity for government-initiated change was at last accepted. I had, of course, forgotten that traditions die hard and that the ability of civil servants to obfuscate is legendary.

Further Government Obstruction

Following the COMA report, a new committee was formed to replace the NACNE committee and to implement the COMA recommendations. This JACNE committee (a "joint" rather than a "national" organization) had a new chairman, Dr John Garrow. After a fierce rearguard action by the BNF, we eventually produced a rather crude health promotional pamphlet which was underfunded because the government in its then monetarist phase was unwilling to provide any further cash to pay for their much vaunted initiative. The report was also blocked by the Department of Health, operating this time under pressure from the Agricultural Ministry, which feared that the pamphlet might be taken to imply that a reduction in milk and meat consumption, regardless of its fat composition, was a good thing.

The JACNE pamphlet was again published after a public outcry and the Chairman's refusal to modify statements which were perceived by the Committee as appropriate. Meanwhile a reformed BNF established its own expert committee on sugar only to find its report delayed endlessly by a battle between nutritionists and the sugar industry over how to specify the need for sugar consumption to fall. Again the issue was whether one specifies a reduction in the average intake of the population or specifies an individual approach. The sugar industry's representatives had to accept that children needed to reduce the frequency of sugar intake and that those who were overweight should reduce their total intake. Thus, they wished to advocate an unrealistic policy exclusively based on health and nutrition education: the educational message would presumably have to change from childhood to adulthood since current sugar intakes in adults were seen to be acceptable, provided individuals were not overweight or from the poorly specified category of those liable to gain weight. Thus, those who perceived themselves as constitutionally thin with a proper approach to dental hygiene and fluoridation need not be advised to reduce their sugar intake! Such is the ability of commercial pressures to push cautious academics into a corner where they can maintain their scientific reputation even if they appear foolish to those struggling to help a confused public to understand nutrition. Before the report finally emerged, after much rewriting, the Department of Health and Social Services (DHSS) had surprisingly set up its own panel on sugar and health, having originally specified that the BNF was dealing with the problem. This probably reflects the desire of government to be seen to be impartial once it is accused of simply pandering to vested interests.

Policy-making in Europe – the Scandinavian Experience

The scientific controversy, intrigue, governmental obstruction, and public debate seen in Britain is somewhat unusual in the rest of Europe, but this may reflect the fact that few other countries have considered the issues in such detail and that the European Economic Community (EEC) still operates an agricultural policy without regard to health issues.

European countries have had food policies for decades, these stemming from the need to ensure adequate food supplies for their populations during and immediately after the Second World War. These policies were usually concerned with ensuring an adequate energy, protein, and mineral (e.g. calcium) and vitamin intake with a prime concern for preventing deficiency diseases. Thus the Report no. 4 of 1963–64 to the Storting in Norway noted that agricultural production was geared to covering the national demand for milk, butter, cheese, and meat, including pork and eggs. This emphasis on dairy and animal products reflected the importance attached to these foods in Europe following, for example, Boyd Orr's pre-war studies on the link between poverty, inadequate food supplies, and children's growth (8). Milk supplements stimulated growth, and the concept of first-class protein from animal sources pervaded nutritional and governmental thinking in the 1930s and 1940s. Yet by 1968 a Nordic committee, representing Norway, Denmark, Sweden, and Finland, had already proposed a set of changes in policy, setting average population limits of 25–35% energy to be derived from fat, and calling for a reduction in sugar intake and the labelling of the fat content of foods. This policy stemmed from the emerging recognition that excess dietary fat was conducive to the development of coronary heart disease.

In the 32nd Report to the Storting in Norway in 1975–76 the Norwegian Ministry of Agriculture – not the Ministry of Health – set out a much more coherent nutrition and food policy and considered the financial and farming implications. They rejected any idea, for example, of growing sugar beet in Norway and considered how best to promote nutritional education. This Norwegian food policy is now famous because it implied that central government had a major role to play in integrating national planning with nutritional education and health promotion.

European Approaches to Food Policy

Other individual countries are, however, developing new initiatives. Italy managed to avoid official endorsement of its new set of dietary guidelines by simply presenting the guidelines with the backing of the National Institute of Nutrition to journalists in 1986. This seems to be a successful way of initiating the debate and stimulating public interest. In contrast, France has established a government committee for considering nutrition and health but, perhaps not surprisingly, nothing has yet happened. The comprehensive food and nutrition policy document produced in the Netherlands by the Ministry of Health seems to have avoided controversy by including a great deal of material on food law and general nutrition relating to EEC food legislation, with the dietary guidelines as a less prominent feature. The Netherlands, with its high consumption of polyunsaturated-rich margarines produced by the dominating industrial giant, Unilever, may, however, be more flexible in its response than Britain.

A New WHO European Approach

To a North American audience the concept of developing a European Health and Nutrition policy will seem strange – not because such a policy is unnecessary – but simply because the diversity of cultures and of economic and political organizations within Europe would argue against such a development. In practice there appears to be only one organization capable of melding the variety of approaches in this field – WHO – and it was this organization which initiated this development in 1984.

Some of the history of this initiative may be of interest. Ms Elisabet Helsing, newly appointed as Nutrition Officer in the WHO European region and based therefore in the Copenhagen office, wondered how best to provide member governments with a coherent view of nutrition, given the pronouncements of recent WHO committees on preventing coronary heart disease. How did these proposals mesh with those reports dealing with the same problem or other aspects of nutrition and health considered by European governmental committees? To this end she convened a panel of experts which selected a quartet of medical nutritionists. Individual opinion of new research was not considered relevant. Instead it was proposed that a document should be produced which would serve to illustrate to government officials the background and implications of the latest concepts of nutrition. Such a document, written by me in conjunction with Prof. A. Ferro-Luzzi of Italy, Prof. B. Isaksson of Sweden, and Prof. V. Szostak of Poland, has now been produced (9). Initial drafts were considered by a variety of individuals involved in nutrition, public health, policy development, and governmental planning. Meetings were held in Denmark, Britain, Finland, and Norway to allow redrafting and a critical analysis of the usefulness of the various drafts.

We now have a document suitable for wide distribution which will allow governments and organizations in both Eastern and Western Europe to consider their policies in a new health-oriented light. This is important because the major outcome of our review was that no East European government had, as yet, recognized that their whole agricultural policy (with huge implications for import/export trade) was based on the same 1930s premises which have conditioned British agricultural practice for decades. Thus, the promotion of meat and dairy product consumption – regardless of fat content – is implicit in the policies of nearly all European countries, thereby imposing a great demand for cereal production and intensive agriculture. In the EEC cereal production is excessive, but in the Comecon countries there is a major deficit. Economists argue that the dietary change to a greater proportion of animal products is an inevitable consequence of developing affluence and that the demand for agricultural land and cereal products inevitably rises. This is certainly happening in some parts of Europe but it may not be inevitable.

The second feature of our analysis of European diets in relation to health was the recognition that European countries in northern latitudes probably had a traditional dietary pattern for strictly climatic reasons. In northern climates it is much easier to survive by using ruminant animals to graze the grass which grows seasonally. Cereal production is also well suited to northern climates. In contrast, Mediterranean countries do not have the pasture for intensive animal and dairy production but have a climate well suited to fruit and vegetable production. It may not therefore be surprising that regional differences in food consumption were apparent. This recognition led us to devise a new approach to policy so that northern European countries could recognize that major agricultural issues are involved in dietary change and to allow progressive and less painful adjustment in agricultural practice.

Table 1 shows a summary of the proposals for a European nutrition policy. The intermediate goals are suitable for northern countries. Each country is advised to assess its current pattern of consumption and choose the intermediate or ultimate (ideal) WHO goals. Countries which already have a low fat diet should ensure that they do not follow the British pattern of agriculture and food production. This is particularly true of Eastern European countries where central planning in theory means that much can be done on a central government policy-making basis. In Italy, Greece, Spain, and Portugal current dietary changes, which seem to be moving away from the traditional Mediterranean diet, are seen as disadvantageous and need to be discouraged. It now remains to be seen whether this new document has the same effect as the British NACNE document and how different governments react to an issue which has huge social, political, and economic implications.

Conclusions

A very personal view of the problem of policy-making has been presented in the hope that it may highlight the complexity of the issues – scientific, health, agricultural, industrial, and political. To generate a new food and nutrition policy is not easy, and as soon as this is done it promptly becomes a major social issue and immediately highlights for each country how changes can be made. In North America there seems to be a greater flexibility because of the power and ef-

Table 1
Intermediate or Ultimate European Nutrient Goals

	Intermediate Nutrient Goals		
	General Population	*High Cardiovascular Risk Group*	*Ultimate Nutrient Goals*
Body Weight	BMI 20 – 25	BMI 20 – 25	BMI 20 – 25
Total fat % energy	35	30	20 – 30
Saturated fat % energy	15	10	10
P: S ratio	0.5	Increase up to 1.0	Increase up to 1.0
Cholesterol mg/4.18 MJ	—	<100	<100
Sugar % Energy	10	10	10
Complex carbohydrates % energy	>40	>45	Increase (45–55)
Dietary Fibre g.d $^{-1}$	30	>30	>30
Nutrient density	Increase	Increase	Increase
Salt g.d. $^{-1}$	7 – 8	5	5
Protein % energy	No change	No change	No change (12–13)
Alcohol	Limit	Limit	Limit
Water fluoride mg/l	0.7–1.2	0.7–1.2	0.7–1.2
Iodine prophylaxis	+	+	+

[1]These goals are based mainly on what is widely considered to be an ideal nutritional pattern for the prevention of cardiovascular diseases. The greater precision in the definition of nutrient goals from those advocated by the WHO committee on cardiovascular diseases is simply to have conformity with the intermediate goals advocated by national and other WHO committees. The body mass index (BMI) values are not necessarily appropriate for the developing world, where the average BMI may be 18. The complex carbohydrate figures are implications of the other recommendations. The intermediate targets are particularly applicable to northern European countries where the average nutrient intakes are far removed from those considered ideal. Those at high risk from cardiovascular disease are advised to have a diet more closely conforming to the ultimate goal. Dietary fibre values are based on analytical methods that measure non-starch polysaccharide and the enzyme-resistant starch produced by food processing or culinary methods. All the values given as a percentage of energy refer to alcohol-free total energy intakes.

fectiveness of consumer organizations. In Europe, however, there are many fewer consumer organizations, and culturally we have a tradition in which central government, with its interplay of vested interests, plays a much more dominant role. This is true of Western European countries as well as of those under a Communist regime. Governmental policy-making in the economic, agricultural, and health fields can be used extremely effectively to promote public awareness of health and dietary change, as was vividly illustrated during the Second World War in Britain. There is still doubt, however, whether European governments will grasp the need for a coherent food and health program, because it does demand that governments reassess a complex range of long-standing policies. The one hopeful sign is that this re-examination of priorities may be precipitated by the need to re-analyze agricultural policy because of its heavy financial burden on the community. It seems likely that only major economic issues are likely to provide the stimulus for governmental change. Without these pressures most of the developments in agricultural and food manufacturing of benefit to health are likely to come from consumer-led changes in demand.

REFERENCES

1 Royal College of Physicians of London, British Cardiac Society. Prevention of coronary heart disease: report of a Joint Working Party. (Chairman: A.G. Shaper). *J R Coll Physicians*, London 1976;10:213–275.

2 Royal College of Physicians of London. *Medical aspects of dietary fibre: summary of a report*. Tunbridge Wells: Pitman Medical, 1980.

3 Royal College of Physicians of London. Obesity: report. *J Roy Coll Physicians*, London 1983;17:5–65.

4 Department of Health and Social Security. *Eating for health: a discussion booklet prepared by the Health Departments of Great Britain and Northern Ireland*. London: HMSO, 1978.

5 Cannon G. *Politics of food*. London: Century Hutchinson, 1987.

6 Health Education Council. *A discussion paper on proposals for nutritional guidelines for health education in Britain*. National Advisory Committee on Nutrition Education. London: HEC, 1983.

7 Department of Health and Social Security. *Diet and cardiovascular disease*. Committee on Medical Aspects of Food Policy. London: HMSO, 1984.

8 Boyd Orr J. *Food, health and income: a survey of adequacy of diet in relation to income*. London: Macmillan, 1937.

9 WHO Regional Office for Europe. *Healthy nutrition: preventing nutrition-related diseases in Europe*. Copenhagen: Nutrition Unit, WHO European Series, no. 24, 1988.

Diet and Cardiovascular Disease

RICHARD J. HAVEL

Dietary and Hereditary Factors in Coronary Heart Disease

Diet may influence coronary heart disease (CHD) in several ways. It can affect lipoprotein levels in blood plasma, as well as the behaviour of cellular elements such as platelets, substances that participate in the development of atherosclerotic plaques and in the ultimate thrombosis that usually causes heart attacks. From many studies in animals fed cholesterol or fat-rich diets, however, it appears that deposition of cholesterol in developing plaques is essential to formation of the complicated lesions that almost invariably underlie the thrombotic event. I shall limit my remarks to the influence of dietary and hereditary factors on plasma lipoprotein levels and the relationship between these levels and CHD.

The general acceptance of a major etiological relationship between plasma lipoprotein levels and CHD is based on several independent lines of evidence. These include epidemiological studies of large population groups, dietary and other studies in experimental animals and in humans, studies of CHD in persons affected by mutant genes that alter plasma lipoproteins, and, most recently, studies of the effects of reducing lipoprotein levels on atherosclerotic plaques and the incidence of CHD.

Discussion as to the proper approach to reducing the burden of CHD in westernized countries in which heart attacks are the most common cause of death is burgeoning. Some people believe that the most effective way of dealing with this problem is to identify and treat those individuals in the population who are at high risk of developing CHD prematurely; others believe that only by intervening against the key etiological factors in the population as a whole will it be possible to eliminate heart attacks as a major cause of death and disability. To facilitate consideration of the underlying issues, I shall briefly review the data that underlie the proposed intervention strategies as well as our current understanding of the regulation of lipoprotein levels in individuals and populations.

Epidemiological Studies of Diet, Plasma Lipoproteins, and CHD

Comparisons of the prevalence of coronary heart disease among populations in different countries, coupled with studies of migrant populations, have provided persuasive evidence that CHD is not an inevitable consequence of aging in any population group. That CHD prevalence in different countries is strongly related to plasma cholesterol levels was clearly shown more than 25 years ago in the seven – countries study of Keys and his associates (1). The average level of plasma cholesterol appeared to be related to diet, primarily the daily intake of saturated fats and cholesterol (2,3). The plasma cholesterol level is a surrogate for the level of cholesterol in a specific lipoprotein class – the low density lipoproteins (LDL); in turn, the LDL-cholesterol level is a surrogate for the concentration of LDL particles in the blood (each LDL particle contains about 2000 molecules of cholesterol). When groups move from a region with a low prevalence of CHD to one with a high prevalence, they take on the risk characteristics of others residing there. In the Ni-Hon-San study (4), Japanese who had migrated from Japan to San Francisco were found to have higher CHD prevalence rates. Those who had migrated to Honolulu had an intermediate prevalence of CHD. In general the prevalence of CHD in these three populations was found to be directly related to their serum cholesterol levels and the extent of acculturation to a "western" life style, including diet.

Studies of CHD incidence within populations have shown a clear relationship to plasma LDL-cholesterol levels measured well in advance of clinical manifestations of coronary artery atherosclerosis. This has been shown for both men and women in the long-term study of the population of Framingham, Massachusetts (5), and in many others. By contrast, the level of high density lipoprotein (HDL)-cholesterol has been found to be a "negative" risk factor – the higher the level of HDL-cholesterol the lower the risk of developing CHD.

It has been difficult to show that individual LDL-cholesterol levels in such populations are related to the habitual intake of saturated fats and cholesterol even though these dietary constituents are known to be important determinants of these levels. This difficulty is thought to be related to the limitations of methods used to estimate the average dietary intake of individuals, to the fact that most individuals within population groups eat similar diets, and to the constitutional (genetic) factors that influence individual LDL-cholesterol levels.

The factors that influence HDL-cholesterol levels in population groups are only partially understood. HDL-cholesterol levels are inversely related to the level of fats (triglycerides) in the blood (6). Triglycerides are transported mainly in very low density lipoprotein (VLDL) particles. In general, the more efficient the transport of VLDL-triglycerides, the higher the level of HDL-cholesterol. The efficiency of triglyceride transport is influenced by many factors, both genetic and environmental. In addition to the relationship to triglyceride transport, alcohol and tobacco use influence HDL-cholesterol levels (6), making it difficult to determine which factors are most important in individuals within populations. Interestingly, in those countries where dietary fat intakes and the prevalence of CHD are low, levels of HDL-cholesterol as well as LDL-cholesterol are lower than in countries with high fat intakes and CHD prevalence (7).

The relationship between LDL-cholesterol level and CHD risk within populations is curvilinear. As levels increase above those found in countries with a low prevalence of developing CHD, the risk of dying from CHD rises slowly at first, and then progressively more rapidly (Fig. 1). From data obtained in the Multiple Risk Factor Intervention Trial (MRFIT) carried out in the United States during the 1970s, there seems to be no prevailing cholesterol level below which risk becomes both low and invariate (8). However, the postulated benefit of a given reduction in serum cholesterol (for example, by 10%) is greater for individuals with high levels (for example, above 240 mg/dl) than for those with lower levels (for example, below 220 mg/dl).

Metabolic Studies of Diet and Plasma Lipoprotein Levels in Humans and Other Mammals

To understand the effect of diet on plasma cholesterol levels, it is necessary to have some familiarity with the pathways of lipid transport in lipoproteins (9). Dietary triglycerides and cholesterol are absorbed in the mucosal cells of the small intestine, where they are packaged into lipoprotein particles called chylomicrons. The chylomicrons are delivered into the blood where the triglycerides are removed

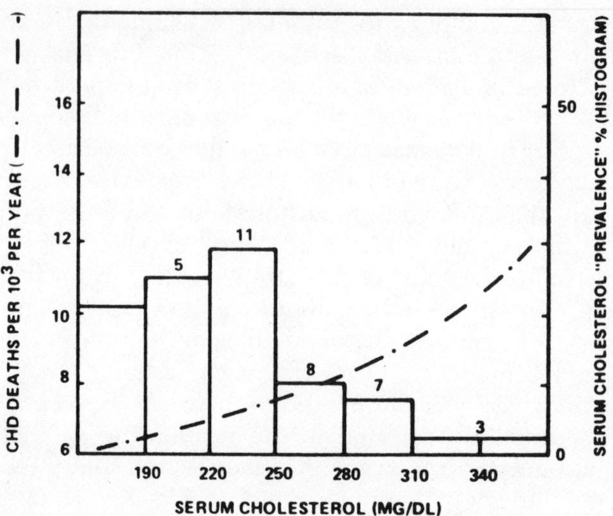

Figure 1. Relative risk of CHD as related to serum cholesterol levels in the population of Framingham, Massachusetts. The histogram shows the distribution of serum cholesterol levels in Framingham, and the curved line is the logistic fit of serum cholesterol levels to the yearly risk of death from CHD. The numbers at the column heads are the excess deaths (above the baseline levels of 6) attributable to each range of serum cholesterol, taking into account the number of people in each range. Note that 47% ($^{16}/_{34}$ × 100) of the deaths attributable to serum cholesterol occur in the range between 190 and 250 mg/dl. From Blackburn H. *Epidemiologic evidence: the causes and prevention of atherosclerosis.* In: Steinberg D, Olefsky JM, eds. New York: Churchill Livingstone, 1987:89, with permission of the publisher.

into various tissues by the action of an enzyme called lipoprotein lipase. This enzyme splits the triglyceride molecule into its component fatty acids and glycerol, which are rapidly metabolized. The remaining chylomicron particle, called a chylomicron remnant, is taken up rapidly into the liver, carrying with it some residual triglyceride and almost all of the dietary cholesterol. For this reason dietary cholesterol does not immediately influence the cholesterol level in blood plasma.

The liver also secretes particles that resemble chylomicrons, but most of these particles are considerably smaller. As with chylomicrons, the triglycerides in VLDL are removed by the action of lipoprotein lipase, and VLDL remnants are formed. Some VLDL remnants, like chylomicron remnants, are taken up efficiently into the liver, but others are further metabolized to form LDL (Fig. 2). LDL are also taken up to a large extent by the liver, but this process is much less efficient,

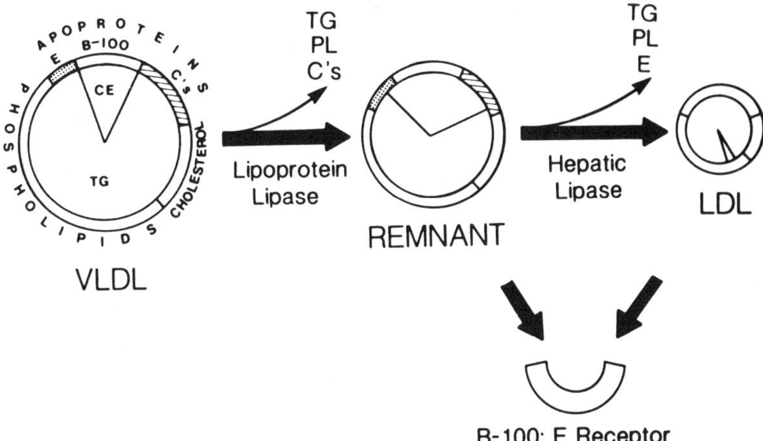

Figure 2. The metabolism of VLDL proceeds in two steps. The first yields VLDL remnants from the action of lipoprotein lipase upon VLDL lipids, mainly triglycerides (TG). The second can proceed in two directions. One involves the further hydrolysis of VLDL lipids and results in the production of LDL particles, rich in cholesterol and cholesteryl esters (CE), in which apolipoprotein B-100 is the sole protein component. The other involves binding of VLDL remnants via apolipoprotein E to LDL (B-100:E) receptors on the surface of hepatocytes and leads to endocytosis and lysosomal degradation of the particles. LDL are also eventually taken up by LDL receptors via apolipoprotein B-100, mainly into hepatocytes, but at a much slower fractional rate than remnant particles. According to this scheme, high receptor levels both reduce the formation and increase the efficiency of removal of LDL. From Havel RJ. Role of the liver in atherosclerosis. *Arteriosclerosis* 1985; 569–580, with permission of the publisher.

so that LDL particles tend to circulate for several days, whereas VLDL remnant particles circulate for only minutes to hours. Consequently, there are normally many more LDL particles than VLDL particles in the blood, and LDL contain about two-thirds of the total circulating cholesterol. About one-fourth of circulating cholesterol is in HDL and the remainder is in VLDL.

The removal of VLDL remnants and LDL into the liver is mediated by a lipoprotein receptor, called the "LDL receptor," on the surface of liver cells. The LDL receptor binds to these lipoproteins specifically via certain protein components called apolipoproteins. The binding leads to uptake of the lipoprotein particle into the cell, where it is rapidly degraded. The number of receptor molecules on the cell surface is regulated by the cell's need for cholesterol. Thus when dietary cholesterol intake is high and the liver cholesterol content tends to rise, liver cells sense this by making fewer LDL receptor molecules. This is particularly the case when the liver's ability to excrete the cholesterol is limited. In some animals, such as the rat, dietary cholesterol is excreted very efficiently into the bile, mainly after conversion to bile acids. In other animals, such as the rabbit, biliary excretion of cholesterol (and its conversion to bile acids) is much more limited, so that dietary cholesterol tends to accumulate in the liver. As a result, the rat liver continues to make LDL receptors when the diet is rich in cholesterol, whereas the rabbit liver virtually stops making receptors. Therefore, rats on cholesterol-rich diets have low plasma cholesterol levels, whereas rabbits develop extremely high levels. In the rabbit, the situation is compounded by the production of VLDL particles that are unusually cholesterol-rich. Humans seem to vary in their response to dietary cholesterol, perhaps in part because they vary in their ability to excrete cholesterol into the bile or to convert cholesterol to bile acids (10). In addition, persons who respond to cholesterol-rich diets with a substantial increase in LDL-cholesterol levels may absorb cholesterol more efficiently than those who do not. In one recent study, individuals who carried an allele for a particular variant of apolipoprotein E (E-4) were found to have higher LDL-cholesterol levels and to be more efficient absorbers of dietary cholesterol (11).

Almost all individuals respond to an increase in dietary saturated fat intake with an increase in LDL (as well as HDL) cholesterol levels (12). From studies in experimental animals, it appears that saturated fat-rich diets reduce the number of LDL receptors on liver cells (13). Although the mechanism of this effect of saturated fat intake is unclear, it is important to note that dietary cholesterol is generally contained in those foods that are also rich in saturated fats, such as dairy products and red meats. Thus, intake of such foods reduces the number of LDL receptors in the liver.

As will be described below, a reduction of the number of LDL receptors on liver cells has two effects, both of which tend to raise LDL levels. First, the removal of LDL becomes less efficient when the receptor number is reduced. Second, fewer VLDL remnants are removed directly by the liver, because they tend to circulate in the blood for longer periods of time and are progressively converted to LDL particles. Thus, with few LDL receptors, not only do LDL particles circulate for longer periods of time, but more LDL particles, which are inherently metabolized less efficiently than VLDL remnants, are produced. A reduction in receptor number therefore has a large effect on the level of LDL in the blood.

It can be predicted that the number of LDL receptors on liver cells is higher in those countries in which the intake of meats (especially red meats) and dairy products is low (14). In such countries, the average individual should remove more VLDL particles efficiently as VLDL remnants. LDL levels are thus low because fewer LDL particles are produced and those that are have a shorter life span in the blood.

Genetic Disorders of the Plasma Lipoproteins and CHD

Not all individuals with high lipoprotein levels are prone to develop CHD prematurely. For example, individuals with genetically determined deficiency of lipoprotein lipase who are unable to make remnant particles (and consequently produce few LDL particles) seem to have little tendency to develop clinical evidences of CHD. As might be expected from the epidemiological relationships described above, individuals who have genetically determined elevations of LDL are prone to premature heart attacks and death from CHD. The best understood of the genetic disorders leading to elevated LDL levels is familial hypercholesterolemia, in which mutations of the gene for the LDL receptor lead to a reduced number of functional receptor molecules (15). Indeed, the LDL receptor was discovered by Brown and Goldstein when they found that cultured skin fibroblasts from patients with the severe, homozygous form of this disease lack high affinity binding sites for LDL and are unable to take up LDL efficiently from tissue culture medium (15). Most individuals with this disorder (about one person in 500 throughout the world) are heterozygous for a mutant gene and hence make about one-half the number of LDL receptors on any given diet. They consequently have somewhat more than twice the normal concentration of LDL particles in the blood. When they live in westernized countries, they tend to develop heart attacks in their 40s or 50s and sometimes even earlier. The rare homozygotes, who have few or no functional LDL receptors, LDL levels several times normal, as well as a substantial accumulation of VLDL remnants, usually develop CHD in childhood.

The pathogenesis of the hyperlipidemia in familial hypercholesterolemia has become better understood as a result of the discovery by Watanabe in Japan of a mutation of the LDL receptor gene in rabbits. This mutation leads to synthesis of an abnormal LDL receptor protein in which five amino acids in the lipoprotein-binding domain of the protein are missing (16). This mutant receptor is not transported normally to the cell surface and it may also bind some lipoprotein particles inefficiently. Inbred rabbits homozygous for this mutant gene have a severe form of hypercholesterolemia resembling that of humans with homozygous familial hypercholesterolemia. Studies of these animals (Watanabe heritable hyperlipidemic (WHHL) rabbits) have shown that they metabolize chylomicrons and chylomicron remnants normally so that dietary cholesterol is delivered efficiently to the liver. However, they take up VLDL remnants and LDL inefficiently. Furthermore, they convert many more VLDL remnant particles to LDL than normal rabbits. As in normal humans, VLDL remnants are normally removed efficiently from the blood of normal rabbits and only about 8% are converted to LDL (17). In normal rabbits, the removal of VLDL remnants is mediated by the binding of a specific protein on the VLDL surface to the LDL receptor. This protein (apolipoprotein E) contains a domain rich in positively charged amino acids which bind to negatively charged binding sites on the receptor molecules. Most VLDL particles contain several molecules of the E protein, so that a single VLDL remnant particle can bind to multiple receptor-binding sites. The resulting binding, which is very tight and irreversible, is thought to underlie the efficient removal of the VLDL remnants from the blood. By contrast, LDL molecules contain no apolipoprotein E molecules or at most only one. They bind to the receptor mainly via a different protein, apolipoprotein B, on the LDL surface. Since each LDL molecule contains only a single molecule of apolipoprotein B, the affinity of binding is much lower than that of VLDL remnant particles. In the WHHL rabbits LDL particles are unable to bind to the few mutant receptors on the surface of liver cells. Some VLDL remnants may bind to some extent, but the net result is that about 40% of VLDL remnants are converted to LDL which circulate for days, building up high levels of LDL (as well as VLDL remnants) in the blood (17). WHHL homozygotes develop visible atherosclerotic lesions in the coronary arteries of the heart and other arteries in a matter of months, and they may die of heart attacks after two to three years (18).

In rabbits and humans with genetically determined deficiency of LDL receptors, there is no other defect that can account for their premature atherosclerosis and heart attacks. The mechanism by which high LDL (or VLDL remnant) levels leads to atherosclerotic plaques is not clearly understood. The atherogenic lipoproteins appear early in scavenger cells (macrophages) in focal regions of the arterial wall (19). In the case of VLDL remnants, these lipoproteins bind to a form of the LDL receptor on the macrophage surface. The receptor concentration in these cells remains high so that they are converted to "foam cells," rich in cholesteryl esters. These cells eventually rupture, spilling large amounts of lipoprotein into the interstitial space of the arterial wall. In the case of LDL, recent studies suggest that uptake into macrophages may require oxidative modification of proteins and lipids on the particle surface. The modified LDL particles are taken up via a special "scavenger" receptor to yield foam cells (20).

Another genetic disorder of the plasma lipoproteins affects apolipoprotein E (21). Mutations of the gene which affect the positively charged binding domain yield a form of this protein that binds poorly to the LDL receptor. About one percent of all individuals in the population, who are homozygous for such mutant forms of apolipoprotein E, tend to accumulate remnants of both VLDL and chylomicrons in the blood. Interestingly, the VLDL remnants are converted poorly to LDL, and LDL levels tend to be lower than in unaffected individuals. Such homozygotes do not appear to be at increased risk of CHD. However, in the presence of other genetic abnormalities that increase VLDL synthesis, they may have high levels of VLDL remnants rich in cholesterol and then develop premature atherosclerotic disease. The lipoprotein abnormality in such affected homozygotes resembles that found in rabbits fed cholesterol-rich diets. However, atherosclerotic plaques develop much more rapidly in cholesterol-fed rabbits than in humans with dysfunctional apolipoprotein E. It is possible that the remnant particles containing dysfunctional apolipoprotein E have less tendency to produce foam cells than the cholesterol-rich particles in rabbits because they bind poorly to macrophage LDL receptors. In any event, it appears that VLDL remnant particles as well as LDL particles are potentially atherogenic.

Intervention against Established CHD

Several recent controlled studies suggest that reducing LDL levels, by diet or by use of drugs, can reduce the rate of progression of established atherosclerotic plaques in the coronary arteries. In the Oslo Study Group Trial, reduction of LDL levels of middle-aged men by dietary means, together with reduced cigarette smoking, was accompanied by a substantially reduced incidence of CHD (22). In the Lipid Research Clinics Primary Prevention Trial, reduction of LDL levels by administration of the bile acid-binding resin, cholestyramine, reduced the incidence of heart attacks and death from CHD. The reduction of death rate from CHD was proportional to the amount of the drug taken and the percentage reduction of LDL-cholesterol level (23). In a recent study, LDL-cholesterol levels were lowered drastically in men with established CHD, who had had coronary bypass graft surgery, by administering another bile acid-binding resin (colestipol) together with large doses of niacin, which reduces VLDL synthesis in the liver. The progression of atherosclerotic lesions in native coronary arteries, as well as in the grafts, was slowed and there was even some suggestion of regression of a few lesions (24). These trials involved men with higher than average LDL-cholesterol levels. On the basis of current knowledge of the pathogenesis of atherosclerosis in experimental animals and humans, and the relationships between LDL-cholesterol levels and the prevalence and incidence of CHD, many investigators in the lipoprotein field believe that the results observed in these and other trials can reasonably be extrapolated to the bulk of the population in westernized countries with plasma cholesterol levels above 180 mg/dl.

Population and Individual Approaches to Lipoproteins and CHD

Not everyone in westernized countries is destined to develop CHD even though CHD is the most common cause of death. If it were possible to identify easily those individuals who are susceptible to atherosclerotic complications (mainly CHD), an individually targeted approach to this problem would seem to be logical and cost-effective (Table 1). Assessment of susceptibility is not simply a matter of determining the ambient level of LDL-cholesterol (or of VLDL remnant or HDL levels). For example, some individuals with heterozygous familial hypercholesterolemia may live to advanced age without developing CHD, or even coronary atherosclerosis demonstrable by angiography. Evidently other factors, about which we know little, determine the likelihood that an individual with a given lipoprotein level will develop occlusive plaques or heart attacks. Under these circumstances, efficient application of the individual approach would appear to require an inexpensive, safe (non-invasive) method to determine the presence and severity of atherosclerotic lesions. Such a method may eventually be developed, but it is unlikely to be available in the next few years. Alternatively, a simple and safe method to reduce the level of atherogenic lipoproteins (for example, with a magic bullet to stimulate the synthesis of LDL receptors or to prolong their lifespan) could conceivably be used in all individuals with an LDL level above some defined set-point. With the current development of specific inhibitors of cholesterol synthesis which secondarily stimulate receptor synthe-

Table 1
The Individual (Genetic) Approach to Hyperlipidemia and Coronary Heart Disease

Current	
– Measurement of lipid levels:	total serum cholesterol
	triglycerides
	HDL cholesterol
Future	
– Identification of major gene abnormalities and protein polymorphisms	
– Non-invasive or minimally invasive evaluation of coronary lesions	
– Prevention by a "magic bullet"	

sis (25), there is some reason to be optimistic about this possibility. Safety would become a paramount consideration in direct relationship to the set-point above which such treatment could be justified, and general experience suggests that it is unlikely that a drug which is safe in virtually everyone will be developed.

The population approach to hyperlipoproteinemia and CHD is predicated upon extrapolation of the results of intervention in hypercholesterolemic men to the general population. The practicality of widespread modification of the diet has been demonstrated to date in only limited studies. However, based upon what is currently known about the regulation of hepatic LDL receptors, the ingredients of an appropriate diet are reasonably simple and straightforward (Table 2). The need for a population approach is based upon the realization that treatment of only those individuals judged to be hypercholesterolemic (for example, the upper 10% of the population) will not reduce the bulk of the burden of premature CHD in westernized countries (Fig. 1). Furthermore, the population approach is based upon the prediction that small reductions in LDL-cholesterol will have substantial effects on the incidence of CHD. The population approach is of necessity confined to the use of dietary modification, and it is important therefore to consider the influence of social, including particularly family, interactions in the implementation of any dietary program. Finally, it must of course be realized that a population approach to dietary modification will only be possible in the long run if the food supply is coordinately modified.

There is no necessary conflict between the individual and population approaches to reducing lipoprotein levels. Individuals at high risk for CHD because of high levels of LDL or VLDL remnants may well require drug treatment as well as extensive dietary modification. Their problem will therefore not be adequately addressed by a mod-

Table 2
The Population Approach to Diet and Coronary Heart Disease

- Single diet is appropriate for almost all purposes
- Small reductions in LDL-cholesterol can yield large overall benefits
- Compliance is enhanced by family and other social interactions
- Change in food supply is facilitated

erate change in the diet of the population as a whole. On the other hand, the individual approach will not help those in the population who are destined to develop premature CHD even though they have "average" lipoprotein levels. If the burden of CHD can be alleviated by modification of lipoprotein levels, both approaches will have to be applied effectively, so that the average cholesterol level is reduced to a value commensurate with a very low incidence of CHD and virtually no one has a level at which CHD risk is inordinately high.

REFERENCES

1 Keys A. Coronary heart disease in seven countries. *Circulation* 1970;41:suppl. 1.

2 Keys A, Anderson JT, Grande F. Serum cholesterol response to changes in diet. II. The effect of cholesterol in the diet. *Metabolism* 1965;14:759–765.

3 Hegsted DM, McGandy RB, Meyers MD, Stare FJ. Quantitative effects of dietary fat on serum cholesterol in man. *Am J Clin Nutr* 1965;17:281–295.

4 Robertson TL, Kato H, Rhoads GG, et al. Epidemiologic studies of coronary heart disease and stroke in Japanese men living in Japan, Hawaii and California: incidence of myocardial infarction and death from coronary heart disease. *Am J Cardiol* 1977;39:239–243.

5 Kannel WB, Castelli WP, Gordon T. Cholesterol in the prediction of atherosclerotic disease: new perspectives based on the Framingham Study. *Ann Intern Med* 1980;90:85–91.

6 Phillips NR, Havel RJ, Kane JP. Levels and interrelationships of serum and lipoprotein cholesterol and triglycerides: association with adiposity and the consumption of ethanol, tobacco, and beverages containing caffeine. *Arteriosclerosis* 1981;1:13–24.

7 Knuiman JT, Hermus RJJ, Hautvast JGAJ. Serum total cholesterol and high density lipoprotein (HDL) cholesterol concentrations in rural and urban boys from 16 countries. *Atherosclerosis* 1982:43:71–82.

8 Stamler J, Wentworth D, Neaton JD. Is relationship between serum cholesterol and risk of premature death from coronary heart disease continuous and graded? *JAMA* 1986;256:2823–2828.
9 Havel RJ. Origin, metabolic fate and metabolic function of plasma lipoproteins. In: Steinberg D, Olefsky JM, eds. *Contemporary issues in endocrinology and metabolism,* Vol. 3. New York: Churchill Livingstone, 1986:117–141.
10 Havel RJ. Dietary regulation of plasma lipoprotein metabolism in humans. *Prog Biochem Pharmacol* 1983;19:111–122.
11 Kesäniemi YA, Ehnholm C, Miettinen TA. Intestinal cholesterol absorption efficiency in man is related to apoprotein E phenotype. *J Clin Invest* 1987;80:578–581.
12 Antonis A, Bersohn I. The influence of diet on serum triglycerides in South African white and Bantu prisoners. *Lancet* 1961;1:3–9.
13 Spady DK, Dietschy JM. Dietary saturated triacylglycerols suppress hepatic low density lipoprotein receptor activity in the hamster. *Proc Natl Acad Sci USA* 1985;82:4526–4530.
14 Goldstein JL, Brown MS. The low-density lipoprotein pathway and its relation to atherosclerosis. *Ann Rev Biochem* 1977;46:897–930.
15 Brown MS, Goldstein JL. A receptor-mediated pathway for cholesterol homeostasis. *Science* 1986;232:34–47.
16 Yamamoto T, Bishop RW, Brown MS, Goldstein JL, Russell DW. Deletion in cysteine-rich region of LDL receptor impedes transport to cell surface in WHHL rabbits. *Science* 1986;232:1230–1237.
17 Yamada N, Shames DM, Havel RJ. Effect of LDL receptor deficiency on the metabolism of apo B-100 in blood plasma: kinetic studies in normal and Watanabe heritable hyperlipidemic (WHHL) rabbits. *J Clin Invest* 1987;80:507–515.
18 Goldstein JL, Kita T, Brown MS. Defective lipoprotein receptors and atherosclerosis. Lessons from an animal counterpart of familial hypercholesterolemia. *N Engl J Med* 1983;309:288–296.
19 Ross R. The pathogenesis of atherosclerosis: an update. *N Engl J Med* 1986;314:488–500.
20 Steinberg D. Lipoproteins and the pathogenesis of atherosclerosis. *Circulation* 1987;76:508–514.
21 Havel RJ. Familial dysbetalipoproteinemia: new aspects of pathogenesis and diagnosis. In: Havel RJ, ed. *Medical clinics of North America on lipid disorders,* vol. 66. Philadelphia: W.B. Saunders, 1982:441–454.
22 Hjermann I, Velve Byre K, Holme I, Leren P. Effect of diet and smoking intervention on the incidence of coronary heart disease: report from the Oslo Study Group of a randomized trial in healthy men. *Lancet* 1981;2:1303–1310.

23 The Lipid Research Clinics Coronary Primary Prevention Trial Results: II. The relation of reduction in incidence of coronary heart disease to cholesterol lowering. *JAMA* 1984;251:365–374.
24 Blankenhorn DH, Nessim SA, Johnson RL, Sanmarco ME, Azen SP, Cashin-Hemphill L. Beneficial effects of combined colestipol-niacin therapy on coronary atherosclerosis and coronary venous bypass grafts. *JAMA* 1987;257:3233–3240.
25 Tobert J. New developments in lipid-lowering therapy: the role of inhibitors of hydroxymethyl-glutaryl coenzyme A reductase. *Circulation* 1987;76:534–538.

SONJA L. CONNOR AND WILLIAM E. CONNOR

Coronary Heart Disease: Prevention and Treatment by Nutritional Change

Diet greatly affects many of the risk factors which cause coronary heart disease. In fact, nutrition itself must be listed as one of the major risk factors because of its tremendous modifying effects on the disease process, atherosclerosis. The most important risk factor in which diet plays the major role, both in causation and in treatment, is hyperlipidemia (See Fig. 1).

Hyperlipidemia is important because it forms the basis for the excessive infiltration of lipid into the arterial intima with atherosclerosis an ultimate consequence. Stage 1 in the development of coronary heart disease is hyperlipidemia or, as depicted in the figure, hypercholesterolemia, but this could indicate any abnormality of the plasma lipids – lipoproteins including cholesterol, low density lipoprotein (LDL), very low density lipoprotein (VLDL), triglyceride, high density lipoprotein (HDL), and the remnants of chylomicrons and VLDL. If hyperlipidemia is not present, then atherosclerosis does not result. Should atherosclerosis be prevented, then stage 3, coronary heart disease, the clinical expression of this underlying and silent disorder, will not occur.

The cause of hyperlipidemia is clearcut for 1% or less of the population. Hyperlipidemia will result regardless of environmental factors because of genetic predisposition. Familial hypercholesterolemia is the classic example of genetic hyperlipidemia, but there are many others. For the other 99% of the population, dietary factors are crucial in the development of hyperlipidemia. Even dietary factors will affect the hyperlipidemia of genetically based disorders but, in most in-

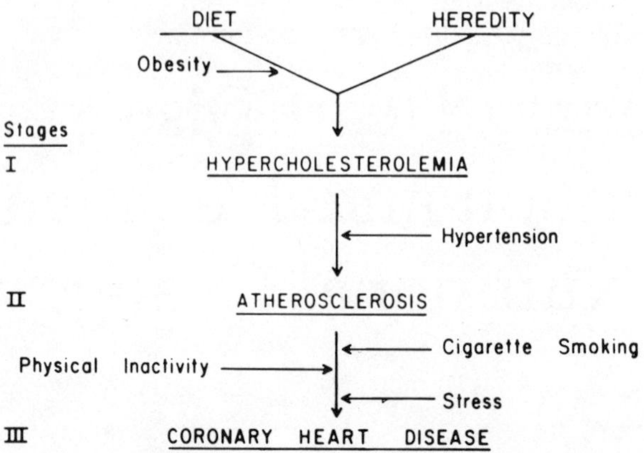

Figure 1. The stages and important factors in the development of coronary heart disease.

stances, will probably not make the situation completely normal. Pharmaceutical agents will be required, but these act synergistically with diet.

The second risk factor affected by diet is thrombosis, a critical event in the evolution of the atherosclerotic plaque to complete coronary occlusion. Certain nutritional factors are thrombogenic, others are antithrombogenic. In both hyperlipidemia and thrombosis, the amount and kind of dietary fat are important.

A third risk factor, one obviously important and affected by nutrition, is obesity, which influences in turn hyperlipidemia, thrombosis and hypertension. Overweight may develop when another risk factor is abolished (i.e. cigarette smoking). Finally, the important risk factor, hypertension, is greatly affected by dietary electrolytes: sodium raises and potassium lowers blood pressure (1). Fortunately, from the point of view of therapeutic simplicity, the same dietary lifestyle can be used to modify all four of these coronary risk factors: hyperlipidemia, thrombosis, obesity and hypertension.

The goals of this paper are 1) to review the precise roles that nutritional factors play in the causation of the atherosclerotic plaque, which is the underlying lesion of coronary heart disease (Fig. 1), and 2) to delineate a practical approach to the dietary prevention and treatment of atherosclerosis. Attention will be given to the two components of the atherosclerotic plaque that lead to the development of overt coronary heart disease – namely, the lipid-rich, fibrous atheroma and the superimposed thrombotic lesion.

Dietary factors affect both the initiation and growth of the atherosclerotic plaque and the final thrombotic episode. The evidence about dietary factors and the genesis of atherosclerosis is best illustrated by the numerous experiments over the past 30 years carried out in subhuman primates. In these experiments dietary cholesterol and fat were the "sine qua non" components necessary to produce hypercholesterolemia and atherosclerosis in many species of monkeys (2–4). The atherosclerosis produced was severe and complicated, culminating in some monkeys in myocardial infarction, stroke and gangrene of an extremity (4). These clinical features have reproduced the spectrum of the consequences of atherosclerotic disease in humans. In all of these experiments, diet exerted its effect on atherosclerosis by raising plasma lipid and lipoprotein concentrations.

The epidemiological evidence is likewise clearcut: populations consuming a low-cholesterol, low-fat diet have little coronary heart disease, whereas in populations of the Western world where the diet concentrates upon animal foods rich in cholesterol and saturated fat, the incidence of coronary heart disease is very high (5). Japan is a classic example of a country with modern technology and a high living standard and yet a low incidence of coronary heart disease. The Japanese consume a low-cholesterol, low-fat diet and habitually have low plasma cholesterol levels. Here, again, the links between diet and clinical expression of coronary heart disease are the lifelong plasma cholesterol and LDL concentrations. In addition, populations with a low incidence of coronary heart disease and a low-fat dietary background also have a low incidence of clinical thrombosis.

The review of information on the vital role of plasma lipid and lipoprotein concentrations in the development of atherosclerosis raises a crucial question: Can dietary change lower elevated plasma lipid and lipoprotein concentrations in patients and in population subgroups of the Western world? The answer is an unequivocal yes. Experiments over the past 20 years have indicated which dietary components have an important effect upon plasma lipid and lipoprotein concentrations in humans. The major dietary factors to be considered include the following:

1 Cholesterol
2 Total fat
  - Saturated fat
  - Monounsaturated fat
  - Polyunsaturated fat (omega-3 and omega-6)

3 carbohydrate, fibre, starch and sugars
4 protein
5 other nutrients (calories, alcohol, lecithin, vitamins and minerals)

Dietary Cholesterol

Dietary cholesterol enters the body via the chylomicron pathway and is removed from the plasma by the liver as a component of chylomicron remnants. Only about 40% of ingested cholesterol is absorbed, the remaining 60% passing out in the stool. Dietary cholesterol is thus added to the cholesterol synthesized by the body, since feedback inhibition of cholesterol biosynthsis in the body only partially occurs in man even when a large amount of dietary cholesterol is ingested (6). Because the ring structure of the sterol nucleus cannot be broken down by the tissues of the body as does occur for fat, protein and carbohydrate, it must be either excreted or stored. Thus, it is easy to see how the body or a particular tissue, i.e. a coronary artery, can become overloaded with cholesterol if there are limitations in cholesterol excretion from the body and from certain tissues. Cholesterol is excreted in the bile and ultimately in the stool, either as such or as bile acids synthesized in the liver from cholesterol. Both of these pathways of excretion are limited and, furthermore, the very efficient enterohepatic reabsorption and circulation returns much of what is excreted into the bile back into the body.

Dietary cholesterol does not directly enter into the formation of the lipoproteins synthesized in the liver, VLDL and LDL, since it is removed by the liver as a component of the chylomicron remnants. It can, however, profoundly affect the catabolism of LDL as mediated through the LDL receptor. Since dietary cholesterol ultimately contributes to the total amount of hepatic cell cholesterol, it can affect the biosynthesis of cholesterol and modify LDL receptor activity in the liver. In particular, an increase in hepatic cell cholesterol will decrease LDL receptor activity and, subsequently, cause an *increase* in the level of LDL cholesterol in the plasma (7–10). Conversely, a drastic decrease in dietary cholesterol will increase the LDL receptor activity in the liver, enhance LDL removal and, hence, lower plasma LDL levels. Table 1 lists the effects of dietary cholesterol.

Over the past 30 years, some 26 separate metabolic experiments involving 196 human subjects and patients have shown decisive effects of dietary cholesterol upon plasma cholesterol and LDL levels (11–14). Even patients with familial hypercholesterolemia respond

Table 1
Effects of Dietary Cholesterol on LDL levels

1 Increased chylomicrons and remnants
2 Increased hepatic cell cholesterol
Consequences:
Decreased cholesterol biosynthesis
Partial compensation in excretion of biliary cholesterol and bile acids to lessen hepatic cholesterol.
Decreased synthesis of LDL receptors
Increased plasma LDL
3 Increased plasma LDL
Consequence:
Deposition of cholesterol into the arterial wall.

greatly to dietary cholesterol. Table 2 shows that the plasma cholesterol level decreased 18% and 21% in two patients with FH (homozygotes) in response to the removal of cholesterol from the diet. This is similar to the mean plasma cholesterol increase of 17% that occurred when 1000 mg dietary cholesterol was added to a cholesterol-free diet in 25 subjects (11 normal, 7 with type II-a mild, 5 with II-a severe, and 9 with type IV hyperlipidemia) (15) (Fig. 2).

LDL increased very significantly in all groups, again showing indirectly the effects of dietary cholesterol upon the LDL receptor. These data further document the importance of dietary factors in hyperlipidemia of any phenotype or genotype. However, as pointed out years ago, the doubling or tripling of the amounts of dietary cholesterol will not necessarily increase the plasma levels if the initial amount of dietary cholesterol is already substantial, i.e. an increase to 950 mg per day from a previous intake of 475 mg per day (12). Despite this earlier literature, such attempts are still being carried out and are highly touted as showing that dietary cholesterol has no effect on the plasma cholesterol levels. There is a review for those who wish to explore the subject more fully (16).

The effects upon the plasma cholesterol as the amount of dietary cholesterol is gradually increased may be depicted in Figure 3, and are supported by both animal and human experiments. With a baseline cholesterol-free diet, the amount of dietary cholesterol necessary to produce an increase in the plasma cholesterol concentration is termed "the threshold amount." Then, as the amount of dietary cholesterol is increased, the plasma cholesterol increases likewise until the second important point on this curve is reached, which is termed

Table 2
The Effect of a Cholesterol-Free Diet on the Plasma Cholesterol Level in Two Patients With Familial Hypercholesterolemia (Homozygotes)

Diet	*Plasma Cholesterol (mg/dl)* DL	DC
Cholesterol, 250 mg/day	737	786
Cholesterol-free	578	644
Change	−21%	−18%
Hyperalimentation	401	418

"the ceiling amount." Further increases in dietary cholesterol do not lead to higher levels of the plasma cholesterol even if phenomenally high amounts may be fed. Each animal or human being probably has its own distinctive threshold and ceiling amounts. Generally speaking, however, and again based on the experimental literature, we would suggest that an average threshold amount for human beings would be 100 mg/day. An average ceiling amount of dietary cholesterol would be in the neighbourhood of 300–400 mg/day. Further experiments will be necessary to provide more precise information about the ceiling. Thus, a baseline dietary cholesterol intake of 500 mg/day from two eggs would, for most individuals, already exceed the ceiling. The addition of two more egg yolks for a total of 1000 mg/day would not then further increase the plasma cholesterol concentration. Yet, beginning with a baseline very low cholesterol diet under 100 mg/day and adding the equivalent of two egg yolks, or 500 mg, to this baseline amount would produce a striking change in plasma cholesterol concentrations, perhaps 60 mg/dl as shown in many experiments.

Recent dietary surveys indicate that the average American intake of dietary cholesterol is about 400 mg/day for women and 500 mg/day for men (17). Decreasing these amounts of dietary cholesterol, as would take place in therapeutic and preventive diets to be amplified subsequently, would then have a profound effect on plasma cholesterol concentrations because operationally one would be on the descending limb of the curve as exemplified in Figure 3.

There has been recent discussion about the wide distribution of individual response to change in dietary cholesterol intake (18) although this finding is not new (11–13, 18–22). Further, variation in individual plasma cholesterol response occurs with other nutrients as well as with lipid-lowering drugs. Katan et al. (18) recently showed

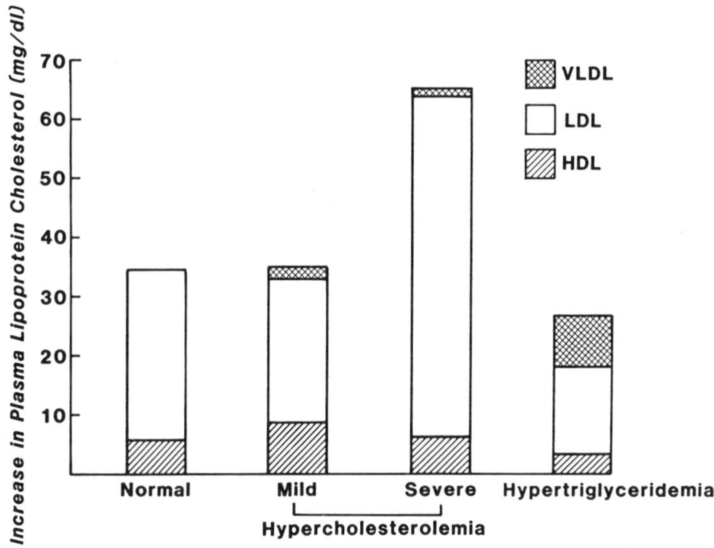

Figure 2. The effects of a 1,000 mg cholesterol diet on the content of cholesterol in the different lipoprotein (LP) fractions.

that 2% of their subjects had a negative or minimal response to dietary cholesterol feeding. Sixteen percent had responses less than half of the mean and 84% had a plasma cholesterol increase greater than half the mean. Therefore, the majority of people could be expected to respond significantly to a decrease in dietary cholesterol from 400–500 mg/day to 100 mg/day or less. Unfortunately, studies to date do not provide a way to predict who would have less than a 10% decrease and who would have greater than 10% decrease in the plasma cholesterol level in response to maximal dietary changes. Studies are needed to provide a means by which one could correctly identify individuals with regard to plasma cholesterol response to decreases in dietary cholesterol and saturated fat intakes.

Also intriguing are the possible metabolic sequelae that could contribute to this individual variation in response, such as the LDL receptor which dietary cholesterol has been shown to down-regulate (8). Mistry et al. suggested that individual differences in plasma lipid and lipoprotein response to dietary cholesterol appear to be related in part to differences in the capacity of peripheral cells to catabolize LDL and to down-regulate cholesterol synthesis (23). Recent data indicate that the various apolipoprotein E alleles may be involved, with

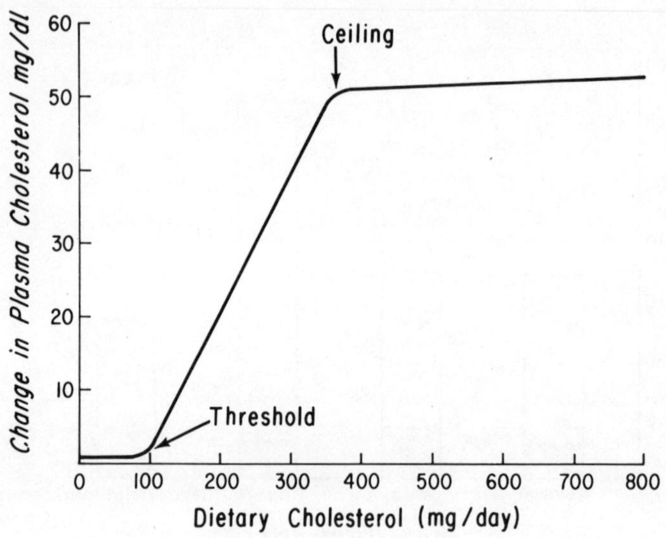

Figure 3. The effects upon the plasma cholesterol level of gradually increasing the amount of dietary cholesterol in human subjects whose background diet is very low in cholesterol content. See the text for discussion of the threshold and ceiling concepts.

the E-2 isoform causing less binding to the LDL receptor (24) and the E-4 isoform possibly increasing VLDL catabolism independently of the LDL receptor (25).

Fat

THE EFFECTS OF DIETARY FATS UPON THE PLASMA LIPIDS AND LIPOPROTEINS

The amount and kind of fat in the diet have a well-documented effect upon the plasma lipid concentrations (26,27). The *total* amount of dietary fat is important in that the formation of chylomicrons in the intstinal mucosa and their subsequent circulation in the blood is directly proportional to the amount of fat which has been consumed in the diet. A fatty meal will result in the production of large numbers of chylomicrons and will impart the characteristic lactescent appearance to post-prandial plasma observed some three to five hours after meal consumption. A typical American diet with 110 gm of fat would produce 110 gm of chylomicron triglyceride per day. "Remnant" production from chylomicrons is proportional to the number of chylomicrons synthesized. Chylomicron remnants are considered atherogenic particles (28). Fat is important in cholesterol metabolism since cholesterol is absorbed in the presence of dietary fat and is transported in chylomicrons.

However, the most important effect of dietary fat upon the plasma cholesterol level relates to the *type* of fat. Fats may be divided into three major classes identified by saturation and unsaturation characteristics. Long-chain, *saturated fatty acids* have no double bonds, are not essential nutrients, and may be readily synthesized in the body from acetate. Dietary saturated fatty acids have a profound hypercholesterolemic effect, increase the concentrations of LDL and have thrombogenic implications (26,27). All animal fats are highly saturated (30% or more of the fat is saturated) except for those which occur in fish and shellfish, these latter being, contrastingly, highly polyunsaturated. The molecular basis for the effects of dietary saturated fat on the plasma cholesterol level is now well understood and rests upon its influence on the LDL receptor activity of liver cells, as described by Brown and Goldstein (29). Dietary saturated fat suppresses hepatic LDL receptor activity, decreases the removal of LDL from the blood and thus increases the concentration of LDL cholesterol in the blood (7). Cholesterol augments the effect of saturated fat by further suppressing hepatic LDL receptor activity and raising the plasma LDL cholesterol level (8). Conversely, a decrease in dietary cholesterol and saturated fat increases the LDL receptor activity of the liver cells, enhances the hepatic pickup of LDL cholesterol and lowers the concentration of LDL cholesterol in the blood (8). Metabolic studies suggest that one can expect an average plasma cholesterol lowering of 10–20% by maximally decreasing dietary cholesterol and saturated fat intake.

Attention has been called to the fact that some saturated fats are not hypercholesterolemic (see Table 3). Medium-chain triglycerides (C8 and C10 saturated fatty acids) are handled metabolically more like carbohydrate and are transported to the liver via the portal vein blood rather than as chylomicrons. These fatty acids do not elevate the plasma cholesterol concentration. Stearic acid, an 18-carbon saturated fatty acid, likewise has a limited effect upon the plasma cholesterol concentration. This is because the body resists the accumulation of stearic acid and the liver converts excessive stearic acid from the diet into oleic acid, a monounsaturated fatty acid, by virtue of the action of a desaturase enzyme. Feeding animals large

Table 3
Effects of Saturated Fatty Acids upon Plasma Cholesterol Levels

C8, C10	Medium chain	Neutral
C12	Lauric	Increase
C14, C16	Myristic, palmitic	Increase
C18	Stearic	Neutral

quantities of a fat such as cocoa butter containing a considerable percentage of its total fatty acids as stearic acid (33%) does not result in the deposition of stearic acid in the adipose tissue as would occur with mono- and polyunsaturated fat feeding (30). This again is because of the action of the desaturase enzyme.

The practical importance of these observations on certain saturated fatty acids is limited because they are not present to any appreciable extent in the diet. The equations developed for the prediction of plasma cholesterol change have been based upon the changes produced by a given fat, including its concentration of stearic acid. Thus, all of the information which has accumulated about the hypercholesterolemic and atherogenic properties of a given fat such as beef fat, butterfat, lard, palm oil, cocoa butter and coconut oil is completely valid. To be emphasized is the fact that palmitic acid, which is the most common saturated fatty acid found in our food supply, is intensely hypercholesterolemic. It has 16 carbons; myristic acid and lauric acid with 14 and 12 carbons respectively are likewise intensely hypercholesterolemic. It is these fatty acids which are present in dietary fats and which cause their unfortunate effects. Amounts of stearic acid in the American diet are not great compared with palmitic acid.

The second class of dietary fats consists of the characteristic *monounsaturated fatty acids* present in all animal and vegetable fats. For practical purposes, oleic acid, having one double bond at the omega-9 position, is the only significant dietary monounsaturated fatty acid. In general, the effects of dietary monounsaturated fatty acids have been "neutral" in terms of their effects on the plasma cholesterol concentrations, neither raising nor lowering them (31). However, reports that Mediterranean basin populations who consume olive oil in relatively large quantities have fewer heart attacks then people in this country has led to further investigations. Recent studies have shown that large amounts of monounsaturated fat, like polyunsaturated oils, lower plasma cholesterol and LDL levels when compared with saturated fat (32,33). Furthermore, unlike polyunsaturated oils, monounsaturated fat did not lower the plasma HDL cholesterol level. However, distinct from omega-3 fatty acids from fish oil, monounsaturated fat does not decrease the plasma triglyceride concentrations (32,33). Furthermore, monounsaturated fat has no known effect upon prostaglandin metabolism or upon platelet function. Omega-3 fatty acids are antithrombotic; monounsaturated fat has no such action.

There are several additional points to be made in regard to these recent studies: 1) The Mediterranean diet is also rich in fish, beans, fruit and vegetables, and is *low* in saturated fat and cholesterol. These could be the decisive factors which influence the lessened incidence of coronary disease and lower plasma cholesterol levels. 2) Olive oil is low in saturated fatty acids (which raise plasma cholesterol levels); this may be why the recent metabolic experiments have shown some cholesterol lowering from large amounts of monounsaturates in the diet. 3) Large amounts of any kind of fat should be avoided to lower the risk of other diseases such as colon or breast cancer and obesity. And all fats, after absorption, form large particles (remnants) which circulate in the blood and are atherogenic. One translation of the latest research on monounsaturated fats is to recommend that patients include them as part of a general lower-fat eating style – use olive oil in salad dressing and Italian dishes. Use peanut oil for special stir-fried dishes. Avocado is delicious but high in fat, so use as a garnish only.

Polyunsaturated fatty acids, the third class of fatty acids, are vital constituents of cellular membranes and serve as prostaglandin precursors (34). Because they cannot be synthesized by the body and are only obtainable from dietary sources, they are "essential" fatty acids. The two classes of polyunsaturated fatty acids are the omega-6 and omega-3 fatty acids (Figure 4). The most common examples of omega-6 fatty acids are linoleic acid, found in food, and arachidonic acid, 20 carbons in length with four double bonds, usually synthesized in the body from linoleic acid by the liver. Since the basic structure of omega-6 fatty acids cannot be synthesized by the body, up to 2–3% of total energy in the diet must be supplied as linoleic acid to meet the requirements of the body for the omega-6 structure, i.e. an essential fatty acid.

Omega-3 fatty acids differ in the position of the first double bond counting from the methyl end of the molecule, this double bond being at the number 3 carbon. Omega-3 fatty acids are also an essential nutrient for human beings since the body is unable to synthesize this

FATTY ACID NOMENCLATURE			DIETARY SOURCES
FAMILY	FATTY ACID	STRUCTURE	
ω 3	Eicosapentaenoic Acid (C20:5 ω3)	H_3C 3 RCOOH	Marine Oils, Fish
ω 6	Linoleic Acid (C18:2 ω6)	H_3C 6 R′COOH	Vegetable Oils
ω 9	Oleic Acid (C18:1 ω9)	H_3C 9 R″COOH	Vegetable Oils; Animal Fats

Figure 4. Fatty acids can be organized into families according to the position of the first double bond from the terminal methyl group. Typical fatty acids from three common families are shown in this figure. Omega-3 fatty acids all have three carbons between the methyl end and the first double bond. Besides eicosapentaenoic acid (C20:5), other common omega-3 fatty acids are linolenic acid (C18:3) and docosahexaenoic acid (C22:6). Linoleic acid (C18:2) and arachidonic acid (C20:4) are the most important omega-6 fatty acids, while oleic acid (C18:1) is the commonest fatty acid in the omega-9 family.

particular structure. Omega-6 and omega-3 fatty acids are not interconvertible. The dietary sources of omega-3 fatty acids are from plant foods – some, but not all, vegetable oils, and leafy vegetables (which are especially rich in omega-3 fatty acids) and, in particular, fish and shellfish. Linolenic acid, C18:3, is obtained from vegetable products. Eicosapentaenoic acid, C20:5, and docosahexaenoic acid, C22:5, are derived from fish, shellfish and phytoplankton (the plants of the ocean) and are highly concentrated in fish oils. Once either the omega-3 or omega-6 structure comes into the body as the 18 carbon linoleic or linolenic acid, the body can synthesize the longer chain and more highly polyunsaturated omega-6 or omega-3 fatty acids (20 and 22 carbons).

There are distinctly different functions in the body for omega-3 and omega-6 fatty acids. Both serve as substrate for the formation of different prostaglandins (34) and are rich in phospholipid membranes. Both omega-3 and omega-6 fatty acids are particularly concentrated in nervous tissue. Omega-3 fatty acids are rich in the retina, spermatozoa, the gonads, and many other organs. Omega-6 fatty acids are concentrated in the different plasma lipid classes (cholesterol esters, phospholipids, etc.) and, in addition, are concerned with lipid transport.

Table 4
Cardiovascular Effects of Omega-3 Fatty Acids

1 Hypolipidemic: decrease plasma lipids-lipoproteins, cholesterol, triglycerides, LDL, VLDL, chylomicrons and remnants.
2 Anti-thrombotic and vasodilatory: decrease platelet stickiness; increase bleeding time.
3 Lower blood pressure.

Polyunsaturated fatty acids in large amounts, of either the omega-6 or omega-3 structure, depress plasma total and LDL cholesterol concentrations (22,31). Omega-3 fatty acids have a second additional action in lowering plasma triglyceride concentrations and, in particular, VLDL, chylomicrons and remnants (35,36).

Already stressed is the wealth of evidence from experimental animals about the important and *sine qua non* necessity of dietary cholesterol and fat being present in the nutrition of animals to produce atherosclerosis. Several important studies in regard to fish oil containing omega-3 fatty acids have indicated much less atherosclerosis developing when fish oil was present in the diet. The species studied to date have been pigs (37) and rhesus monkeys (38). Both coronary and aortic atherosclerosis have been greatly reduced by fish oil. This reduction in experimental atherosclerosis from omega-3 fatty acids is not necessarily explainable by changes in the plasma lipid-lipoprotein concentration. Since these were lowered only partially or not at all during the experimental atherosclerosis period, other mechanisms, possibly involving prostaglandins, must be postulated to explain the anti-atherogenic effects of fish oil. Table 4 lists possible effects of omega-3 fatty acids from fish oil upon coronary heart disease.

It is not known exactly how the evidence about omega-3 fatty acids should translate in eating behaviour. However, one study from the Netherlands showed that men who included fish in their diet twice a week had fewer deaths from heart disease (39). Even very low-fat seafood contains an appreciable amount of omega-3 fatty acids. Eating a total of 12 oz. of a variety of fish and shellfish each week would provide 1000 to 5000 mg of omega-3 fatty acids as well as protein, vitamins and minerals. The patient with hyperlipidemia could be expected to have only beneficial effects from following this dietary advice, especially if the fish replaced meat in the diet.

Most of the comparisons of the effects of saturated and polyunsaturated fat upon the plasma lipids have indicated that gram for gram, saturated fat is up to two times greater at raising plasma cholesterol than is polyunsaturated fat in depressing it (40,41). Regression equations have been calculated to indicate the plasma cholesterol changes from dietary manipulations of saturated fat, polyunsaturated fat and cholesterol. These will be discussed later in the development of the cholesterol-saturated fat index of foods.

Many, but not all, of the currently marketed vegetable oils, shortenings, and margarines are only partially hydrogenated and thus retain the basic unsaturated characteristics of vegetable oils. Coconut oil, cocoa butter (the fat of chocolate) and palm oil are common "saturated" vegatable fats consumed in quantities; they have a hypercholesterolemic effect. The ratio of polyunsaturated to saturated fatty acids in a given fat or oil is termed the P/S value. Fats with a high P/S value of 2 and above, compared to 0.4 and less, are generally recognized as being hypocholesterolemic. The typical Western diet has a P/S value of 0.4. In the suggested low-fat, high-carbohydrate diet to prevent coronary disease, the P/S value is above 1.0.

DIETARY FAT AND THROMBOSIS

Table 5 lists possible dietary effects on thrombosis and platelet aggregation. These effects are based upon both experimental and epidemiological evidence. As may be appreciated, firm documentation in this arena may not always be possible and no clinical trials have been conducted to support the suggested relationships. However, both in vitro and in vivo, saturated fatty acids of a chain length C12 and above appear to be thrombogenic, activating the coagulation cascade and aggregating platelets (42–45). Any circumstance which elevates the levels of free fatty acids in the plasma such as starvation, diabetic acidosis, myocardial infarction, or certain hormonal stimulation must be considered as having a thrombotic effect as well (46–50). For example, in starvation, free fatty acids are released into the plasma from adipose tissue triglyceride. The mechanism of this effect may occur from a level of free fatty acids exceeding the two tight binding sites on the albumin molecule, the usual transport form of free fatty acids (51). This, then, allows the free fatty acids to interact with various coagulation proteins and with platelets.

Polyunsaturated fat, in general, has an antithrombotic effect. This effect is best documented by dietary studies in human beings (34) and by the epidemiological evidence in the Greenland Eskimos who have a low incidence of thrombotic disease (52). They consume fish and

Table 5
Dietary Factors Affecting Thrombosis and Platelet Function

1 Thrombotic factors
  Saturated fatty acids
  Free fatty acids
2 Anti-thrombotic factors
  Low-fat, high CHO diet
  Polyunsaturated fat
    omega-6 fatty acids (linoleic) from vegetable oils
    omega-3 fatty acids (eicosapentaenoic) from fish oil

seal, both rich in the omega-3 fatty acids, eicosapentaenoic and docosahexaenoic fatty acids (53). The feeding of fish and fish oil to humans or their presence in a natural diet not only has a hypolipidemic effect but also increases the bleeding time and reduces platelet aggregation (54,55). On the other hand, the ingestion of a low-fat diet high in carboydrate and fibre is associated with a low incidence of thrombosis in certain population groups, such as the Ugandans (56–58). These populations ingest a low-fat diet and consume most of their fat in the form of polyunsaturated fatty acids with a very low intake of saturated fat.

Accordingly, an antithrombotic diet for human beings would be low in total fat and saturated fat and might contain fish. It should also be a high-carbohydrate, high-fibre diet. High circulating levels of the plasma-free fatty acids should also be avoided. This is particularly important in obese patients with vascular disease who are given low calorie diets. Such diets should avoid ketosis, which would be an indication that plasma-free fatty acid concentrations are greatly increased. They should contain sufficient calories in general, about 700–1000 kcalories day, in which the chief sources of calories would be carbohydrate and protein.

Carbohydrate

If the total fat content of an anti-coronary diet is reduced from the current American intake of 40% to 20% of the total calories and if protein is to be kept constant, the difference in caloric intake between a high-fat diet and a low-fat diet must be made up by increasing the carbohydrate content of the diet. As already indicated, both the epidemiological evidence and experimental studies buttress this basic concept, since populations ingesting a high-carbohydrate diet, usually from complex carbohydrates, have a low incidence of coronary disease and other thrombotic conditions.

Over 25 years ago it was demonstrated that a sudden increase in the amount of dietary carbohydrate in Americans accustomed to a high-fat diet would increase the plasma triglyceride concentration rather dramatically (59). However, after many weeks, adaptation occurs, and the hypertriglyceridemia regresses (60,61). We regard this situation as metabolically normal, since it is a universal occurrence in Americans given a high-carbohydrate diet. It is analogous to the hyperglycemia which results in individuals who have previously been consuming a reduced number of calories or a low-carbohydrate diet and are given a glucose load. In order to obtain a valid glucose tolerance curve, an individual must eat a diet reasonably high in carbohydrate for at least three days before the test.

High-carbohydrate diets have been used in diabetic patients over a long period of time without impairment of glucose tolerance and without the occurrence of hypertriglyceridemia (60). Since any lasting dietary change is adopted gradually, as will be emphasized in the behavioural modification approach taken to educate patients about dietary change, it is highly unlikely that any patient with coronary disease asked to follow the low-cholesterol, low-fat, high-carbohydrate diet would develop hypertriglyceridemia. There would be ample time for adaptation as he passed through the three or more phases of this dietary approach.

We recently increased the dietary carbohydrate intake gradually from 45% kcal to 65% kcal over a 28-day period in seven mildly hypertriglyceridemic subjects. There was a significant lowering of the mean plasma cholesterol level from 226 to 190 mg/dl, −16% ($p < 0.001$), whereas the mean plasma triglyceride level remained constant, 217 mg/dl to 222 mg/dl (62).

Studies in rats have indicated that sucrose and fructose have a hypertriglyceridemic effect in contrast to starch or glucose (63). The evidence in human beings that even very large amounts of sucrose (over 50% of the total calories) produce hyperlipidemia is not completely convincing. However, even if large quantities of sucrose have a mild hypertriglyceridemic and perhaps also a hypercholesterolemic effect, this does not bear particularly upon the dietary design of the anti-coronary diet as envisioned. In the low-fat, high-carbohydrate diet the vast majority of the carbohydrate is in the form of cereals and legumes, not sucrose. Americans commonly consume about 20% of the total calories as sucrose or about half of their carbohydrate intake. In the dietary changes being suggested, sucrose would fall to 10–15% of the total calories, and so any effect from sucrose would be diminished rather than accentuated by the dietary change.

Fibre

Dietary fibre is a broad nondescript term which includes several carbohydrates thought to be indigestible by the human gut. These include cellulose, hemicelluloses, lignin, pectin and beta glucans. Dietary fibre is only found in plants and is commonly present in unprocessed cereals, legumes, vegetables and fruits. In ruminant animals, dietary fibre is completely digested by the microbial flora of the rumen, so that fibre provides a major source of energy for these animals. In man, however, dietary fibre contributes little to the caloric content of the diet, promotes satiety through its bulk, and affects colonic function greatly. A high-fibre diet produces larger stools and a more rapid intestinal transit, factors which may prevent certain diseases of the colon (i.e. diverticulitis, colon cancer). A high-fibre diet increases the emptying time of the stomach, thereby promoting slower absorption of nutrients, especially glucose.

Fibre experiments date back at least 30 years (64,65). Fibre added to semisynthetic diets fed to rats has usually had a plasma cholesterol lowering effect. In humans, fibre fed predominantly in the insoluble form was not hypocholesterolemic (66). A study in which large amounts of soluble fibre (17 gms/2000 kcal) from oat bran and beans were fed to people produced a 20% lowering of the plasma total and LDL cholesterol levels (67). Other studies have produced similar results (68,69). Rich sources of soluble fibre include fruits, pectin being a soluble fibre, oats and other cereals, legumes and vegetables. One way soluble fibre acts is to bind bile acids in the gut, prevent their reabsorption and thus lower cholesterol levels much like the bile acid-binding resins like cholestyramine.

A high-fibre diet is integral to the dietary concepts for the treatment of hyperlipidemia. The consumption of more foods from vegetable sources will automatically mean a higher consumption of both total and soluble fibre.

Protein

The dietary treatment of hyperlipidemia involves, in general, a shift from the consumption of protein derived from animal sources, such as meat and dairy products, to the consumption of more protein from plants. The nutritional adequacy of such protein shifts is assured, because mixtures of vegetable proteins, plus the provision of ample low-fat animal protein sources, provide abundantly for essential amino acid requirements. Ranges of protein intake from 25 to 150 grams have been tested over the years for effects upon blood lipids and have been found to have no effect within amounts commonly consumed by Americans. However, experiments in animals have suggested that an animal protein such as casein (from milk) is definitely hypercholesterolemic and that a vegetable protein such as soy protein has the opposite effect. There have been few definitive experiments in humans to test the hypocholesterolemic effect of vegetable proteins vis à vis animal proteins. As might be expected, it is difficult to control all the variables, including the cholesterol and fat content. However, there are suggestions that the consumption of vegetable protein may have some hypocholesterolemic action. Thus, it may be postulated that a shift in protein intake to include more vegetable protein carries no harm and may confer some benefit to the hyperlipidemic individual.

Calories

Excessive caloric intake and adiposity can contribute also to both hypertriglyceridemia and hypercholesterolemia by stimulating the liver to overproduce VLDL. The plasma triglyceride and VLDL concentrations of hypertriglyceridemic patients greatly improve after weight reduction and are increased by the hypercaloric state (70–72). There is little direct evidence, however, that the LDL receptor and plasma cholesterol and LDL concentrations are directly affected by caloric excess. Nonetheless, it is known that obese individuals have a total body cholesterol production which is higher than in individuals of normal weight. Weight reduction and fasting, which involve a decrease in the consumption of cholesterol and saturated fat from the diet, could certainly upregulate the LDL receptor and could be expected to improve LDL levels in patients with familial hypercholesterolemia. It is, therefore, reasonable to advise caloric control and the avoidance of obesity in the dietary management of hyperlipidemia. The role of increased physical activity is most important in weight control.

Alcohol

Results from large population studies have shown that people who report consuming alcohol have a lower incidence of coronary heart disease than people who do not drink (73,74). These studies, while indicating trends in large populations, need to be reinforced by the much stronger evidence provided by controlled experiments in which other factors that influence the plasma HDL cholesterol level such as body weight, smoking, exercise habits and diet are accounted for. Many such studies testing the effect of alcohol consumption on HDL cholesterol levels have been conducted. These studies have shown significant increases in HDL cholesterol after alcohol consumption ranging from an equivalent of two beers to seven beers per day over three to six weeks compared to a similar abstention period. The type of alcohol given (beer, wine, spirits) did not appear to influence results. Alcohol appears to increase the HDL_3 component of HDL which is less related to protection against coronary heart disease (75). It is HDL_2, affected by exercise but not alcohol, which is more protective (76). Because of these results, and since the increased levels of HDL have been linked to lower rates of atherosclerosis, some drinkers have been tempted to drink more, claiming that alcohol is "good for the heart." Should alcohol consumption be encouraged to protect against coronary heart disease?

Specific recommendations are not easy to make, because the effects of alcohol consumption are complex, affecting other components of the plasma in addition to HDL cholesterol. Most of the metabolic studies have involved people with plasma cholesterol values below 190 mg/dl, and these results may not translate directly to patients with hyperlipidemia. The effects of alcohol on the levels of HDL_2 (linked to reduced coronary disease) and HDL_3 (no relationship to coronary disease) are controversial. Alcohol is packed with calories. There are about 290 kcalories in two 12-ounce beers or two 6-ounce glasses of wine. On the average, up to 8% of calories consumed by adult Americans come from alcohol. This may be one of the reasons why so many people who drink heavily are overweight and have alcohol-related problems. Theoretically, the amount of alcohol it would take to increase a person's HDL cholesterol from below 30 to above 40 mg/dl is five to six drinks per day. Other consequences of alcohol consumption – admittedly when excessive – include cirrhosis of the liver, certain cancers, gastritis, mental deterioration, neuropathies and, of course, the personal and social ravages of chronic alcoholism.

We do not think that alcohol should be part of a daily diet, rather – for those who enjoy an occasional drink – we suggest a limit of one to two drinks on any given day and up to four to five drinks per week. The inclusion of alcohol in the diet to increase HDL cholesterol levels is not recommended.

Lecithin

This phospholipid derived from soybeans is commonly sold in health food stores and is widely publicized as a popular remedy for hypercholesterolemia. Aside from its high content of linoleic acid, the consumption of lecithin has little or no effect upon lipid metabolism. Contrary to popular belief, lecithin is not absorbed as such from the digestive tract but is hydrolyzed into its constituent fatty acids and choline. Choline is a lipotrophic substance which was tested in the treatment of hypercholesterolemia 30 years ago and found to be of no value (77). The plasma phospholipid levels have not been affected by the addition of lecithin to the diet; the circulating plasma phospholipids are largely synthesized by the liver. Parenthetically, high levels of plasma phospholipids are found in patients with familial hypercholesterolemia.

Minerals and Vitamins

Under the assumption that the minimum daily requirements have been met in the diet, there is no information to indicate that additional vitamins and minerals above and beyond the content of a nutritionally adequate diet will have any effect upon the plasma lipid concentrations. This comment applies equally to vitamin C (78) and vitamin E (79), both enthusiastically consumed by the public without there being any proof of benefit. On the contrary, massive doses of vitamin A may produce liver damage (80). The sole exception is niacin, a B-vitamin used in massive doses for the treatment of hyperlipidemia.

Design of a Dietary Approach for Treating and Preventing Coronary Heart Disease

In view of the evidence about dietary factors, hyperlipidemia, thrombosis and coronary heart disease, it should now be possible to indicate the features of an appropriate and effective preventive diet against coronary heart disease in patients with hyperlipidemia and for the public at large. In general terms, such a diet, from what has already been indicated in this chapter, should be hypolipidemic and antithrombotic. It should be nutritionally adequate and meet the necessary nutritional requirements during childhood and adult life. This feature is essential because the dietary approach is less likely to succeed unless it is familial. Coronary heart disease occurs in families.

Many in the family who have not yet developed overt symptomatology of coronary heart disease are undoubtedly at risk for subsequent coronary heart disease. Another criterion of the dietary approach is that it should be no more costly than the current Western diet. Finally, its use should be facilitated and supported by recipes and menu plans to make it possible for interested patients and their families to incorporate the proposed dietary changes into their lifestyle after a suitable educational and training period. The dietary approach presented here, i.e. the low-fat, high-carbohydrate diet, is intended to produce a maximal lowering of plasma total and LDL cholesterol concentrations, to reduce excess body weight when this is present, and to respond to all of the evidence concerning antithrombotic dietary factors. This diet can be used to treat the many different types of hyperlipidemia. No longer is it necessary to have a different diet for each phenotype of hyperlipidemia. The same diet with slight modification can be used for any type of hyperlipidemia. This single diet concept has been delineated in detail elsewhere (81, 82).

THE CHOLESTEROL-SATURATED FAT INDEX (CSI) OF FOODS (83)

The major plasma cholesterol elevating effects of a given food reside in its cholesterol and saturated fat content. To help understand the contribution of these two factors in a single food item and to compare one food with another, we have computed a cholesterol-saturated fat index (CSI) for selected foods (Figure 5 and Table 6). This index was based on a modification of the regression equation used earlier to calculate the cholesterol index of foods (84). Since the objective of the low-fat, high-carbohydrate diet is to maintain, but not to increase, the current intake of polyunsaturated fat, we chose not to include the polyunsaturated fat component of the equation in assessing an individual food item. The cholesterol index of foods was thus modified and is called the cholesterol-saturated fat index (CSI): CSI $=$ ($1.01 \times$ gm saturated fat) $+$ ($0.05 \times$ mg cholesterol), where the amounts of saturated fat and cholesterol in a given amount of a food item are entered into this equation.

In this context it is particularly instructive to compare the CSI of fish versus moderately fat beef. A 100 gm portion of cooked fish contains 66 mg of cholesterol and 0.20 gm of saturated fat. This contrasts to a 96 mg cholesterol content and 8.1 gm of saturated fat of 20% fat beef. The CSI for 100 gm (3.5 oz) fish is 4, while that of beef is 13. The caloric value of these two portions also differs greatly (91

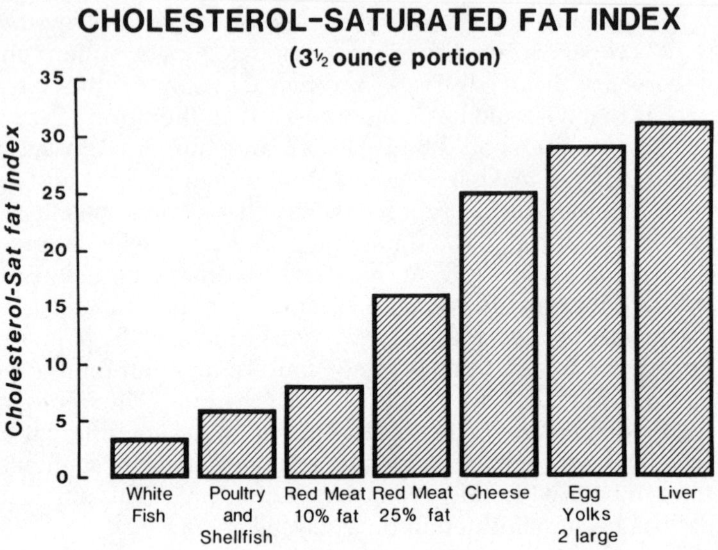

CHOLESTEROL-SATURATED FAT INDEX

(3½ ounce portion)

Cholesterol-Sat fat Index

White Fish | Poultry and Shellfish | Red Meat 10% fat | Red Meat 25% fat | Cheese | Egg Yolks 2 large | Liver

Figure 5. The cholesterol-saturated fat index (CSI) of 3½ oz. of fish, poultry, shellfish, meat, cheese, egg yolk, and liver. The CSI for poultry is the average CSI for cooked light and dark chicken without skin. The CSI for shellfish is the average CSI of cooked crab, lobster, shrimp, clams, oysters and scallops. The CSI for cheese is the average CSI of cheddar, Swiss and processed cheese.

for fish and 286 for beef). The CSI of cooked chicken and turkey (without the skin) is also preferable to beef and other red meats. Again, the total fat content is quite a bit lower and the saturated fat per 100 gm is 1.3, with the cholesterol 87 mg. The CSI of poultry is 6. Table 6 lists the CSI for various foods.

Shellfish have low CSIs because their saturated fat content is extremely low, despite the fact that their cholesterol or total sterol content is 2.5 to 3 times higher than fish, poultry or red meat. This means that, when considering both cholesterol and saturated fat, shellfish have a CSI of 6, very much like poultry, and are a better choice than even the leanest red meats. Salmon also has a low CSI and is preferred to meat.

THE LOW-FAT, HIGH-CARBOHYDRATE DIET

The relationship between nutrients and coronary heart disease presents both responsibility and opportunity. The challenge is to define

Table 6
The Cholesterol-Saturated Fat Index (CSI) and Kilocalorie Content of Selected Foods

	CSI	*kcalories*
Fish, Poultry, Red Meat (3½ ounces or 100 grams cooked)		
Whitefish-snapper, perch, sole, cod, halibut, etc.	4	91
Salmon	5	149
Shellfish (shrimp, crab, lobster)	6	104
Poultry, no skin	6	171
Beef, Pork and Lamb:		
10 per cent fat (ground sirloin, flank steak)	9	214
15 per cent fat (ground round)	10	258
20 per cent fat (ground chuck, pot roasts)	13	286
30 per cent fat (ground beef, pork, and lamb, steaks, ribs, pork and lamb chops, roasts)	18	381
Cheeses (3½ ounces or 100 grams)		
Low-fat cottage cheese, tofu (bean curd), pot cheese,	1	98
Cottage cheese, Lite-Line, Lite'n Lively, part-skim ricotta, reduced calorie Laughing Cow	6	139
Imitation Mozzarella, Cheezola, Min Chol (Swedish low fat), Hickory Farm Lyte, Saffola American*	6	317
Olympia Low Fat, Green River, Keil Kase (lower fat Cheddars), part-skim mozzarella, Neufchatel (lower fat cream cheese), Skim American,	12	256
Cheddar, roquefort, Swiss, brie, jack, American, cream cheese, Velveeta, cheese spreads (jars), and most other cheeses	26	386
Eggs		
Whites (three)	0	51
Egg Substitute (equivalent to two eggs)	1	91
Whole (two)	29	163
Fats (¼ cup or 4 tablespoons)		
Peanut Butter	6	380
Mayonnaise	8	404
Most vegetable oils	6	491
Soft vegetable margarines	8	420
Soft shortenings	13	464
Bacon grease	20	464
Butter	36	409
Coconut oil, palm oil	38	491
Frozen Desserts (1 cup)		
Water ices	0	245
Sherbet or frozen yogurt	2	290
Ice milk	6	214
Ice cream, 10% fat	13	272
Rich ice cream, 16% fat	18	349
Specialty ice cream, 22% fat	34	768

*Cheeses made with skim milk and vegetable oils.

Table 6, Cont.

	CSI	kcalories
Milk Products (1 cup)		
Skim milk (0.1% fat), or skim milk yogurt	<1	88
1% milk, buttermilk	2	115
2% milk or plain lowfat yogurt	5	144
Whole milk (3.5% fat) or whole milk yogurt	10	159
Liquid non-dairy creamers: Mocha Mix, Poly Rich	7	376
Liquid non-dairy creamers: store brands, Cereal Blend, Coffee Rich	22	344
Sour cream	39	468
Imitation sour cream (IMO)	43	499

dietary objectives in specific and very practical terms relating to shopping, food preparation and eating (84). One of the first low-cholesterol, low-fat cookbooks was produced by Dobbin et al. in 1957 (86). Our own such diet plan and cookbook is called *The New American Diet* (85). The first objective of all low-fat diets must be to reduce cholesterol consumption from 500 to less than 100 mg per day. This requires keeping egg yolk consumption to a minimum since 45% of dietary cholesterol comes from egg yolk, with approximately half from visible eggs and half from eggs incorporated into foods (Figure 6) (86). Meat and poultry and fish are limited as well as the use of lower-fat dairy products.

The second objective is to reduce fat intake by one-half, from 40 to 20% of calories. This can be done by avoiding fried foods, reducing the fat used in baked goods by one-third and using low-fat dairy products. Added fat should be limited to three teaspoons per day for women and children and five teaspoons per day for teenagers and men. Peanut butter should be used as part of a meal and not as a snack, and nuts used sparingly as condiments.

Another objective is to decrease the current saturated fat intake by two-thirds, from 14 to 5–6% of calories. This requires eating red meat or cheese no more than twice a week, using lower-fat cheeses (20% fat or less), avoiding products containing coconut and palm oil, limiting ice cream and chocolate to once a month and using soft margarines and oils sparingly.

When people are advised to decrease the amount of fat in their diets, they usually think only of visible fat and are surprised to learn that fat added at the table represents only 22% of their fat intake (Figure 7) (87). Decreasing dietary fat would be very difficult without

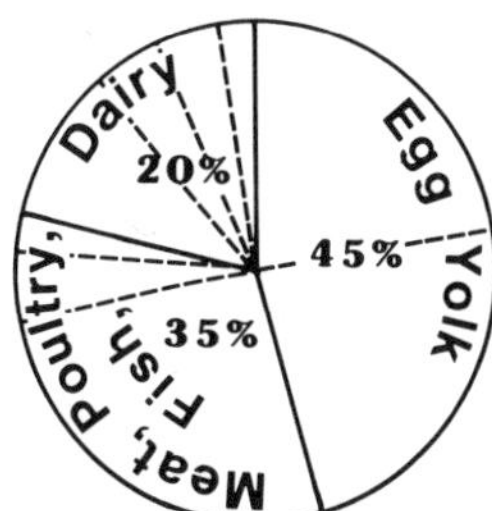

Figure 6. The sources of dietary cholesterol for people in the United States. Forty-five percent of the dietary cholesterol is derived from egg yolk, with half of that being from visible eggs (1–2 eggs per week) and half from eggs used in food preparation (the broken line in the egg yolk segment). Twenty-eight percent of the cholesterol is from red meats, poultry (4%), and fish (2%). Twenty percent is from dairy products: 8% from milk, 5% from cheese, 4% from butter, and 2% from ice cream.

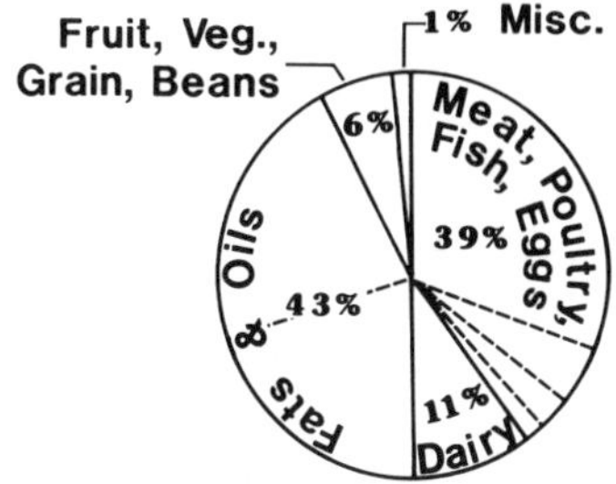

Figure 7. The sources of dietary fat for people in the United States. Thirty percent of the dietary fat is derived from red meats (30%), poultry (5%), eggs (3%), and fish (1%), as per the broken lines dividing that segment of the circle. Eleven percent is from dairy products. Forty-three percent is directly from fats and oils, 21.5% being from visible fat (spreads and dressings) and 21.5% from fat used in cooking and baking. Six percent is from fruits, vegetables, grains, and beans, and 1% is from miscellaneous sources.

knowing that 78% is invisible, with the majority coming from red meat, cheese, ice cream and other dairy products, and fat used in food preparation.

If dietary fat is reduced from 40 to 20% of calories and protein kept constant at 15% of calories to maintain weight, carbohydrate intake must be increased from 45 to 65% of total calories. What this means practically is that at least two complex carbohydrate-containing foods should be eaten at each meal. For example, eating toast *and* cereal for breakfast, a sandwich (two slices of bread) or bean soup and low-fat crackers at lunch, and 1–2 cups of rice, pasta, potatoes, corn, etc. *with* bread at dinner, in addition to selecting complex carbohydrate snacks such as popcorn or low-fat crackers and low-fat cookies. This is a significant change, as most Americans currently limit carbohydrate foods to no more than *one* per meal. To reach the increased carbohydrate objective, the patient must also eat two to four cups of legumes per week and two to four cups of vegetables per day. While research supports the value of a high-carbohydrate diet, many people are reluctant to adopt it because "starchy" foods are falsely associated with gaining weight and are viewed as the food of the poor. Another objective is to eat three to five pieces of fruit per day with a concomitant decrease in refined sugar intake from 20% of calories to 10%. This means that sweets (pop *or* candy *or* desserts) must be limited to no more than one serving per day.

THE PHASES OF THE LOW-FAT, HIGH-CARBOHYDRATE DIET

Even well-motivated patients do not make abrupt changes in their dietary habits that are maintained over time. It will take many months and even years to make permanent changes in food consumption patterns. Therefore, we suggest that the recommended changes be approached in a gradual manner, with each phase introducing more changes toward the low-fat, high-carbohydrate diet pattern (82,85,89). The manner in which patients are guided through these phases can be individualized. An example of three phases is summarized in Table 7.

Phase I

The aim of Phase I is to decrease the consumption of foods high in cholesterol and saturated fat (Table 6). This can be accomplished by deleting egg yolk, butterfat, lard, and organ meats from the diet and by using substitute products when possible: soft margarine for butter, vegetable oils and shortening for lard, skim milk for whole milk, and egg whites for whole eggs. Many alternative foods can replace foods that contain large amounts of cholesterol and saturated fat. Increasing numbers of new products low in cholesterol and saturated fat are now marketed: low-fat cheeses, egg substitutes, soy meats, and frozen yogurt are a few examples.

Many recipes currently in use can easily be altered. For example, most recipes, including baked items, can be made without egg yolks. Usually 1½ to 2 egg withes can be used successfully in place of one whole egg in making cakes, cookies, custards, potato salad and many other products without changing their quality.

Phase II

The goal of Phase II is a reduction of meat and cheese consumption with a gradual transition from the Western ideal of up to a pound of

Table 7
Summary of the Three Phases of the Low-Fat, High-Carbohydrate Diet

Phase		
Phase I: Substitutions	This is accomplished by:	
	avoiding egg yolks, butterfat, lard and organ meats (liver, heart, brains, kidney, gizzards);	trimming fat off meat and skin from chicken
	substituting soft margarine for butter;	choosing commercial food products lower in cholesterol and fat (low-fat cheeses, egg substitutes, soy meat substitutes, frozen yogurt, etc.)
	substituting vegetable oils and shortening for lard;	modifying favorite recipes by using less fat or sugar and vegetable oils instead of butter or lard;
	substituting skim milk and skim milk products for whole milk and whole milk products;	
	substituting egg whites for whole eggs;	
Phase II: New recipes	This step involves:	
	reducing amounts of meat and cheese eaten and replacing them with chicken and fish;	eating more grains, beans, fruit and vegetables;
	eating meat, chicken or fish only once a day;	when eating out, make low-fat, low-cholesterol choices;
	cutting down on fat; as spreads, in salads, cooking and baking;	finding new recipes to replace those which cannot be altered
Phase III: A new way of eating	The final phase means:	
	eating meat, cheese, poultry and fish as "condiments" to other foods, rather than as main courses;	drinking 4–6 glasses of water per day;
	eating more beans and grain products as protein sources;	keeping extra meat, shellfish, regular cheese, chocolate, candy, coconut, and richer home-baked or commercially prepared food for special occasions (once a month or less
	using no more than 3–5 teaspoons of fat per day as spreads, salad dressings, or in cooking and baking	enjoying a wide variety of new food and repertoire of totally new and savory recipes

meat a day to no more than 6–8 ounces per day (Table 7). The use of lean, well-trimmed meat will help to decrease greatly the amount of saturated fat. Fatter meats such as lunch meats, bacon, sausage, wieners, spareribs and others should be saved for very special occasions. Meat or cheese should be used no more than *once* a day. One significant point is the change in the composition of the traditional sandwich. Meat and cheese are not necessarily essential parts of a sandwich, nor is a sandwich always necessary for lunch. In addition, less fat and cheese should be used. Broiling, baking, steaming or braising should be the methods of cooking instead of frying. Fewer foods should be used which contain a lot of fat. Only cheeses with part or all skim milk (20% fat or less) should be selected for daily cooking. Cheeses made from whole milk should be used sparingly, one ounce of cheese being substituted for three ounces of lean meat.

At this point, new recipes will be needed to replace the recipes which cannot be altered to meet these new requirements. Recipes centred about meat or high-fat dairy products (cream cheese, butter, sour cream, cheese) can be replaced with recipes that use larger amounts of grains, legumes, vegetables and fruits. Furthermore, because of the world-wide concern for the conservation of natural resources and the use of economical foods as well as the current interest in gourmet cooking and exotic foods, a large number of new recipes can be found in current cookbooks, magazines and newspapers. Many of these stress the use of non-animal food products.

Many other cultures have developed delicious meals which are low in cholesterol and in fat. A wide variety of spices and different products and foods from the cuisines of other countries can be used. Oriental dishes emphasize fresh vegetables and rice products; Mexican dishes make use of tortillas, peppers and beans. The Mediterranean countries (Greece, Italy and Spain) incorporate pastas and vegetable sauces. The cuisine of the Middle Eastern countries employs a variety of wheat products and legume dishes.

Phase III

In Phase III the final goals of the low-fat, high-carbohydrate diet are attained. The cholesterol content of the diet is reduced to 100 mg per day and the saturated fat lowered to 5 or 6% of the total calories. These changes mean that consumption of meat and cheese, in particular, must be reduced. For most patients this will present a considerable challenge. We take an historical approach to the consumption of meat. Man has always eaten meat. What he has not done is to eat meat every day, let alone several times a day. Even today, *daily* meat consumption is only possible for the affluent minority of the world's population. It is not to our advantage, from the standpoints of either health or the wise use of resources, to consume large amounts of meat every day.

We propose, therefore, in Phase III, that meat, fish and poultry be used as "condiments" rather than "aliments." With this philosophy, no longer will the meat dish occupy the centre of the table. Instead, meat in smaller quantities will spice up vegetable-rice-cereal-legume based dishes, much as in Oriental, Indian and Mediterranean cookery. The use of low-fat, low-cholesterol cheeses is also an important component of Phase III.

The total of meat, shellfish (shrimp, crab, lobster) and poultry should average three to four ounces per day. Poultry and especially fish should be stressed instead of meat because of their lower saturated fat content. In lieu of meat or poultry, fish and molluscs (clams, oysters, scallops) may be included in the diet in amounts up to six ounces per day because of the omega-3 fatty acids.

By this time, new recipes will be emphasizing whole grains and legumes. In Phase II of the low-fat, high-carbohydrate diet, lunch, the smaller meal of the day, was changed by using beans, grains and low-fat animal products in place of meat. In Phase III the larger meal of the day becomes very different. A large variety of new flavours and spices will be introduced. An example of entrées for dinner over a week include lean beef or pork for 1–2 days, poultry for 2–3 days, fish for 2–3 days, and meatless for 1–2 days. During Phase III, the transition from the current Western diet to the low-fat, high-carbohydrate diet will have been completed (Table 7). Sample menus for one week are provided in Table 8.

Special Occasions: Eating away from Home, and Entertainment

Many restaurants serve a variety of the foods recommended in Phase III of the low-fat, high-carbohydrate diet. Oriental, Italian, Mexican and Middle Eastern restaurants all have tasty foods to choose from. In the inevitable situation where the food choices are minimal, such as at parties or when eating in friends' homes, one can concentrate upon the salad, vegetable, fruit and cereal foods and take small amounts of the animal foods to be used as condiments. Guests entertained at home can be introduced to a new way of eating which they will discover to be attractive, tasty and healthful. Obviously, meeting the goals for Phase III is very difficult when eating out of the home. Therefore, one needs to eat meals at home which are as low-fat as possible to meet the goals. Then, by being selective about the frequency of eating out and by making choices, one can afford to have special occasions or feasts which include extra meat, cheese, chocolate and coconut.

Table 8
Low Fat, High Carbohydrate Sample Menus

Day 1	*Day 2*	*Day 3*	*Day 4*	*Day 5*	*Day 6*	*Day 7*
Cantaloupe Raisin Bran cereal Skim milk English muffin with jam	Orange Juice Whole Wheat pancakes topped with unsweetened applesauce	Plain low-fat yogurt with banana, Cereal Bran Muffins*	Berries Shredded wheat Skim Milk Whole grain toast	Grapefuit half Potatoes (Hashbrowned with small amount of oil in non-stick pan) Whole grain toast with marmalade	Blueberries Hot whole grain cereal Skim milk English muffin	Fresh melon German oven pancakes*
Tuna sandwich (water-packed tuna mixed with tangy dressing* or imitation mayonnaise) Carrot sticks Fresh fruit	Chili bean salad* in whole wheat pocket bread Tomato soup (Campbell's Low-sodium) Fresh fruit Graham crackers	Lentil soup* Low-fat crackers Laughing cow reduced calorie cheese, Fresh fruit	Bean burritcs Lettuce and sliced tomato Fresh fruit	Salad bar (greens topped with kidney beans, tomato, radishes, garbanzo beans, and cucumbers) Low-calorie commercial or Western dressing* Bagel Fruit	Peanut butter and jelly sandwich Vegetable sticks (carrot, celery, etc) Fresh orange Whole wheat fig bar	Minestrone soup Wheat berry rolls Low-fat cottage cheese, Fresh fruit
Bean lasagna* Tossed salad with Western dressing* French bread Fresh berries	Cashew chicken* Steamed rice Fresh pineapple slices Wheat berry rolls Hot fudge pudding cake*	Easy Tuna noodle casserole* Steamed broccoli Confetti Appleslaw*, Wheat rolls Strawberry ice*	Pizza Rice casserole* Green peas Green salad with low-calorie dressing Sourdough rolls Gingersnaps	Baked herbed fish* Baked potato with mock sour cream* Steamed zucchini Waldorf salad* Caraway puffs*	Corn chips* with bean dip* Creamy enchiladas* Meatless Spanish rice Shredded lettuce & tomato Fresh fruit	Spaghetti with marinara sauce* Tossed salad with low-calorie dressing Steamed green beans seasoned with lemon and pepper, French bread, Fresh fruit

*recipes from (85)

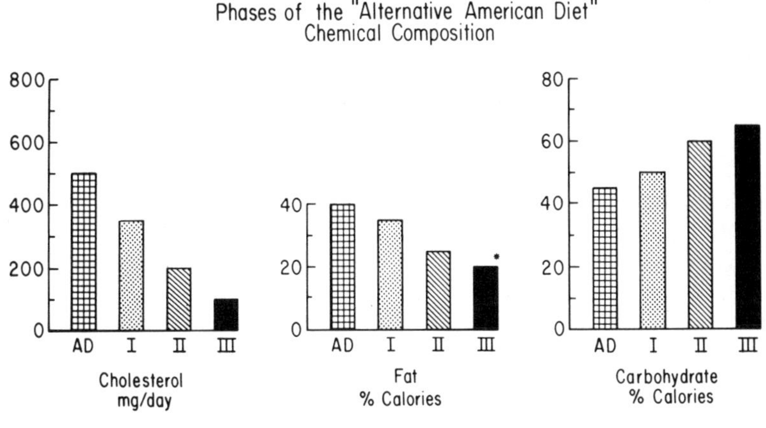

Figure 8. The cholesterol, fat, and carbohydrate content of the Western diet (AD) and the phases of the low fat, high carbohydrate diet (I, II, III).

Chemical and Nutrient Content

The chemical composition of the Western diet and the three phases of the low-fat, high-carbohydrate diet are given in Figure 8. The Western diet contains approximately 500 mg cholesterol per day. This is decreased in Phase I to 350 mg, in Phase II to 200 mg, and in Phase III to 100 mg per day. The fat content decreases from 40% of calories in the Western diet to 35% in Phase I, to 25% in Phase II, and to 20% in Phase III, with special consideration given to the decrease of saturated fat. In order to have sufficient calories to meet body needs we propose a gradual increase in carbohydrate, with emphasis on the use of the fibre-containing complex carbohydrates found in whole grains, cereal products and legumes. The increase in carbohydrate content to 65% in Phase III increases the bulk of the diet considerably, a feature which induces satiety sooner per unit of calories and helps to promote weight loss. The dietary fibre content of the low-fat, high-carbohydrate diet increases from 10 to 12 gm per day to 35 to 50 gm per day. Increasing the complex carbohydrate as fruits, vegetables, grains and beans will ensure that 30% of the fibre intake is soluble fibre (11 to 15 gm). Even though the total carbohydrate is increased, the refined sugar content is actually decreased, from 20 to 10% of calories, and a greater emphasis is placed on eating more fruit.

Using the Low-Fat, High-Carbohydrate Diet for Patients Who Are Also Hypertensive or Diabetic

A persistent problem in the dietary treatment of disease has been the use of a separate and individual diet for each disease. A good example would be the hyperlipidemic patient who also has high blood pressure and has been advised to follow a low-sodium, high-potassium diet. Such a diet is completely compatible with the low-fat, high-carbohydrate diet, which has incorporated into its design a phased approach to a low-sodium and high-potassium intake (81,82,85). Should caloric reduction be required to treat obesity, the low-fat, high-carbohydrate diet in reduced calories can be utilized. This diet has also been used in the treatment of diabetic patients (60). The high intakes of complex carbohydrate and fibre are in keeping with the latest trends in diabetic diets.

Predicted Plasma Cholesterol Lowering from the Three Phases of the Low-Fat, High-Carbohydrate Diet

As has been emphasized, both dietary cholesterol and saturated fat elevate plasma cholesterol levels, whereas polyunsaturated fat has a mild depressing effect. By steps, the cholesterol and saturated fat of each phase of the low-fat, high-carbohydrate diet are progressively reduced, with Phase III providing for the lowest intakes. According to calculations derived from Hegsted and coworkers (40), one would expect a 6 to 7% decrease, on the average, in the plasma total and LDL cholesterol level for each dietary phase (Table 9). If a patient were to reach Phase III goals there would be, on the average, an 18 to 21% lowering of the plasma cholesterol level. Approximately one-half of the plasma cholesterol lowering would result from decreasing dietary cholesterol intake from 500 to 100 mg/day and one-half of the lowering would result from decreasing saturated fat intake from 14 to 5% of calories.

For example, a patient with a plasma cholesterol level of 300 mg/dl when consuming the typical Western diet would have a plasma cholesterol level of 237 to 246 mg/dl if Phase III goals were to be achieved. Then a small dose of one of the hypocholsterolemic drugs would be used to decrease the plasma cholesterol further to below 200 mg/dl.

The scenario just described represents a mean plasma cholesterol response to dietary change. Based on the data from Katan et al. (18),

Table 9
Predicted Plasma Cholesterol Lowering from the Three Phases of the Low Fat, High Carbohydrate Diet

	*Total Fat**	*Saturated Fat**	*Poly-saturated Fat**	*P/S*	*Cholesterol (mg/day)*	*Predicted total change in plasma cholesterol from Western Diet to each phase (percent)*	*Predicted change in plasma cholesterol from phase to phase (percent)*
Western Diet	40	15	6	0.4	500		
Low Fat, High Carbohydrate Diet							
Phase I	35	14	9	0.6	350	−6	−6
Phase II	25	8	8	1.0	200	−13	−7
Phase III	20	5	8	1.3	100	−19	−6

*per cent of the total calories

calculated per the formula of Hegsted, McGandy, Myers, and Stare (40)

$$\text{Chol} = 2.16\ \ S - 1.65\ \ P + 6.77\ \ C - 0.53$$

Where Chol = the change in plasma cholesterol in mg/dl
S = the change in saturated fat as per cent of total calories
P = the change in polyunsaturated fat as per cent of total calories
C = dietary cholesterol intake in decigrams/day

The baseline diet from which changes have been made is the Western Diet.

one would estimate that 75 to 85% of people who achieved maximal dietary changes would have a plasma cholesterol decrease of 9% or greater and 50% of those people would have an 18% or greater reduction in the plasma cholesterol level. Extrapolation from the Lipid Research Clinics Primary Prevention Trial results, which showed a 2% reduction in risk for coronary disease for every 1% reduction in plasma cholesterol (90), one might then expect that 50% of individuals maximally reducing their plasma cholesterol level by diet would decrease their coronary risk by 36% and 75 to 85% of individuals having such reductions would decrease their coronary risk by 18%.

Summary and Conclusions

The dietary treatment and prevention of the atherosclerotic lesions underlying coronary heart disease have a logical and well-established rationale which has been developed over the past three decades. The low-fat, high-carbohydrate diet for these purposes is designed to prevent and treat hyperlipidemia and to have an antithrombotic action. The proposed low-cholesterol, low-fat diet is safe, inexpensive, and can become habitual through the process of gradual change, practice and patience. It offers a practical means of dealing with some of the key risk factors in coronary heart disease, especially hyperlipidemia. Furthermore, the same dietary philosophy may be applied to hyperlipidemias of differing severity, of different etiologies and of different lipoprotein types.

This dietary approach may be used with therapeutic benefit at any stage in the development of coronary heart disease. Atherosclerosis is inevitably progressive but focal. The same coronary artery may have occlusive lesions in one location and in neighbouring locations only beginning lesions. Likewise, in other coronaries the lesions may be minimal, severe or variable. Thus, the complete therapy of coronary heart disease must concentrate upon the removal or alleviation of those factors causing plaques to worsen and upon enhancing those factors promoting regression of atherosclerosis.

The primary prevention of coronary heart disease is clearly the ultimate goal to deal most effectively with the current epidemic of coronary heart disease. The dietary changes suggested for the coronary patient are completely safe and are prudent measures to be followed by any population (i.e., Western) at serious risk for coronary disease. These nutritional changes should be instituted early in life when they will have the greatest impact. This is a familial disease and its control and treatment can best be approached on a family basis. The primary prevention of coronary heart disease is dependent upon the prevention of diet-induced hyperlipidemia.

Acknowledgements

Special thanks are accorded to Patricia McCormick for the meticulous preparation of this manuscript.

Permission has been granted by the publishers to reproduce material from references 81,82,83.

REFERENCES

1 Intersalt Cooperative Research Group. Intersalt: an international study of electrolyte excretion and blood pressure. Results for 24 hour urinary sodium and potassium excretion. *Brit Med J* 1988;297:319–28.

2 Armstrong ML, Warner ED, Connor WE. Regression of coronary atheromatosis in Rhesus monkeys. *Circ Res* 1970;27:59–67.
3 Armstrong ML, Connor WE, Warner ED. Xanthomatosis in Rhesus monkeys fed a hypercholesterolemic diet. *Arch Path* 1967;84:226–37.
4 Taylor CB, Cox GE, Counts M, et al. Fatal myocardial infarction in Rhesus monkeys with diet-induced hypercholesterolemia. *Circulation* 1959;20:975. (Abstract)
5 Connor WE, Connor SL. The key role of nutritional factors in the prevention of coronary heart disease. *Prev Med* 1972;1:49–83.
6 Lin DS, Connor WE. The long-term effects of dietary cholesterol upon the plasma lipids, lipoproteins, cholesterol absorption, and the sterol balance in man: the demonstration of feedback inhibition of cholesterol biosynthesis and increased bile acid excretion. *J Lipid Res* 1981;21:1042–52.
7 Spady DK, Dietschy JM. Dietary saturated triacylglycerols suppress hepatic low density lipoprotein receptor activity in the hamster. *Proc Natl Acad Sci USA* 1985;82:4526–30.
8 Spady DK, Dietschy JM. Interaction of dietary cholesterol and triglycerides in the regulation of hepatic low density lipoprotein transport in the hamster. *J Clin Invest* 1988;81:300–9.
9 Kovanen PT, Brown MS, Basu SK, Bilheimer DW, Goldstein JL. Saturation and suppression of hepatic lipoprotein receptors: a mechanism for the hypercholesterolemia of cholesterol-fed rabbits. *Proc Natl Acad Sci USA* 1981;78:1396–1400.
10 Mahley RW, Hui DY, Innerarity TL, Weisgraber KH. Two independent lipoprotein receptors on hepatic membranes of dog, swine and man. *J Clin Invest* 1981;68:1197–1206.
11 Beveridge, JMR, Connell WF, Mayer GA, Haust HL. The response of man to dietary cholesterol. *J Nutr* 1960;71:61–5.
12 Connor WE, Hodges RE, Bleiler RE. The serum lipids in men receiving high cholesterol and cholesterol-free diets. *J Clin Invest* 1961;40:894–900.
13 Connor WE, Stone DB, Hodges RE. The interrelated effects of dietary cholesterol and fat upon the human serum lipid levels. *J Clin Invest* 1964;43:1691–6.
14 Steiner A, Howard EJ, Akgun S. Importance of dietary cholesterol in man. *J Am Med Assoc* 1962;181:186–90.
15 Connor WE, Connor SL. Dietary cholesterol and fat and the prevention of coronary heart disease: risks and benefits of nutritional change. In: Hallgren B, et al., eds. *Diet and Prevention of Coronary Heart Disease and Cancer*. New York: Raven Press, 1986:113–47.
16 Roberts SL, McMurry M, Connor WE. Does egg feeding (i.e. dietary

cholesterol) affect plasma cholesterol levels in humans? The results of a double-blind study. *Am J Clin Nutr* 1981;34:2092–9.

17 Gordon T, Fisher M, Ernst N, Rifkind BM. Relation of diet to LDL cholesterol, VLDL cholesterol and plasma total cholesterol and triglycerides in white adults. *Arteriosclerosis* 1982;2:502–12.

18 Katan MB, Beynen AC, De Vries JHM, Nobels A. Existence of consistent hypo- and hyperresponders to dietary cholsterol in man. *Am J Epidemiol* 1986;123:221–34.

19 Connor WE, Rohwedder JJ, Hoak JC. The production of hypercholesterolemia and atherosclerosis by a diet rich in shellfish. *J Nutr* 1963; 79:443–50.

20 Flaim E, Ferreri LF, Thye FW, Hill JE, Ritchey SF. Plasma lipid and lipoprotein cholesterol concentrations in adult males consuming normal and high cholesterol diets under controlled conditions. *Am J Clin Nutr* 1981;34:1103–8.

21 Connor WE, Hodges RE, Bleiler RE. The effect of dietary cholesterol upon the serum lipids in man. *J Lab Clin Med* 1961;57:331–42.

22 Connor WE, Witiak DT, Stone DB, Armstrong ML. Cholsterol balance and fecal neutral steroid and bile acid excretion in normal men fed dietary fats of different fatty acid composition. *J Clin Invest* 1969;48:1363–75.

23 Mistry P, Miller NE, Laker M, Hazzard WR, Lewis B. Individual variations in the effect of dietary cholesterol on plasma lipoproteins and cellular cholesterol homeostatsis in man. *J Clin Invest* 1981;67:493–502.

24 Mahley RW, Innerarity T, Rall SC, et al. Plasma lipoproteins: apolipoprotein structure and function. *J Lipid Res* 1984;25:1277–94.

25 Gregg RE, Brewer HB Jr. The role of apolipoprotein E in modulating the metabolism of apolipoprotein B-48 and apolipoprotein B-100 containing lipoproteins in humans. In: Angel A, Frohlich J, eds. Lipoprotein deficiency syndromes. *Adv Exp Med Biol* 1986;201:289–98.

26 Ahrens EH, Hirsch J, Insull W. The influence of dietary fats on serum lipid levels in man. *Lancet* 1957;1:943–53.

27 Keys A, Anderson JT, Grande F. Serum cholesterol response to dietary fat. *Lancet* 1957;1:787.

28 Zilversmit DB. Atherogenesis: a postprandial phenomenon. *Circulation* 1979;60:473–85.

29 Brown MS, Goldstein JL. A receptor-mediated pathway for cholesterol homeostasis. *Science* 1986;232:34–47.

30 Lin DS, Spenler CW, Connor WE. The effects of different dietary fatty acids upon the fatty acid composition of adipose tissue: saturated, monounsaturated and n-3 and n-6 polyunsaturated fatty acids. Unpublished observations.

31 Becker N, Illingworth DR, Alaupovic P, Connor WE, Sundberg EE. Effects of saturated, monounsaturated, and omega-6 polyunsaturated fatty acids on plasma lipids, lipoproteins and apoproteins in humans. *Am J Clin Nutr* 1983;37:355–60.
32 Grundy SM. Comparison of monounsaturated fatty acids and carbohydrates for lowering plasma cholesterol. *N Eng J Med* 1986;314:745–8.
33 Mattson FH, Grundy SM. Comparison of effects of dietary saturated, monounsaturated and polyunsaturated fatty acids on plasma lipids and lipoproteins in men. *J Lipid Res* 1985;26:194–202.
34 Goodnight SH Jr, Harris WS, Connor WE, Illingworth DR. Polyunsaturated fatty acids, hyperlipidemia and thrombosis. *Arteriosclerosis* 1982; 2:87–113.
35 Harris WS, Connor WE. The effects of salmon oil upon plasma lipids, lipoprotein and triglyceride clearance. *Trans Assoc Am Phys* 1980;93:148–55.
36 Harris WS, Connor WE, Alam N, Illingworth DR. The reduction of postprandial triglyceridemia in humans by dietary n-3 fatty acids. *J Lipid Res* 1988;29:1451–60.
37 Weiner BH, Ockene IS, Levine PH, et al. Inhibition of atherosclerosis by cod liver oil in a hyperlipidemic swine model. *N Engl J Med* 1986;315:841–6.
38 Davis HR, Bridenstine RT, Vesselinovitch D, Wissler RW. Fish oil inhibits development of atherosclerosis in Rhesus monkeys. *Arteriosclerosis* 1987;7:441–9.
39 Kromhout D, Bosschieter EB, Coulander CdeL. The inverse relation between fish consumption and 20-year mortality from coronary heart disease. *N Engl J Med* 1985;312:1205–9.
40 Hegsted DM, McGandy RB, Myers ML, Stare FJ. Quantitative effects of dietary fat on serum cholesterol in man. *Am J Clin Nutr* 1965;17:281–95.
41 Keys A, Anderson JT, Grande F. Prediction of serum-cholesterol responses of man to changes in fats in the diet. *Lancet* 1957;2:959–66.
42 Haslam RJ. Role of adenosine diphosphate in the aggregation of human blood-platelets by thrombin and by fatty acids. *Nature* 1964;202:765–8.
43 Hoak JC, Warner ED, Connor WE. Platelets, fatty acids and thrombosis. *Circ Res* 1967;20:11–17.
44 Mahadevan V, Singh MH, Lundberg WO. Effects of saturated and unsaturated fatty acids on blood platelet aggregation in vitro. *Proc Soc Exp Biol Med* 1966;121:82–5.
45 Renaud S, Kinlough RL, Mustard JF. Relationship between platelet aggregation and the thrombotic tendency in rats fed hyperlipemic diets. *Lab Invest* 1970;22:339–43.

46 Beckett AG, Lewis JG. Mobilization and utilization of body fat as an aetiological factor in occlusive vascular disease in diabetes mellitus. *Lancet* 1960;2:14–18.
47 Fredrickson DS, Gordon RS Jr. Transport of fatty acids. *Physiol Rev* 1958;38:585–630.
48 Gjesdal K. Platelet function and plasma free fatty acids during acute myocardial infarction and severe angina pectoris. *Scand J Haematol* 1976;17:205–12.
49 Gjesdal K, Nordoy A, Wang H, Berntsen H, Mjos OD. Effects of fasting on plasma and platelet-free fatty acids and platelet function in healthy males. *Thromb Haemost* 1976;36:325–33.
50 Kurien VA, Oliver MF. Serum free fatty acids after myocardial infarction and cerebral vascular occlusion. *Lancet* 1966;1:122–7.
51 Connor WE, Hoak JC, Warner ED. Plasma free fatty acids, hypercoagulability and thrombosis. In: Sherry S, Brinkhous KM, Genton ED, Stengle JM, eds. *Thrombosis*. Washington, D.C.: Nat Acad Sci, 1969:355–73.
52 Bang HO, Dyerberg J. Lipid metabolism and ischemic heart disease in Greenland Eskimos. In: Draper HH, ed. *Advanced Nutrition Research*, vol 3. New York: Plenum Press, 1980:1–22.
53 Bang HO, Dyerberg J, Hjorne N. The composition of food consumed by Greenlandic Eskimos. *Acta Med Scand* 1973;200:69–73.
54 Dyerberg J, Bang HO. Hemostatic function and platelet polyunsaturated fatty acids in Eskimos. *Lancet* 1979;2:433–5.
55 Goodnight SH Jr, Harris WS, Connor WE. The effects of dietary omega-3 fatty acids upon platelet composition and function in man: a prospective, controlled study. *Blood* 1981;58:880–5.
56 Burkitt DP. Varicose veins, deep vein thrombosis, and hemorrhoids. *Brit Med J* 1972;2:556–61.
57 Davies JNP. Pathology of central African natives. IX Cardiovascular diseases. *East African Med J* 1948;25:454–67.
58 Latto C. Hemorrhoids, diverticular disease and deep vein thrombosis. In: Trowell HC, Burkitt DP, eds. *Western Diseases: Their Emergence and Prevention*. Cambridge, MA: Harvard University Press, 1981:421–4.
59 Ahrens EH, Hirsch J, Oette K, Farquhar JW, Stein Y. Carbohydrate-induced and fat-induced lipemia. *Trans Assoc Amer Phys* 1961; 74:134–46.
60 Stone DB, Connor WE. The prolonged effects of a low cholesterol, high carbohydrate diet upon the serum lipids in diabetic patients. *Diabetes* 1963;12:127–32.
61 Weinsier RL, Seeman A, Herrera MG, Assul J-P, Soeldner JS, Gleason RG. High and low carbohydrate diets in diabetes: study of effects on

diabetic control, insulin secretion and blood lipids. *Ann Int Med* 1974;80:332–41.
62 Ullmann D, Connor WE, Hatcher LF, Connor SL, Flavell DP. The absence of carbohydrate-induced hypertriglyceridemia during a phased high carbohydrate diet. *Circulation* 1988;78(suppl.):II73.
63 Nikkila EA, Ojala K. Induction of hypertriglyceridemia by fructose in the rat. *Life Sci* 1965;4:937–43.
64 Keys A, Grande F, Anderson JT. Fiber and pectin in the diet and serum cholesterol concentration in man. *Proc Soc Exp Biol Med* 1961;106:555–8.
65 Grande F, Anderson JT, Keys A. Effect of carbohydrates of leguminous seeds, wheat and potatoes on serum cholesterol concentration in man. *J Nutr* 1965:86:313–17.
66 Raymond, T.L., Connor, W.E., Lin, D.S., Warner, S., Fry, M.M., and Connor, S.L. The interaction of dietary fibers and cholesterol upon the plasma lipids and lipoproteins, the sterol balance, and bowel function in human subjects. *J. Clin. Invest.* 1971;60:1429–1437.
67 Anderson JW, Story L, Sieling B, Chen WJL, Petro MS, Story J. Hypocholesterolemic effects of oat-bran or bean intake for hypercholesterolemic men. *Am J Clin Nutr* 1984;40:1146–55.
68 Kay RM, Truswell AS. Effect of citrus pectin on blood lipids and fecal steroid excretion in man. *Am J Clin Nutr* 1977;30:171–5.
69 McLean Ross AH, Eastwood MA, Anderson JR, Anderson DMW. A study of the effects of dietary gum arabic in humans. *Am J Clin Nutr* 1983;37:368–75.
70 Galbraith WB, Connor WE, Stone DB. Weight loss and serum lipid changes in obese subjects given low-calorie diets of varied cholesterol content. *Ann Int Med* 1966;64:268–75.
71 Olefsky J, Reaven GM, Farquhar JW. Effects of weight reduction on obesity. *J Clin Invest* 1974;53:64–76.
72 Schwartz RS, Brunzell JD. Increase of adipose tissue lipoprotein lipase activity with weight loss. *J Clin Invest* 1981;67:1425–30.
73 Castelli WP, Gordon T, Hjortland MC, et al. Alcohol and blood lipids. *Lancet* 1977;2:153–5.
74 St Leger AS, Cochrance AL, Moore F. Factors associated with cardiac mortality in developed countries with particular reference to the consumption of wine. *Lancet* 1979;1:1017–20.
75 Haskell WL, Camargo C, Williams PT, et al. The effect of cessation and resumption of moderate alcohol intake on serum high-density-lipoprotein subfractions. *N Eng J Med* 1984;310:805–10.
76 Wood, PD, Haskell WL, Blair SN, et al. Increased exercise level and plasma lipoprotein concentrations: a one-year randomized, controlled study in sedentary middle-aged men. *Metabolism* 1983;32:31–9.

77 Katz LN, Stamler J, Pick R. *Nutrition and Atherosclerosis*. Philadelphia: Lea and Febiger, 1958:98.
78 Peterson VE, Crapo PA, Weininger J, et al. Quantification of plasma cholesterol and triglyceride levels in hypercholesterolemic subjects receiving ascorbic acid supplements. *Am J Clin Nutr* 1975;28:584–7.
79 Beveridge JMR, Connell WF, Mayer GA. The nature of the substances in dietary fat affecting the level of plasma cholesterol in humans. *Can J Biochem Physiol* 1957;35:257–70.
80 Muenter MD, Perry HO, Jurgen L. Chronic vitamin A intoxication in adults. *Am J Med* 1971;50:129–36.
81 Connor WE, Connor SL. The dietary treatment of hyperlipidemia: rationale, technique and efficacy. In: Havel RJ, ed. Lipid Disorders. *Med Clin North Am* 1982;66:485–518.
82 Connor WE, Connor SL. The dietary prevention and treatment of coronary heart disease. In: Connor WE, Bristow JD, eds. *Coronary Heart Disease: Prevention, Complications and Treatment*. Philadelphia: Lippincott, 1985:43–64.
83 Connor SL, Artaud-Wild SM, Classick-Kohn CJ, et al. The cholesterol saturated fat index: an indication of the hypercholesterolemic and atherogenic potential of food. *Lancet* 1986;1:1229–32.
84 Zilversmit DB. Cholesterol index of foods. *J Am Dietet Assoc* 1979; 74:562–5.
85 Connor SL, Connor WE. *The New American Diet*. New York: Simon & Schuster, 1986.
86 Dobbin LV, Gofman HF, Jones L, et al. *The Low Fat, Low Cholesterol Diet*. New York: Doubleday, 1957.
87 Brewster L, Jacobson MF. *The Changing American Diet*. Washington, D.C.: Center for Science in the Public Interest, 1978.
88 Welsh SO, Marston RM. Review of trends in food use in the United States, 1909 to 1980. *J Am Dietet Assoc* 1982;81:120–5.
89 Connor WE, Connor SL, Fry MM, Warner S. *The Alternative Diet Book*. Iowa City: University of Iowa Press, 1976.
90 Lipid research clinics programs: the lipid research clinics coronary primary prevention trial results: I. Reduction in incidence of coronary heart disease. *JAMA* 1984;251:351–64.

J. ALICK LITTLE

Coronary Heart Disease Prevention Trials

Dr Richard Havel has described the influence of plasma lipoproteins and nutrients on atherogenesis and coronary heart disease earlier in this conference (1) and Dr William Connor has explained how the diet can be altered to decrease the risk of coronary disease (2). Over the last three decades there have been a number of clinical trials using diet and/or lipid lowering medications aimed at reducing the high incidence of coronary heart disease. This paper will review the results from some of these intervention trials.

Atherosclerosis is a kind of "hardening of the arteries" causing thickening of the wall and narrowing or occlusion of the passageway or lumen. Coronary heart disease (CHD) is almost always due to atherosclerosis with thrombosis or blood clot. The major clinical complications of this are: heart attacks or myocardial infarction (MI) (death of heart muscle), usually from complete occlusion, and angina pectoris (transient chest pain), usually from partial occlusion. We should also consider why human clinical coronary heart disease is used as the model for experiments to test the hypothesis that lowering plasma lipids will slow atherogenesis and prevent clinical complications. Foremost is the fact that in our society coronary heart disease is very common, accounting for about one-third of all deaths in North Americans. It is more common in middle-aged men than in premenopausal females, which is why intervention studies are conducted using men. The clinical manifestations are easily and accurately detected by history, electrocardiography, and biochemical tests, and without invasive techniques. For practical purposes there is only one pathological cause of coronary ischemia and that is atherosclerosis. Elevated plasma cholesterol levels, along with hypertension and smoking, are the major risk factors for coronary disease. Elevated plasma cholesterol is a less important risk factor for cerebral and peripheral vascular disease. Therefore heart attacks and other complications of coronary disease are better end points than strokes or lower limb ischemic claudication for the study of the effect of lowering plasma cholesterol on atherogenesis.

Despite the high incidence of coronary heart disease in our population and the relative absence of other interfering diseases, its prevention is still difficult to study. Unlike some other diseases, such as acute infections, that develop quickly and respond in an all or none way to treatment, atherosclerosis develops slowly and insidiously. The earliest pathologic lesions are the fatty streaks in the endothelial lining of the arteries shortly after birth. These clinically insignificant lesions may regress and leave a normal coronary artery or may go on to larger, coalescent accumulations of cholesterol in the thickened artery wall (Figure 1) surrounded by areas of tissue reaction, scarring, calcification, and hemorrhage into the artery wall. Often there is an associated thrombus or blood clot to narrow or occlude the lumen further. The clinical manifestations from this process, in the case of the coronary arteries, are angina pectoris from partial occlusion and periodic ischemia of heart muscle, or a heart attack from myocardial infarction (MI) (either non-fatal or fatal) from complete coronary occlusion. Infarction means death of tissue, and in the heart it means death of part of the muscular wall, resulting in a serious loss of function. However, the clinical manifestations of atherosclerosis do not occur usually until after age 70 unless the patient has a bad risk profile such as elevated plasma cholesterol and/or blood pressure and/or smoking.

Not only is atherogenesis in man slow, it appears to have multiple causes besides increasing age. These include the concentration of the lipoproteins in the blood, increasing blood pressure, the use of smoking tobacco, the presence of diabetes mellitus, and obesity. It is convenient to think of these causative factors as acting concomitantly in hastening the rate of atherogenesis and the risk of clinical complications. It is not my purpose to discuss the details of the mechanisms for the interaction of the various causes of atherosclerosis other than to suggest that they act by increasing lipid infiltration of the artery wall through injury or increased plasma lipid concentrations or impaired removal of lipids or increased tendency for thrombosis. How-

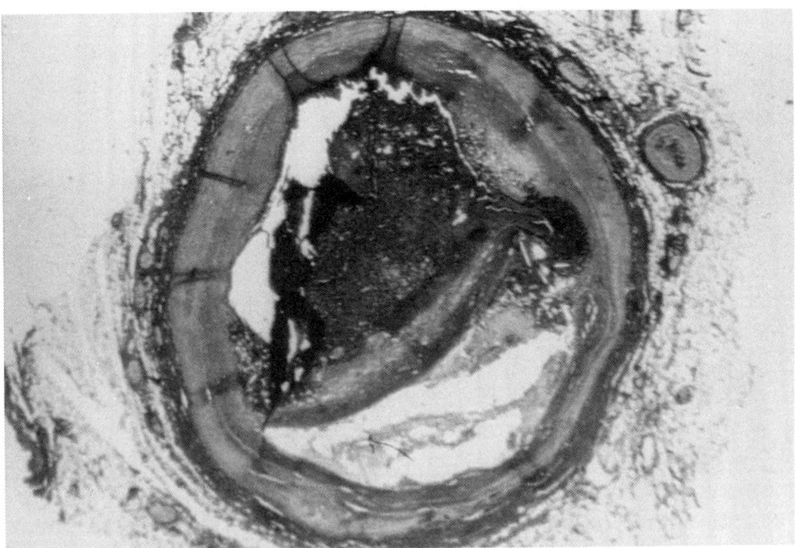

Figure 1. A microphotograph of the cross-section of a human coronary artery containing, in the lower half, an atheromatous plaque that is cracked at the junction of the atheroma capsule with the original artery wall resulting in hemorrhage into the plaque and thrombosis occluding the vessel lumen above.

ever, it is important for this discussion to recognize their presence as co-variables in the design, follow-up, and interpretation of the results of intervention trials. Other variables of an adverse nature have recently been discovered. These are the elevating effects on plasma lipid levels by commonly used medications for hypertension and angina, such as the beta blockers and thiazide diuretics and oral contraceptive drugs.

In this regard, the various lipid and lipoprotein fractions which can be measured also have to be considered. Total plasma cholesterol, total triglycerides, low density lipoprotein cholesterol (LDL-C), and very low density lipoprotein cholesterol (VLDL-C) all have positive associations with the development of coronary heart disease, meaning the higher the concentrations the greater the risk, whereas high density lipoprotein cholesterol (HDL-C) has a negative association, meaning the lower the concentration the greater the risk (3). Despite the fact that total cholesterol contains HDL-C, it remains as a significant and useful positive risk factor for coronary heart disease because HDL-C is small (approximately 25%), relative to total cholesterol, and the variations of HDL-C levels are also relatively small. Because of their opposite risks, the ratio of total cholesterol to HDL-C is a potent risk index (4). Because lipids like cholesterol, triglycerides, and phospholipids do not exist as free molecules in the plasma but rather as components, along with a number of apoproteins, of various lipoprotein fractions, it seems more logical to measure their concentrations only in the different lipoprotein fractions. This is now being done to a limited extent, and the results indicate that the components have special significance for risk of atherosclerosis (5). Fortunately, the concentration of total plasma cholesterol is a good index of LDL-C, which is the major atherogenic lipoprotein fraction. Because of this and the relative simplicity and accuracy of its measurements, total cholesterol was, and still is, a very useful atherogenic index.

Lipoprotein metabolism and the levels of the plasma lipoproteins can be influenced by dietary factors, as described by Drs Havel and Connor (1, 2). They can also be affected by certain drugs in selective ways. Figure 2 shows the lipid metabolic pathways, and the numbers indicate sites where various drugs may act and alter plasma lipoprotein and lipid patterns. One needs to recognize that whereas a drug can improve the plasma lipoprotein pattern of a person with one type of lipoprotein disorder, it can worsen the pattern of another type of dyslipoproteinemia. Drugs should not be prescribed without follow-up to ensure that the desired effect is occurring. Some early prevention trials without the benefit of this knowledge prescribed drugs without regard for the lipoprotein phenotype of the subjects, and this could have adversely influenced the outcome.

Coronary prevention trials were undertaken to test the hypothesis that lowering plasma lipids would delay or prevent atherogenesis and thus coronary heart disease. This seemed reasonable as a result of the huge body of knowledge derived from animal experiments and clinical observations that proved conclusively that elevated plasma cholesterol was causative for atheroma formation and premature clinical coronary disease (6). Furthermore, animal studies showed that lowering previously elevated plasma cholesterol levels resulted in regression of atheromata (7). However, there was no certainty that this could be done in man, in whom the disease takes several decades to develop, and for whom adherence to a study protocol must be voluntary.

Several primary prevention trials were completed between 1968 and 1979 (8–13). Primary prevention means an attempt to prevent the initial heart attack, as opposed to secondary prevention, which is

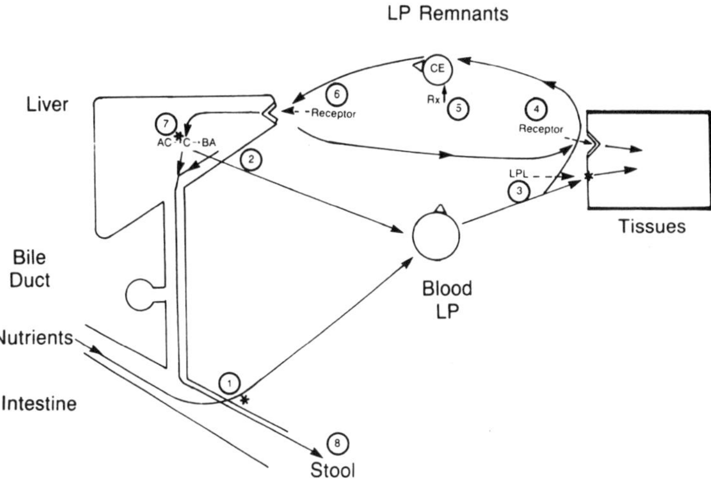

Figure 2. Schematic representation of the metabolism of lipoproteins (LP) showing sites where various drugs can modify the process: 1. absorption of lipid from the intestine; 2. synthesis by the liver; 3. stimulation of catabolism by lipoprotein lipase (LPL); 4. and 6. increasing receptors for apolipoprotein ligands (△); 5. drugs combining with remnant lipoproteins to modify their catabolism; 7. interfering with cholesterol (C) synthesis from acetate (AC); 8. combining with bile acids (BA) in the stool to promote excretion.

preventing recurrence of a heart attack. Out of necessity, middle-aged males were the subjects, in order to provide a sufficient number of ischemic events within a reasonable time period and a cohort of reasonable size. The diet to lower plasma lipids had limited amounts of saturated fat and cholesterol and increased amounts of polyunsaturated fat. Good adherence to diet resulted in 5–10% lowering of plasma cholesterol. In some trials, adding lipid-lowering medications sometimes resulted in another 10–30% lowering as compared to the control group. The end points for coronary heart disease were definite or "hard," such as a fatal or a non-fatal heart attack. Softer end points were probable heart attacks and angina pectoris. Other ischemic events were strokes and peripheral vascular disease. In these trials the general tendency was a decreased incidence of coronary end points in the experimental group compared with the controls, but this did not always reach significance. Not surprisingly, considering the limited statistical power, deaths from all causes were not reduced in any of these or subsequent prevention trials.

Several secondary prevention trials were completed between 1966 and 1978 (14–17). The most impressive of these secondary trials was the 15-year study in Oslo of 412 male infarction patients, with half randomized to a strict diet and half to a conventional diet (14). Plasma cholesterol was 14% lower on the experimental diet, and there were significantly fewer myocardial reinfarctions (34 vs 54), especially in men under age 60, but total cardiovascular deaths were not significantly different (38 vs 52).

Since 1981 there have been four primary prevention trials in different countries (18–21). These were multiple risk factor intervention trials, because two or more intervention programs were involved including diet and exercise, and reduction in smoking, blood pressure, and weight. The tendency for fewer coronary end points in the experimental groups continued, but these did not always reach the 0.05 level of significance. In the U.K. Heart Disease Prevention Project (20) in 18,210 men over five years there was only slight lowering of plasma cholesterol, weight, blood pressure, and smoking, and no objective decrease in coronary heart disease. However, using more aggressive intervention in the same protocol, the Belgian Heart Disease Prevention Project in 19,409 men achieved significant lowering of plasma cholesterol, smoking, and blood pressure, and a reduction of coronary heart disease incidence by 24.5%, $p = 0.031$ (21). This difference in the results of the two trials indicates dramatically that it is not the treatment itself, but the lowering of the risk factors that prevents heart attacks.

In 1972 the forerunner of the U.S. National Heart Lung and Blood Institute organized 12 Lipid Research Clinics (LRC) in North America to undertake the Coronary Primary Prevention Trial (CPPT) that would test the hypothesis that lowering plasma cholesterol would prevent coronary heart disease. It had been decided earlier, as a result of the National Diet Heart Trial involving 1211 men for one year, that a double blind dietary intervention alone was impractical because of only 5–10% lowering of plasma cholesterol, a 10% drop-out rate annually, and the requirement of up to 150,000 volunteers followed for up to 40 years at a prohibitive cost (22). Therefore, the CPPT needed a more practical plan. The number of expected coronary end points in the control group was increased by selecting middle-aged males at high risk because of elevated plasma cholesterol. Cholesterol lowering of the experimental group was increased by combining with the diet the non-toxic bile acid sequestrant drug, cholestyramine, which at a full dose of 24 g daily would lower cholesterol 25–30%. A suitable

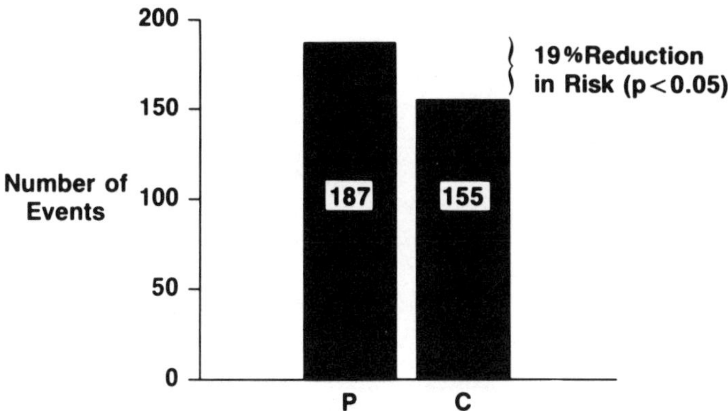

Figure 3. The incidence of myocardial infarction in the placebo (P) and cholestyramine (C) groups during the Lipid Research Clinics' Coronary Primary Prevention Trial.

placebo was available for a double blind design. Recruitment over a two-year period provided 3806 male volunteers, 35–59 years of age, with plasma cholesterol levels exceeding 265 mg% on three visits over a three-month period. They were randomized into two groups for 7–10 years of follow-up every two months.

The results, published in 1984 (23, 24), showed an average lowering of plasma cholesterol and LDL-C of 8.5% and 13% respectively in the cholestyramine compared with the placebo group. Figure 3 shows that the incidence of fatal and non-fatal myocardial infarctions was 19% lower in the active treatment group ($p < 0.05$). Other softer coronary disease end points, including positive exercise ECG tests, angina pectoris, and coronary bypass surgery, were reduced 25% ($p < 0.001$), 20% ($p < 0.01$), and 21% ($p < 0.06$) respectively. The average dose of cholestyramine during the trial was 70% of the prescribed 24 g daily, and this was associated with an 8% reduction in cholesterol and 19% reduction in coronary risk. However, the subjects who took the full dose had a 25% reduction in cholesterol and a 49% reduction in coronary risk. The latter statistic can be remembered from the simplification that each 1% reduction in plasma cholesterol resulted in approximately a 2% reduction in risk of myocardial infarction in this group of subjects.

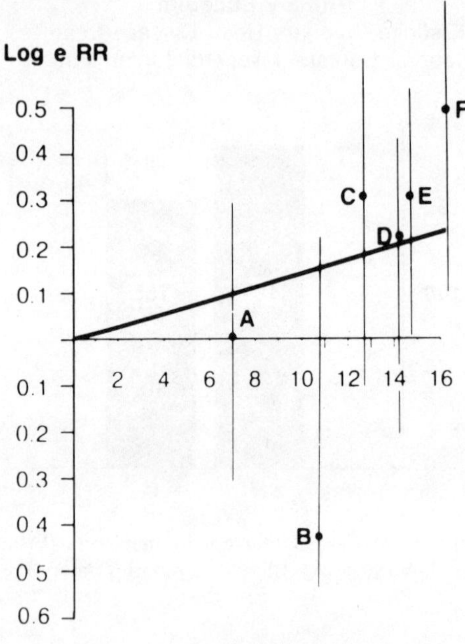

Figure 4. The relative coronary heart disease risk and confidence limits in relation to reduction in cholesterol levels in six randomized dietary prevention trials. A = MRC study (26), B = Rose et al. (27), C = Dayton et al. (10), D = MRC (28), E = Leren (14), F = Turpeinin et al. (8).

Richard Peto of Oxford University has provided a statistical method for evaluating the combined results of the major randomized trials that have been conducted. He pointed out the considerable margin of error in the result from each individual trial. Therefore, he determined the confidence limits of the relative risks for each trial and plotted these against the difference in plasma cholesterol level between the experimental and control groups for each trial. Figure 4, adapted from Mann and Marr (25), shows the best regression line passing through zero for a number of dietary trials. The small numbers in each study caused the wide confidence limits, which explained the inconsistent and conflicting results. However, using the regression we find that a 10% reduction in plasma cholesterol by diet resulted in a 15 ± 6% reduction in coronary heart disease risk, which was highly significant ($p < 0.01$).

Similarly, an analysis of five drug prevention trials resulted in a regression line where 10% lowering of plasma cholesterol gave a 21 ± 5% reduction in CHD risk (25). The consistency of the data from these two sets of prevention trials, one with diet and the other with drugs, suggested that cholesterol reduction by a variety of methods in middle-aged men did indeed prevent coronary disease events.

Using this method of analysis did not show, however, that with the combined power of all the trials there was a significant reduction in deaths from all causes. This would require much larger numbers of men followed over many more years. The very high cost and long duration means that such trials will never be done. For the same reason, coronary prevention trials cannot be done in women, young adults, and children. However, this should not provide a licence for the purists to deny the benefits of coronary prevention programs to younger men and to women.

Peto concludes, from a more recent analysis of this type (29), that the estimated benefit of a 10% reduction in cholesterol is fairly consistent for different types of trials. Primary prevention studies have a 13% decrease in coronary risk, and secondary prevention trials a 17% decrease. Using fatal CHD as the end point, the reduction in risk is 19%. Drug trials have a 16% drop in risk and dietary trials a 13% decrease in risk. He concludes that the decrease in coronary risk depends on the size of the reduction in plasma cholesterol and not on any of the present methods of reducing cholesterol.

However, I believe it is possible that future research will reveal more specific risk indices than total cholesterol, LDL-C, and HDL-C, and will provide more specific drugs and diets to help correct the risk profile. Certain of the HDL subfractions and components, such as HDL_2, HDL-triglycerides (HDL-TG), Apo AI, the major protein of HDL, and Apo B, the major protein of LDL, may prove to have stronger associations with atherogenesis in population studies. The combined use of some of these indices may prove even more powerful. Furthermore, the combined use of diet with combinations of safe and potent lipid-lowering drugs will likely add to our ability to lower plasma lipoproteins selectively and to modify the risk profile more specifically.

In the meantime, a number of countries, including the U.S. (30) and European countries (31), using our present knowledge, have developed a consensus regarding what kinds of patients and what segments of the population should receive advice for modifying their risk profiles for coronary heart disease, and what the goals of the program should be. The Canadian Atherosclerosis Society, in collaboration with Health and Welfare Canada and the Heart Foundation, is planning a conference for March 9–11, 1988, to consider these issues in relation to the specific needs of the Canadian people. I anticipate that we are on the verge of significantly reducing the incidence of coronary heart disease still further.

REFERENCES

1 Havel RJ. Overview of dietary and hereditary factors in coronary heart disease. In this collection.

2 Connor WE. Dietary approaches. In this collection.

3 Gordon T, Castelli WP, Hjortland MC, Karmel WB, Dawber TR. High density lipoprotein as a protective factor against coronary heart disease: The Framingham Study. *Am J Med* 1977;62:707–714.

4 Castelli WP. HDL in assessing risk of CHD. *Metab Ther* 1977;6:1–00.

5 Little JA, Kakis G, Feather T, Breckenridge CW. Plasma high density lipoprotein triglyceride as a risk factor for ischemic vascular disease in a prospective study. *Clin Invest Med* 1984;7:Suppl 2, 68 (abstr).

6 Stamler J. Population studies. In: Levy RI, Rifkind BM, Dennis BH. *Nutrition, lipids and coronary heart disease.* New York: Raven Press, 1977:25–88.

7 Wissler RW, Vesselinovitch D. Studies of regression of advanced atherosclerosis in experimental animals and man. *Ann NY Acad Sci* 1976; 275:363–378.

8 Turpeinin O, Karvonen MJ, Pekkarinin M, Miettinen M, Elosuo R, Paavilainen E. Dietary prevention of coronary heart disease: the Finnish Mental Hospital Study. *Int J Epidemiol* 1979;8:99–118.

9 Rinsler SH. Primary prevention of coronary heart disease. *Bull NY Acad Med* 1968;44:936–949.

10 Dayton S, Pearce ML, Hashimoto S, Dixon WJ, Tomivasu UA. A controlled trial of a diet high in unsaturated fat in preventing complications of atherosclerosis. *Circulation* 1969;39–40:Suppl 2, 1–63.

11 Kresno LR, Kidera GJ. Clofibrate in coronary heart disease. *J Am Med Assoc* 1972; 219:845–851.

12 Dorr AE, Gundersen K, Schneider JC, Spencer TW, Martin WB. Colestipol hydrochloride in hypercholesterolemic patients – effect on serum cholesterol and mortality. *J Chronic Dis* 1978;31:5–14.

13 Committee of Principal Investigators. A co-operative trial in the prevention of ischaemic heart disease using clofibrate. *Br Heart J* 1978;40:1069–1118.

14 Leren P. The Oslo Diet Heart Study: eleven year report. *Circulation* 1970;42:935–942.
15 Group of Physicians of the Newcastle upon Tyne Region. Trial of clofibrate in the treatment of ischaemic heart disease. *Br Med J* 1971;4:767–775.
16 Research Committee of the Scottish Society of Physicians. Ischemic heart disease: a secondary prevention trial using clofibrate. *Br Med J* 1971;4:775–784.
17 The Coronary Drug Project Research Group. The Coronary Drug Project: clofibrate and niacin in coronary heart disease. *J Am Med Assoc* 1975;231:360–381.
18 Hjermann I, Velve Byer K, Holme I, Leren P. Effect of diet and smoking intervention on the incidence of coronary heart disease: Report of the Oslo Study Group of a randomized trial in healthy men. *Lancet* 1981;2:1303–1310.
19 Multiple Risk Factor Intervention Trial Research Group. Coronary heart disease death, nonfatal acute myocardial infarction and other clinical outcomes in the Multiple Risk Factor Intervention Trial. *Am J Cardiol* 1986;58:1–13.
20 Rose G, Tunstall-Pedoe HD, Heller RF. The UK Heart Disease Prevention Project: incidence and mortality results. *Lancet* 1983;1:1062–1065.
21 Kornitzer M, Dramaix M, Thilly C, et al. Belgian Heart Disease Prevention Project: incidence and mortality results. *Lancet* 1983;1:1066–1070.
22 *Arteriosclerosis: a report by the National Heart & Lung Institute Task Force on Arteriosclerosis*. Washington DC: National Institutes of Health, 1971, vol. 1. Dept. of Health, Education & Welfare publication (NIH) 72–137.
23 The Lipid Research Clinics Program. The Lipid Research Clinics Coronary Primary Prevention Trial Results. I. Reduction in incidence of coronary heart disease. *J Am Med Assoc* 1984;251:351–364.
24 The Lipid Research Clinics Program. The Lipid Research Clinics Coronary Primary Prevention Trial Results. II. The relationship of reduction in incidence of coronary heart disease to cholesterol lowering. *J Am Med Assoc* 1984;251:365–374.
25 Mann JI, Marr JW. Coronary Heart Disease Prevention Trials of diets to control hyperlipidemia. In: Miller NE, Lewis B, eds. *Lipoproteins, atherosclerosis and coronary heart disease*. Amsterdam: Elsevier/North-Holland Biomedical Press, 1981:197–000.
26 Research Committee to the Medical Research Council. Low-fat diet in myocardial infarction – a controlled trial. *Lancet* 1965;2:500–504.
27 Rose G, Thomson WB, Williams RT. Corn oil in the treatment of ischemic heart disease. *Br Med J* 1965;1:1531–1533.

28 Research Committee to the Medical Research Council. Controlled trial of soya-bean oil in myocardial infarction. *Lancet* 1968;2:693–700.
29 Peto R. *Cholesterol, the epidemiological evidence. International symposium, lipoproteins and atherosclerosis: current views, future trends*, Helsinki Finland, Oct 17, 1986. Rahway NY: Merck and Co Inc.
30 Consensus Conference. Lowering blood cholesterol to prevent heart disease. *J Am Med Assoc* 1985;253:2080–2086.
31 Study Group, European Atherosclerosis Society. Strategy for the prevention of coronary heart disease, a policy statement of the European Atherosclerosis Society. *Eur Heart J* 1987;8:77–88.

PIRJO PIETINEN

A Public Health Program for Prevention of Cardiovascular Disease

Cardiovascular diseases (CVD) form the major public health problem in Finland. The province of North Karelia has proved to have the highest occurrence of CVD within Finland. From 1969 to 1971 CVD accounted for 43% of total mortality among North Karelian men aged 35–64 years. Awareness of this severe problem in North Karelia led to the development of a community-based prevention program for CVD, the North Karelia Project (1). The North Karelia Project was the first systematic attempt to implement the community approach to reduce the high CVD rates in the entire population of that area. The project was originally set up for five years starting in 1972, but was subsequently continued and, after ten years, has been gradually expanded to cover also prevention of some other major non-communicable diseases.

Intervention

The intervention goal was to reduce disease rates by reducing the population levels of the major coronary heart disease risk factors: smoking, serum cholesterol, and blood pressure. The framework for the intervention included improved preventive services, information, persuasion, training, community organization, and environmental change (2).

The nutrition sub-program aimed at reducing the generally high level of serum cholesterol in the population through general dietary changes. Internationally well-established principles of cholesterol-lowering diet were adapted to local conditions. Reduction of the extremely high consumption of dairy fat was the major aim, and especially the reduction of the amount of butter on bread and the change to favour low-fat milk products were recommended. This main aim was supplemented by encouraging people to use vegetable oil and to increase the consumption of vegetables.

The implementation of the comprehensive program was integrated in the health services and social organization of the province. The elements of the intervention included the following aims, channels, and methods:

1 Information to educate people about the relationship between behaviours and their health. This was disseminated via newspapers, radio, leaflets, posters and stickers, health education meetings, public campaigns, schools, working places, etc.
2 Organization of services: systematic integration of the necessary measures with the existing health services and creation of necessary new ones, via primary community health services (health centres), special supportive services, and services by other organizations.
3 Training of personnel, especially in the practical tasks of the program. The groups trained were health personnel, social workers, teachers, workers in voluntary organizations, journalists, and community leaders.
4 Environmental services to encourage better life styles: smoking restrictions, promoting use of low-fat dairy products and low-fat sausages, growing of vegetables, etc.
5 Internal information services to assist in the practical work: patient cards, files, registries (hypertension, infarction, stroke), follow-up surveys, other information.

Evaluation

The aim of the evaluation was to demonstrate the feasibility and the effect of the program, to estimate the costs and obtain a comprehensive picture of the process that took place in the community during the five-year period from 1972 to 1977. We were also able to evaluate the long-term effects of the program over ten years from 1972 to 1982.

A baseline survey for assessing changes in risk factors was carried out in the spring of 1972 in North Karelia and a matched reference area – another province in eastern Finland. A random 6.6% sample was drawn from the populations of the two provinces using the national population register. The five-year follow-up survey was carried out in 1977 and the ten-year follow-up survey in 1982 in the two areas. The survey methods were the same as those in the baseline survey (3,4). Other data used for the evaluation include, for example, mortality and morbidity statistics (5–7).

Results

The results of the North Karelia Project showed that serum cholesterol levels fell by 11% among middle-aged men and women in North Karelia over ten years. The reduction was significantly greater in North Karelia than in the reference area among men for the period from 1972 to 1977 and from 1972 to 1982. Among women no significant difference was observed between the two areas (4).

The findings of dietary fat intake obtained by questionnaire showed a remarkable reduction in the intake of saturated fats from milk and spreads used on bread. These changes in saturated fat intake were relatively similar among men and women. The major net reduction in North Karelia took place during 1972 to 1977. During the second five-year period favourable changes started to take place also in the reference area, which is understandable, because national implementation of the activities found feasible in North Karelia started after 1977. Although the intake of saturated fats remained higher among rural populations, the changes showed a similar trend both in urban and rural areas.

The proportion of current smokers among 30- to 59-year-old men in North Karelia decreased from 52% in 1972 to 44% in 1977, and to 38% in 1982. In the reference area the respective smoking rates were 50, 45, and 45%. About 27% of male smokers in North Karelia stopped smoking during the project period, while in the reference area the proportion was 10%. Among women the initially low smoking rates increased in both areas by 7% – because of new birth cohorts with higher smoking rates entering the age group of the study. At the same time, the prevalence of ex-smokers among women increased markedly, especially among the younger females (8).

By 1982, mean diastolic blood pressure had declined 5.6% among men and 8.5% among women of this age group (4). The net reduction in blood pressure was significantly bigger both among men and women in North Karelia than in the reference area, and the hypertension program seemed to reach all the different socio-economic strata of the community equally.

Overall, the ten-year results supported the evidence that the decrease in risk factor levels in North Karelia was an effect of the intervention program. We were also able to demonstrate significantly decreased mortality from coronary heart disease during the ten-year period. The average fall in coronary heart disease mortality was about 29% among men during the ten-year period in North Karelia. At the same time the decrease on the national level was about 23% (7).

Also, cancer mortality started to fall in North Karelia as well as in the whole country during the observation period. The average decline was almost 2% per year.

Conclusions

The experiences and results of the North Karelia project show that a well-conceived, community-based program can have a meaningful impact on the life styles, risk factors, cardiovascular disease rates, and general health status of the population, and that through this kind of systematic action the modern epidemic of our times – heart disease – can be effectively fought.

REFERENCES

1 Puska P, Tuomilehto J, Salonen JT, et al. *Community control of cardiovascular diseases – the North Karelia Project: evaluation of a comprehensive community programme for control of cardiovascular diseases in 1972–77 in North Karelia*. Copenhagen: WHO/EURO, 1981.

2 McAlister A, Puska P, Salonen JT, Tuomilehto J, Koskela K. Theory and action for health promotion: illustrations from the North Karelia project. *Am J Publ Health* 1982;72:43–50.

3 Puska P, Tuomilehto J, Salonen J, et al. Changes in coronary risk factors during comprehensive five-year community programme to control cardiovascular diseases (North Karelia Project). *Br Med J* 1979;2:1173–1178.

4 Puska P, Salonen JT, Nissinen A, et al. Change in risk factors for coronary heart disease during ten years of a community intervention programme (North Karelia Project). *Br Med J* 1983;287:1840–1844.

5 Salonen J, Puska P, Mustaniemi H. Changes in morbidity and mortality during comprehensive community programme to control cardiovascular diseases during 1972–77 in North Karelia. *Br Med J* 1979;2:1178–1183.

6 Salonen JT, Puska P, Kottke TE, Tuomilehto J, Nissinen A. Decline in mortality from coronary heart disease in Finland from 1969 to 1979. *Br Med J* 1983;286:1857–1860.

7 Tuomilehto J, Geboers J, Salonen JT, Nissinen A, Kuulasmaa K, Puska P. Decline in cardiovascular mortality in North Karelia and other parts of Finland. *Br Med J* 1986;293:1068–1071.

8 Vartiainen E, Puska P, Koskela K, Nissinen A, Tuomilehto J. Ten-year results of a community-based anti-smoking program (as part of the North Karelia Project in Finland). *Health Educ Res* 1986;1:175–000.

Diet and Selected Health Problems

NORMAN M. KAPLAN

Diet and Hypertension

Diet is probably involved in the causation of most hypertension and should be involved in the treatment of virtually all hypertension. For simplicity, I shall consider the major dietary components separately, providing a bit about their role in causation, which remains uncertain, and more about their role in treatment, which is fairly well established.

Calories

About half of hypertensives are overweight, and the prevalence of hyptertension rises progressively at all ages with increasing degrees of obesity. The tendency for the blood pressure to rise with weight gain probably reflects the interaction of multiple factors, including hormones, fluid volume, and cardiac function. One unifying concept places increased blood levels of insulin resulting from insulin resistance as a central mechanism since both hypertension and obesity are often accompanied by high plasma insulin levels (1). The concept invokes progressively more insulin resistance with weight gain, particularly when it is distributed primarily in the abdomen. Higher insulin levels may cause hypertension by directly stimulating sympathetic nervous activity or increasing renal reabsorption of sodium.

Just as hypertension becomes more prevalent with increasing weight, so does blood pressure usually fall with weight loss. Moreover, weight loss not only usually lowers the blood pressure but will also improve the blood lipid profile (Figure 1) (2). During this study,

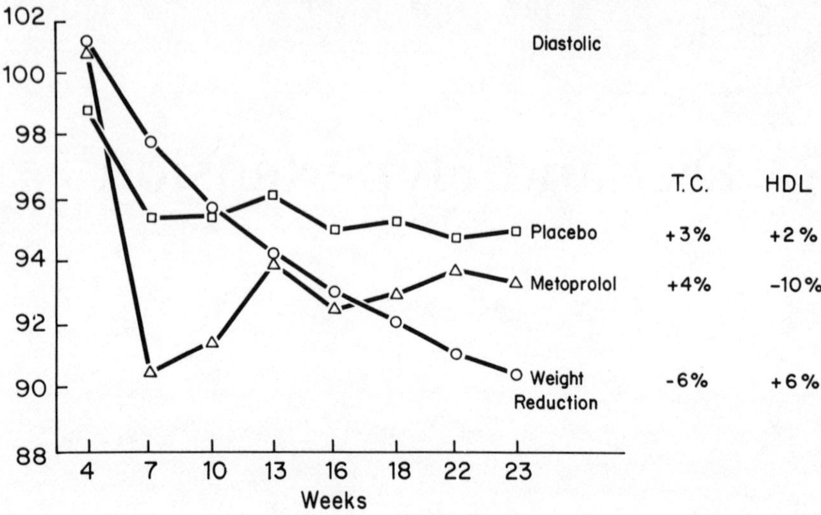

Figure 1. The course of the diastolic blood pressure, and changes in total cholesterol and HDL-cholesterol during 21 weeks of treatment with placebo, or metoprolol 100 mg twice a day, or weight reduction averaging 7.4 kg accomplished by a diet reduced by 1000 calories per day. The therapies were randomly assigned to the 56 overweight subjects with mild hypertension (2).

young overweight hypertensive patients were randomly assigned to weight-reduction, a beta-blocker drug, or a placebo. Those on weight reduction, who lost an average of 8.3 kg, not only had a greater fall in blood pressure than did those on the beta-blocker but also had a fall in total cholesterol and a rise in high-density lipoprotein (HDL) cholesterol, both of which provide further protection from coronary disease.

Beyond the fall in blood pressure that will probably accompany weight loss in those who are already hypertensive, weight loss may be the only proved and practical way to prevent the development of hypertension. In an 11-year longitudinal survey of 2925 school children in Muscatine, Iowa, those who lost weight tended to have a fall in blood pressure, those who gained weight, a rise (3). The magnitude of the change in blood pressure was related directly to the change in body weight and was not dependent on the initial blood pressure.

It seems appropriate then that weight loss should be encouraged for all hypertensives who are overweight. Thereby, the blood pressure will probably fall and, as an extra benefit, the plasma lipid profile may also improve. The regimen for weight loss should be whatever the patient will accept and follow. For some, a structured, carefully monitored, very low calorie program may be best. For others, a more gradual reprogramming of daily dietary practices based on behavioural modification may be more effective. With caution against the use of diet pills containing sympathomimetics, which may raise the blood pressure, any weight loss regimen that works should be tried, remembering that with persistence, success is more likely than many have assumed.

Dietary Fat

Hypertensives are more likely than normotensives to have elevated blood cholesterol levels and lower levels of cardioprotective HDL-cholesterol. Moreover, the two most widely used classes of antihypertensive drugs, diuretics and beta-adrenergic blocking agents, may further worsen lipid profiles, diuretics by raising cholesterol, beta-blockers by lowering HDL-cholesterol.

Therefore, hypertensives need to reduce dietary saturated fat and cholesterol as much or more than normotensives to overcome the hazards of premature vascular disease induced by both their hypertension and their most frequent hyperlipidemia. In limited trials, reduced amounts of dietary saturated fat and increased amounts of polyunsaturated fat have been found to lower the blood pressure. An additional antihypertensive effect may be achieved by ingestion of omega-3 fatty acids, as shown in one controlled trial (4).

Despite the apparent wisdom of following the "prudent" diet to reduce the risks of hypercholesterolemia, ingestion of such a low (20%) fat/high (60%) carbohydrate diet for 15 days has been shown to raise both plasma glucose and insulin levels in a group of non-obese hypertensive patients compared to the effects of a 40% fat/40% carbohydrate diet (5). These changes could diminish if not ablate the reduction in cardiovascular risk provided by a beneficial effect on lipids. They are particularly worrisome in view of the previously noted high plasma insulin levels in hypertensives.

Beyond fat, changes in the consumption of the other two food categories, carbohydrates and protein, have not been found to influence blood pressure meaningfully.

Sodium

Dietary sodium excess is probably a principal cause of primary (essential) hypertension. The evidence is largely circumstantial but quite

Table 1
Estimated Diet of Late Palaeolithic Man vs That of Modern Americans (7)

	Late Palaeolithic diet (assuming 35% meat)	*Current American diet*
Total dietary energy (%)		
Protein	34	12
Carbohydrate	45	46
Fat	21	42
Polyunsaturated: saturated fat ratio	1.41	0.44
Sodium (mg)	690	3500
Potassium (mg)	11000	2400
K/Na ratio	16.1	0.7:1
Calcium (mg)	1580	740

persuasive (6). Simply stated, sodium intake in excess of the quite small amounts needed for physiologic needs is probably a necessary but not sufficient component of the hemodynamic cascade that eventuates in hypertension. Even if it were not, reduction of sodium intake to the levels consumed by humans throughout most of history should not be looked upon as an "unnatural" move, since our physiology is presumably constructed to handle the lower sodium diet that was natural until fairly recent times (Table 1) (7). The hypothesis that our current high sodium intake is involved in the pathogenesis of hypertension is supported by the recognition that hypertension is more prevalent in blacks than in whites in the United States. American blacks largely came from areas in Africa where sodium was quite scarce, so their body physiology probably adapted to a low sodium intake. After their migration to the United States, their sodium intake must have risen, and this may be a factor in their high prevalence of hypertension.

Although the sensitivity of the blood pressure to both increases and decreases of sodium intake has been found to vary considerably among hypertensive patients, I believe that moderate dietary sodium restriction, to a level of 2 g per day (5 g of sodium chloride), is both practical and useful, at least for a trial period, for all patients. The evidence as recently summarized (8) shows an average 5 mm Hg fall in systolic and diastolic blood pressure in most hypertensives over age 40 after a reduction of dietary sodium intake down to a level of 2 g per day.

Potassium

Part of the roles ascribed to sodium excess in the pathogenesis of hypertension and to sodium restriction in the treatment of hypertension may, in fact, be played by potassium instead. As noted in Table 1, the diets eaten by Palaeolithic man were both lower in sodium and higher in potassium than those now consumed. When dietary sodium restriction is achieved by reducing the consumption of processed foods in favour of natural forms, potassium intake often rises as sodium falls. Therefore, the antihypertensive effect of such an altered diet could reflect the addition of potassium. Vegetarians tend to have lower blood pressures than non-vegetarians and this, too, may reflect their high potassium intake.

Potassium supplements have been given to reduce the blood pressure with only modest effect, probably less than that observed with sodium restriction, although the number of controlled trials with potassium remains fairly small. The appropriate advice for most hypertensives is simply to increase dietary intake of fresh foods, which are almost all high in potassium. If potassium depletion is present, usually from diuretic therapy, potassium supplements may be needed, and they may cause the blood pressure to fall (9).

Calcium

An increased concentration of calcium within cardiac and vascular smooth muscle cells is a feature of most currently held models for the development of hypertension. Intracellular calcium may increase in various ways (Figure 2) (10), thereby increasing the tone and contractility of smooth muscle and raising the blood pressure by both cardiac and vascular mechanisms.

Despite the probable involvement of too much calcium within cells as a cause of hypertension, there has been considerable interest in the use of calcium supplements to lower the blood pressure. This interest arises, in part, from reports that dietary calcium intake may be lower in hypertensive than in normotensive people. The most complete analysis of the best data relating calcium intake to blood pressure, however, failed to show a relation (11).

Some hypertensives excrete more than normal amounts of calcium into the urine, probably as a consequence of a renal response to an expanded body fluid volume. As shown on the right side of Figure 2, this renal leak could lower blood levels of calcium, in turn stimu-

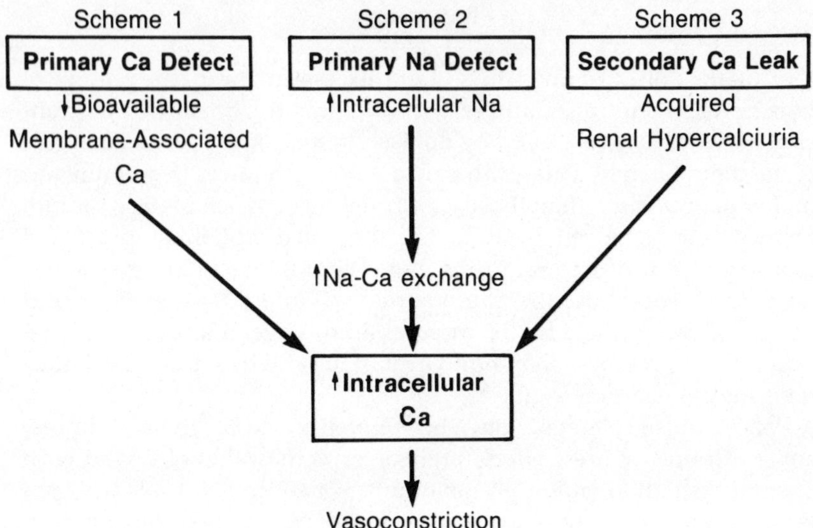

Figure 2. Three possible defects in calcium metabolism, all of which could eventuate in increased intracellular calcium (10).

lating the release of parathyroid hormone, the main hormonal regulator of calcium balance. Increased parathyroid hormone levels, shown to be present in those hypertensives who have a renal leak of calcium, will increase calcium movement from extracellular fluid across cell membranes, leading to an increased intracellular calcium concentration.

This mechanism may be simply an accompaniment to volume-expanded forms of hypertension or may be a primary mechanism for the rise in blood pressure with volume expansion. Regardless, in the largest study yet published on the effects of giving calcium supplements to hypertensive patients, those whose blood pressure fell were those who started with lower blood calcium levels and higher blood parathyroid hormone levels (12).

Present evidence suggests that calcium supplements will lower the blood pressure in one-third to one-half of hypertensives. Whether the calcium leak/parathyroid hormone mechanism is responsible for the favourable effects is uncertain. However, some of those given calcium supplements have a further rise in blood pressure. Therefore, until it is possible to identify beforehand those who will respond favourably, calcium supplements should not be used indiscriminately in hopes of lowering the blood pressure.

Moderation of Alcohol

Although not usually considered as a part of the diet, alcohol in excess is a problem for many hypertensives, not only because of the dangers of alcoholism but also because it may impair control of their hypertension and increase their likelihood of having a stroke. Alcohol, even in smaller amounts – any amount over that contained in three drinks a day – may exert a direct pressor effect. This pressor effect has been clearly documented when about two ounces (0.76 g/kg body weight) of alcohol were consumed over 15 minutes, raising the blood alcohol level to a peak of 91 mg per 100 ml (20 mmol/L) (13). When compared to the unchanged blood pressures during the placebo therapy in this randomized, double-blind cross-over trial, the systolic levels rose significantly, the diastolic less so after alcohol; in three of the nine patients, the rise in systolic pressure was greater than 25 mm Hg.

Chronic consumption of lesser amounts of alcohol probably does not raise the blood pressure, although the evidence is not clear. In a review of 30 cross-sectional studies, it was found that the blood pressure of those who drank fewer than three drinks per day was greater than that of non-drinkers in seven cases, no different in 11, and lower in 12 (14). Since such light drinking has been shown to be associated with less coronary heart disease, the best advice would seem to be: keep alcohol intake to no more than 30 g or 40 ml, the amount contained in three usual drinks a day (one drink = 12 ounces of beer, 4 ounces of wine, 1 ounce of distilled spirits). Those who drink more should be strongly encouraged to cut down for numerous reasons, including a probable fall in their blood pressure. There seems little reason to recommend total abstinence, either for the blood pressure or for overall health.

Other Dietary Changes

Almost everything from acupuncture to zinc, with a heavy pinch of garlic, has been claimed to lower the blood pressure. However, most have not lived up to the hopes that attended their introduction. No modalities other than those previously covered have been proved to be effective in properly conducted trials of sufficiently large numbers of people to justify their use.

Prohibitions against the intake of caffeine-containing beverages have been repeatedly advocated in the management of hypertension. Although caffeine will acutely raise the blood pressure of non-users, tolerance to its pressor action rather quickly develops, and there is

Table 2
Dietary Therapy for Hypertension

If obese, weight reduction
Dietary sodium restricted to 2 g (88 mmol) per day
Supplemental potassium, magnesium, and calcium if deficiency exists
More fibre and less saturated fat
Alcohol limited to 1 ounce per day

no convincing evidence that cutting it out will lower the blood pressure.

Overall Dietary Recommendations

All hypertensives should be encouraged to follow as many of the dietary manipulations listed in Table 2 as applicable and possible. The appropriate timing for their use is usually sooner rather than later. For example, an obese hypertensive probably will be more easily motivated to stay with a low-calorie diet if weight reduction is accompanied, as is likely, by a fall in blood pressure. If, while starting the diet, the patient also monitors the blood pressure, the usual fall in pressure will be noted to accompany the fall in weight that almost always occurs at the beginning of a new diet. If, after a few weeks, the patient stops the diet, a rise in blood pressure probably will accompany the rise in body weight. The recognition of parallel change in pressure may help motivate the patient to return to effective weight reduction. On the other hand, if medications are given at the outset, the fall in blood pressure they induce may detract from the motivation the patient would have to lose weight. Further, if subsequent weight loss occurs and lowers the blood pressure, the medication may need to be discontinued.

Certainly, many will not accept these non-drug approaches, and some who use them will not respond with a fall in blood pressure. However, for most hypertensives at least a four- to six-month trial before instituting drug therapy is appropriate. During this time, repeated checks on the blood pressure are needed to ensure that the patient is truly hypertensive and in need of drugs. If diet, exercise, and the other non-drug approaches help to lower the pressure below the level needing drug therapy, a considerable number of patients will be saved the expense, monetary, psychological, and physical, of many drugs used to treat the disease.

The long-term effectiveness of dietary changes in lowering blood pressure has not been clearly established. However, one four-year study of a group of hypertensives previously treated with drugs who then stopped their medications and were given, in a random fashion, either a lower-calorie, lower-sodium diet or no nutritional change showed that 39% of those on the dietary program remained normotensive after four years, whereas only 5% of those who simply stopped their medications remained normotensive (15).

Although more such information is needed on the long-term effectiveness of various non-drug therapies, enthusiastic use of the various dietary approaches described should provide additional control of the blood pressure in many hypertensive patients with little or no discomfort or impairment in the quality of life. Along with the blood pressure, other cardiovascular risk factors should also be reduced. Moreover, for the population at large, there is at least a possibility that the development of hypertension may thereby be postponed or even prevented.

REFERENCES

1 Modan M, Halkin H, Almog S, et al. Hyperinsulinemia: a link between hypertension obesity and glucose intolerance. *J Clin Invest* 1985;75:809–817.

2 MacMahon SW, Macdonald GJ, Bernstein L, et al. Comparison of weight reduction with metoprolol in treatment of hypertension in young overweight patients. *Lancet* 1985;1:1233–1236.

3 Clarke WR, Woolson RF, Lauer RM. Changes in ponderosity and blood pressure in childhood: the Muscatine study. *Am J Epidemiol* 1986; 124:195–206.

4 Singer P, Berger I, Lück K, Taube C, Naumann E, Gödicke W. Long-term effect of mackerel diet on blood pressure, serum lipids and thromboxane formation in patients with mild essential hypertension. *Atherosclerosis* 1986;62:259–265.

5 Parillo M, Coulston A, Hollenbeck C, et al. Effect of a 'prudent' diet on risk factors for coronary artery disease in patient with hypertension. *Clin Res* 1987;35:188A (abstr).

6 Kaplan NM. Chapter 3: Primary (essential) hypertension: pathogenesis. In: Kaplan NM, ed. *Clinical hypertension*, 3rd ed. Baltimore: Williams and Williams, 1986:56–122.

7 Eaton SB, Konner M. Paleolithic nutrition. *N Engl J Med* 1985;312:283–289.

8 Grobbee DE, Hofman A. Does sodium restriction lower blood pressure? *Br Med J* 1986;293:27–29.

9 Kaplan NM, Carnegie A, Raskin P, Heller JA, Simmons M. Potassium supplementation in hypertensive patients with diuretic-induced hypokalemia. *N Engl J Med* 1985;312:746–749.

10 Pak CYC. Calcium and hypertension. In: Horan MJ, Blaustein M, Dunbar JB, Kachadorian W, Kaplan NM, Simopoulos AP, eds. *NIH workshop on nutrition and hypertension: proceedings from a symposium*. New York: Biomedical Information Corporation, 1985:155–165.

11 Sempos C, Cooper R, Kovar MG, et al. Dietary calcium and blood pressure in national health and nutrition examination surveys I and II. *Hypertension* 1986;8:1067–1074.

12 Grobbee DE, Hofman A. Effect of calcium supplementation on diastolic blood pressure in young people with mild hypertension. *Lancet* 1986; 2:703–707.

13 Potter JF, Macdonald IA, Beevers DG. Alcohol raises blood pressure in hypertensive patients. *J Hypertension* 1986;4:435–441.

14 MacMahon SW, Norton RN. Alcohol and hypertension: implications for prevention and treatment – editorial. *Ann Intern Med* 1986;105:124–126.

15 Stamler R, Stamler J, Grimm R, et al. Nutritional therapy for high blood pressure: final report of a four-year randomized controlled trial – the Hypertension Control Progam. *JAMA* 1987;257:1484–1491.

THOMAS M.S. WOLEVER AND DAVID J.A. JENKINS

Diet and Diabetes

The name diabetes mellitus originates from two Greek words: *diabetes*, passing through, and *meli*, honey; so called because, when the disorder is poorly controlled, the urine contains much suger and is like honey. Diabetes is a metabolic disorder characterized by a deficiency or lack of effectiveness of insulin, a hormone produced by the beta-cells in the pancreas. An important function of insulin is to stimulate the uptake of glucose from the blood into the tissues. A lack of insulin therefore leads to the presence of raised blood glucose levels and the presence of glucose in the urine, the two hallmarks of diabetes. There are two major types of diabetes, now known as insulin dependent (IDDM) and non-insulin dependent (NIDDM) diabetes mellitus. The features of these are shown in Table 1.

Diabetes was described over 3000 years ago. Before the discovery of insulin in 1921, diet was the only form of therapy. During the seventeenth and eighteenth centuries little was known about diabetes except that the urine tasted sweet because of the presence of sugar. This led to two schools of thought about treatment. One was that the sugar lost in the urine was essential to the body and should be replaced with a high carbohydrate diet. The other was that the sugar lost in the urine was toxic to the body, and therefore the diet should contain no carbohydrate.

In the early 1900s it was found that a very low calorie diet could prevent the development of diabetic ketoacidosis, which in those days was rapidly fatal. However, the quality of life for these semi-starved patients was poor. After insulin was introduced in 1921 there was a

Table 1
Typical Features of Insulin and Non-insulin Dependent Diabetes

	Insulin Dependent	*Non-insulin Dependent*
% of diabetic population	less than 20%	over 80% of total
Age of onset	early (under 30)	late (over 50)
Body weight	normal weight	80% are overweight
Ketosis proneness	ketosis prone	not ketosis prone
Blood insulin level	low or zero	normal or raised
Treatment	requires insulin	diet ± oral agents ± insulin

careful reintroduction of carbohydrate into the diabetic diet, but it was generally considered that carbohydrate was harmful, and the amounts in the diet were strictly controlled. This led to the development of carbohydrate rationing schemes based on food tables giving the carbohydrate content of foods. In the 1930s Himsworth showed that dietary carbohydrate could be increased from about 20% of calories to 40% without increasing the amount of insulin needed. Nevertheless, during the next 40 years, the dietary management of diabetes varied widely; in 1953 about 25% of diabetic clinics in Britain were still prescribing 20% carbohydrate diets. By the 1970s it was generally held that the diabetes diet should contain about 40% of energy as carbohydrate, similar to a typical North American diet. However, unlike other aspects of diabetes treatment, the rationale behind dietary practice was based on assumptions rather than research.

During the past decade there has been renewed research interest into the dietary management of diabetes. The rapid accumulation of data means that guidelines for the management of diabetes should always carry the statement that they are based on the best evidence available at present and are subject to change. Concern over the increased risk of cardiovascular disease in the diabetic population (1) has resulted in advice to reduce saturated fat and cholesterol intake and hence increase carbohydrate consumption. However, the emphasis on increasing carbohydrate consumption has posed a number of questions. Which type of carbohydrate foods should be selected: should they be foods which are high in dietary fibre? Should they be foods which are digested slowly and result in low blood glucose responses (low glycaemic index foods)? What is the status of sucrose, the nutritive sweeteners (e.g. fructose), and the non-nutritive sweet-

Table 2
Summary of Recommended Daily Intakes in Diabetes: ADA 1986

Carbohydrate	55–60% calories
Protein	0.8 g/kg bodyweight
Fat	<30% calories
PUFA	6–8% calories
Saturated	<10% calories
Cholesterol	<300 mg/day
Sodium (elemental)	<3 g/day

eners in the dietary management of diabetes? In addition, there are new considerations with respect to protein and fat. Current ideas about the relationship between a high protein intake and the progression of kidney disease may apply in diabetes, where renal damage is one of the common complications. The effect of omega-3 fatty acids in reducing blood lipids is also of relevance. Finally, the benefits of exercise *per se*, or as a part of a weight reduction program is being debated.

The beginning of this year saw the publication of new Dietary Guidelines from the American Diabetes Association (ADA) (2), which have been supported in the past by recommendations in Canada (3), Britain (4), and elsewhere. Also this year will see the publication of an NIH Consensus Conference on Diet and Exercise in Type 2 Diabetes held in December 1986 (5). The conclusions of this conference were sometimes rather different than those of the ADA. Current dietary recommendations will therefore be discussed here from the point of view of the ADA guidelines, which are both compehensive and practical. Points of contention with the NIH report will be highlighted.

Current Dietary Recommendations for Diabetes

Current dietary recommendations for diabetes are shown in Table 2. Carbohydrate should comprise 55–60% of energy, protein 0.8 g/kg bodyweight, and fat less than 30% of calories. The reduction in fat would be accomplished by a reduction in saturated fat intake to less than 10% of energy, maintaining polyunsaturated fat (PUFA) at 6–8% of energy. This results in a modest increase of the PUFA to saturated fat ratio (P/S ratio). Cholesterol intake should be restricted to less than 300 mg per day and salt reduced so that elemental sodium is less than 1000 mg/1000 kcal, and no more than 3000 mg per day (Table 2). Alcohol should be consumed in moderation because of its unpredictable effect on glycaemic control, including hypoglycaemia, and the tendency of alcohol to raise serum triglyceride levels. Raised triglyceride (TG) levels are an apparent risk factor for the development of cardiovascular disease in the diabetic population. About half of all diabetics have raised TG levels, in part due to obesity and poor glycaemic control.

No clear advice has been given with respect to vitamin and mineral supplements. On a balanced diet the need for these is not clearly established. However, those on diets containing less than 1000 kcal may well need supplements in order to meet minimum daily requirements.

SPECIFIC RECOMMENDATIONS FOR IDDM AND NIDDM

IDDM: It is generally agreed that the timing of meals in relation to injected insulin is of great importance. A consistent habit of regularly distributed meals and snacks throughout the day may allow better control while reducing the risk of hypoglycaemia.

NIDDM: 80% of patients with NIDDM are overweight. For these individuals, weight reduction is a major aim of therapy. Central adiposity has been associated with insulin resistance, glucose intolerance, hyperlipidaemia, and increased risk of cardiovascular disease (6). General recommendations are to reduce caloric intake by 500–1000 kcal per day, which would lead to 1–2 pounds of weight loss per week. However, it is considered that diets containing 500–800 kcal or less should be monitored by a physician and the appropriate supplements provided to ensure an adequate intake of nutrients.

IMPLEMENTATION OF DIETARY RECOMMENDATIONS

It is generally considered important, to enhance compliance, that each patient be given a diet plan individualized to suit his or her specific tastes and lifestyle. If the diet is to have long-term impact, a team approach should be used in which the patient, physician, nurse, and dietitian discuss the diet plan, along with, when possible, relevant family members. The team approach should be evident in a detailed initial phase of education of the patient and family, and be maintained with frequent follow-up.

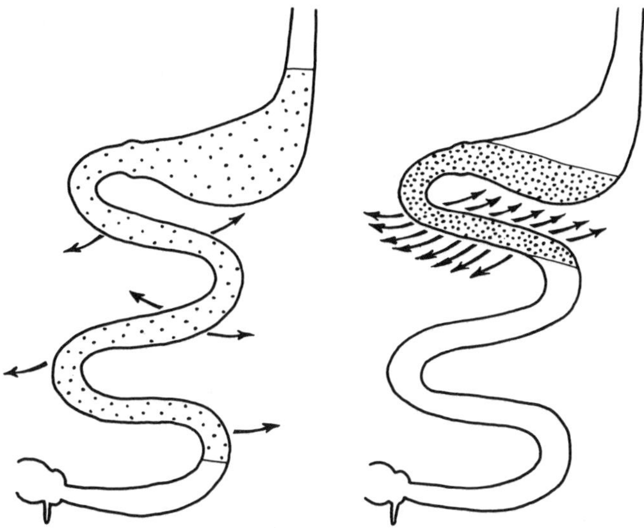

Figure 1. Hypothetical effect of a diet high in fibre on the rate of absorption of carbohydrate (left) compared with that of a refined diet (right).

AREAS OF DISAGREEMENT AND DEBATE

With the emergence of new data, there has been debate and vigorous disagreement about many aspects of the diabetes diet. The issues debated include the desirability of protein restriction and the use of omega-3 fatty acids. There is marked disagreement on the value of dietary fibre, the glycaemic index, and sucrose restriction. Even the value of one of the classic cornerstones of diabetes management, exercise, is now being challenged.

DIETARY FIBRE

The original rationale for the use of fibre was that, by forming a barrier to the digestion and absorption of foods (Figure 1), the rate of absorption of glucose would be reduced, and this would result in flatter responses of blood glucose and insulin (Figure 2) (7). Interest in the use of dietary fibre in the management of diabetes arose in the 1970s on the basis of two lines of evidence. In studies where a range of purified dietary fibres was added to test meals, some fibres caused smaller rises of blood glucose and insulin levels postprandially. The

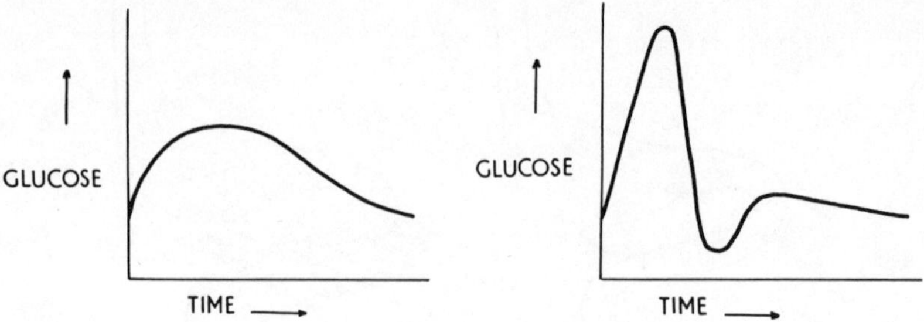

Figure 2. Hypothetical effects of slowly absorbed (left) and rapidly absorbed (right) carbohydrate on blood glucose responses.

degree to which fibre reduced the postprandial glycaemia was directly related to the viscosity of fibre solutions *in vitro*. Thus guar, which forms a viscous gum, was most effective, while bran, which does not increase the viscosity of water, had little effect on blood glucose responses. When guar was given to diabetic patients in the longer term, urinary glucose losses were reduced. In addition, increasing fibre intake with high carbohydrate, high fibre foods markedly improved diabetes control. Unfortunately, the fibre supplement used, guar, was not readily available in palatable form, and the high-carboyhydrate, high-fibre diet was rigorous and not immediately suited for general application. Nevertheless, over subsequent years a number of centres have produced similar results (8), although the gains have not always been as dramatic, and in some cases negative results have been obtained. Therefore, the general application to the diabetic population of dietary fibre has been called into question, most notably by the NIH Consensus Conference which came to fairly negative conclusions (Table 3).

One of the reasons for the uncertainty about the use of dietary fibre is that there are two broad classes of fibre, soluble and insoluble, which have quite different physiological effects (Table 4). As can be seen, it is the soluble fibres which have the metabolic effects that are desirable to achieve in diabetes. Failure to differentiate between studies in which the predominant increase in dietary fibre has been from foods containing insoluble fibre (9) as opposed to those containing soluble fibre (10) is one of the reasons for the lack of unanimity in the purported effects of fibre on carbohydrate and lipid metabolism (Table 5 gives examples of foods which contain soluble and insoluble fibre). This difference was recognized by the ADA, which came to more positive conclusions about the use of dietary fibre (Table 6).

Table 3
Summary of NIH Consensus Conference Position on Dietary Fibre

1 Studies showing benefits – inconclusive
2 Unpalatable
3 Negative effects not defined
4 Contra-indicated in autonomic neuropathy
5 If the patient desires fibre, give soluble fibre
6 Fibre supplements not recommended

Table 4
Summary of the Effects of Soluble and Insoluble Dietary Fibres

	Soluble	*Insoluble*
Faecal bulking	0	+ + +
Colonic fermentation	+ + +	±
Cholesterol reduction	+ +	0
Reduced postprandial glycaemia	+ +	±
Longer term improvement in carbohydrate metabolism	+	±
Satiety	+	±
Weight reduction	±	±

Table 5
Examples of Foods High in Soluble and Insoluble Dietary Fibre

Soluble	*Insoluble*
Legumes	Whole wheat
Oats	Wheat bran
Barley	Whole rye
Okra	Brown rice
Persimmon	Millet

Table 6
Summary of ADA Position on Dietary Fibre

1 Double the intake
2 Use soluble types especially
3 Use legumes, whole-grain cereals, root vegetables, tubers, leafy vegetables
4 Advantages: i Carbohydrate metabolism improved
ii Blood lipids decreased
5 Cautions: i Mineral deficiency; e.g. Ca + +
ii Gastric bezoars
iii Abdominal discomfort

DELETERIOUS EFFECTS OF DIETARY FIBRE

The adverse effects of fibre range from making the diet unpalatable to causing abdominal discomfort, flatulence, gastric bezoars, and mineral deficiency.

High fibre foods are not part of a traditional "Western" diet and rather than being unpalatable, simply may be unfamiliar to the North American population. On the other hand, high fibre foods are part of the traditional diet in many cultures whose cuisine is becoming popular in North America (e.g. Indian, Middle Eastern, Chinese). Palatability is a personal matter, and the selection of high fibre foods will be according to individual taste and background. This is in line with the goal of individualizing the diet and the recognition of the possible value of many "ethnic" foods.

Abdominal discomfort and flatulence will usually be experienced during the introduction of high fibre foods into the diet because of colonic fermentation of the unavailable carbohydrate. The risk of this can be reduced by increasing the fibre intake gradually; symptoms usually disappear with more prolonged use.

Gastric bezoars have been reported as a rare complication of taking high fibre foods. When they are biopsied, cabbage has been found as a causative agent, and large amounts of underripe persimmon have been found to be associated with intussusception. In addition, the effectiveness of fibre has been questioned in patients with severe autonomic neuropathy of the gut. In this situation, gastric emptying, gut motility, and the rate of small intestinal absorption is already reduced.

Mineral deficiency has been a major cause for concern. It is true that insoluble types of fibre such as wheat bran have been associated with increased losses of Ca^{++}, Zn^{++}, and Fe^{++}. Such effects have not been clearly documented with the more soluble types of fibre (11). Caution may therefore be required in prescribing large amounts of insoluble fibre to those whose mineral status may be compromised, such as the elderly. General concern for healthy people over possible dangers from doubling the mean population intake of dietary fibre from mixed sources does not appear warranted (11).

Although there is no clear-cut evidence for a major therapeutic effect of fibre, its addition to the diet may contribute to overall health and have some specific metabolic advantages for those with diabetes.

THE GLYCAEMIC INDEX

The available carbohydrate in foods has classically been grouped into "simple" and "complex" carbohydrates. "Simple" carbohydrates include mono- and disaccharides (i.e. the sugars), and "complex" carbohydrates include the digestible polysaccharides amylose and amylopectin (i.e. starch). Traditionally, diabetics have been advised to avoid "simple" carbohydrates. It was suggested that sugars caused higher rises in blood glucose after their consumption because they were broken down and absorbed more rapidly than the "complex" starch molecules which have to undergo hydrolysis by pancreatic amylase. However, it is now known that there is a wide range of glycaemic responses to different sugars and that this range overlaps and is virtually indistinguishable from the range of glycaemic responses to different starchy foods. Since the classification of foods according to their chemical nature (i.e. simple and complex carbohydrate) does not allow prediction of their glycaemic effects, a classification of foods according to their biological effect on the blood glucose response was developed (12). This classification was called the glycaemic index (GI) where:

$$\text{GI} = \frac{\text{Incremental glycaemic response to 50 g carbohydrate from test food} \times 100}{\text{Incremental response to 50 g carbohydrate from reference food}}$$

Either bread or glucose has been used as a reference to "standarize" an individual's response to a test food. Effectively, the glycaemic response of the test food is expressed as a percent of that for the reference food taken by the same subject, and the results from different individuals are averaged to give the GI for that food. It was reasoned that such a classification could be used to select carbohydrate foods for inclusion in the diabetic diet. The GI established in normal, NIDDM, and IDDM subjects was found to be similar for the same foods, and there was a broad measure of agreement in results between different centres (12,13). This has prompted the suggestion that at a future stage this form of classification could form part of the "exchange system" for carbohydrate foods. Many factors may be responsible for differences in postprandial responses to carbohydrate foods, including not only the fat and protein content of a food, but also fibre, the food form (e.g. particle size of grains and degree of compactness –

Table 7
Summary of ADA Position on the Glycaemic Index

1	Classification may facilitate management
2	Consistencies suggest future use as exchange
3	Inconsistencies suggest delaying general application
4	Area for more research
5	Meanwhile use tables to identify foods to offer patients on a trial basis

bread as opposed to pasta), the method of processing (parboiled as opposed to polished rice), cooking, and, in the case of fruit, the degree of ripeness. These factors need to be more carefully documented and comprehensive tables of values established and validated before the practical utility of the GI can be assessed. However, in the meantime, the current recommendations of the ADA suggest that individual patients could be offered low GI foods on a trial basis (Table 7). In addition, the Canadian Diabetes Association specifically recommends the use of what are, in effect, low GI foods. Table 8 gives the GI ranking of some common starchy foods. While the ADA recommendations can be summed up as supportive of the GI concept, the opposite point of view was expressed by the NIH (Table 9). However, their data base for drawing conclusions was considerably narrower than that of the ADA. The panel felt that the factors responsible for differences in glycaemic effect were unpredictable, failing to acknowledge evidence to the contrary. Above all, they considered that the differences in glycaemic effects of different single foods were abolished when the foods were fed in the context of a mixed meal, and therefore that the concept lacked clinical utility. Again, data contrary to this view were ignored. The application of this concept therefore remains a matter for debate, and studies of the longer term effects of low GI foods on metabolic control in diabetes are required. Individual physicians and dietitians may nevertheless wish to try its application for themselves, especially where it increases the variety of starchy foods found acceptable by the patient.

SWEETENERS IN THE DIABETIC DIET

Traditionally the use of sugar by the diabetic was forbidden. However, evidence of deleterious effects of sucrose from controlled trials is not strong (14). In addition, the effect of sucrose on the postprandial glycaemia is no worse than that of many starchy foods (12). The latter

Table 8
Glycaemic Index (GI) Ranking of Some Common Starchy Foods into Higher (Class I), Intermediate (Class II), and Lower (Class III) Groups

Class I *GI > 90*	*Class II* *GI 70–90*	*Class III* *GI < 70*
Most breads	All bran	Pumpernickel bread
Plain crackers	Oatmeal	Most pasta
Most breakfast cereals	Most cookies or biscuits	Parboiled rice
Most potatoes	Rice	Most dried legumes
Millet	Buckwheat	Nuts
Corn chips	Sweet corn	Barley
	Boiled new potatoes	Bulgur (cracked wheat)
	Yams	
	Sweet potatoes	

Table 9
Summary of NIH Consensus Conference Position on Glycaemic Index

1 Many factors alter glycaemic effect:
- processing
- cooking
- food storage
- mastication
- diurnal variation in absorption
- racial and ethnic differences

2 No effect in mixed meals
3 Conclusion: Not recommended

has recently been confirmed in the context of mixed meals and has nevertheless caused considerable surprise (15). There appears, therefore, to be no reason to prohibit the use of sugar as a sweetening agent in high-carbohydrate, low-fat diets except for two cautions. First, it is assumed that it will be used as a sweetening agent and not as a means of increasing carbohydrate intake, since there are many starchy foods with lower glycaemic responses and greater nutritional qualities than sucrose. Secondly, when taken with a higher saturated fat diet, sucrose has been shown to enhance the rise in blood lipids (16).

Fructose, sorbitol, and other nutritive sweeteners have been proposed for the diabetic, since they may be taken up and metabolized with little additional requirement for insulin and with little effect on the blood glucose level (17). Much interest has focused on fructose, since it may raise both serum triglyceride (TG) and uric acid levels. In a recent study, diabetic volunteers were given 60 g fructose daily in place of sucrose as a sweetener (18). Those subjects with normal TG showed no change in serum TG. However, patients with raised TG levels showed a further increase in fasting TG on fructose. More experience is needed with both sucrose and fructose to define the ideal amounts that could be used and the individuals to whom they are most suited.

Non-nutritive sweeteners such as aspartame may also be used in the diabetic diet. No deleterious effects have been seen in the short term with large doses of aspartame (19). However, a number of good trials are still required to show that non-nutritive sweeteners do in fact enhance weight reduction and improve diabetic control. Logical though this might appear, these trials have not been forthcoming. The benefits of the use of non-nutritive sweeteners must therefore also be open to question.

PROTEIN

It has been suggested by some that increasing the protein content of the diabetic diet may be beneficial in that protein stimulates insulin secretion, and, in test meal situations, has been associated with lower postprandial blood glucose responses (20). This must be balanced against the facts that (i) the Western diet contains protein in excess of requirements and (ii) a common long-term complication of diabetes is renal failure. In the 1960s low-protein diets were advocated for patients with chronic renal failure by Giovanetti and Giordano. With the more routine use of dialysis and renal transplantation the importance of these diets was minimized. More recently, studies by Brenner and associates have highlighted the possible disadvantages of high protein intakes in situations of minimal renal damage (21). This issue is of importance in diabetes, for both IDDM and NIDDM. The theory is that increased protein intake causes increased intrarenal blood pressure, renal hyperperfusion, and mesangial cell loss. The preliminary results of longer term trials in man of the effects of protein restriction early in the course of renal disease look hopeful (22). The nature of the protein sources which it may be most advantageous to eliminate have not been defined. Preliminary short-term studies in IDDM suggest that lower protein intake may be of advantage in terms of some measures of renal function (23). In the future, specific guidance with respect to protein may be given. At present, the ADA recommends that protein intake should be held at about 0.8 g/kg, which is lower than current mean intakes.

OMEGA-3 FATTY ACIDS

There is much current interest in the use of polyunsaturated fatty acids of the omega-3 series derived from fish oils (eicosapentaenoic acid, e.g. "MaxEpa") in the treatment of raised blood lipids (24). This has implications for the treatment of diabetes. Evidence suggests that the inclusion of 20 g omega-3 fatty acids daily may have potent effects in lowering raised serum TG levels. This is not a feature of the omega-6 fatty acids (e.g. linoleic acid) derived from plant sources, whose primary effect is to reduce serum cholesterol. The omega-3 fatty acids have many other effects, including the alteration of membrane fluidity, the activity of membrane-bound enzymes and cell recognition, and a reduction of platelet activity and leucocyte function (25). There is some suggestion that the omega-3 series may be ketogenic and may raise LDL cholesterol levels. Despite their promising effects in reducing serum lipids in non-diabetic, hyperlipidaemic patients, the place of these fatty acids in diabetic therapy remains to be defined by direct experimentation.

Exercise

Exercise can be considered under the heading of nutrition because it forms part of the overall equation of energy balance. For this reason exercise has long been one of the cornerstones of diabetes therapy: diet, exercise, and medication. The value of exercise has been called into question by the NIH Consensus Conference, which felt that the benefits of a reduction in body weight far outweighed the putative metabolic benefits of exercise. In addition, since the effects of exercise are short-lived, it would have to be sustained over a lifetime. The panel was not impressed with the evidence that exercise may modify the progression of cardiovascular disease in NIDDM, but cautioned that it may result in increased caloric intake above energy expenditure, lead to retinal detachment, vitreous haemorrhage, and even sudden death. A thorough medical examination was therefore required by those diabetics who contemplated an exercise program (Table 10). Nevertheless, there is evidence for improved glucose tolerance in athletes and also evidence that both fasting and postprandial blood glucose can be reduced in NIDDM (26,27). The immediate advantage

Table 10
Summary of NIH Consensus Conference Position on Exercise

1 Effect on metabolic control is small
2 May benefit coronary heart disease – but no evidence
3 Body fat reduction far outweighs "putative" benefits of exercise
4 May cause increased caloric intake, sudden death, retinal detachment, vitreous haemorrhage
5 Thorough medical examination required
6 Effects short-lived
7 Needed for a lifetime

Table 11
Summary of ADA Position on Exercise

	NIDDM	IDDM
1 Exercise should be taken regularly every day		
2 Aerobic exercise is best		
3 If >30y of age or >10y of diabetes, should obtain a physician's approval		
4 Benefits for diabetes:	NIDDM	IDDM
a. Cardiovascular	x	x
b. Weight maintenance	x	x
c. Blood lipids	x	x
d. Blood glucose	x	

in terms of overall glycaemic control is less clear in poorly controlled diabetics whose glycaemic control may be worsened. Furthermore, in patients taking insulin, the increased blood flow during exercise may increase insulin mobilization from the injection site. This, and increased sensitivity to the action of insulin, may precipitate hypoglycaemia. Despite these potential drawbacks, it seems imprudent to dismiss the value of regular exercise tailored to the individual needs and abilities of the diabetic. This is especially so because it is advocated in the non-diabetic population as an adjunct to diet in the control of obesity, as a prophylactic measure for the prevention of cardiovascular disease, and as a means of enhancing the retention of calcium and the maintenance of bone mass (28). With these points in mind and with specific cautions, the ADA statement endorsed the use of exercise (Table 11).

Conclusions

The differences between the conclusions of the recent ADA guidelines for the dietary management of diabetes, which are supported by most major Western Diabetes Associations, and those of the recent NIH

Table 12
Diet and Exercise in the Management of Type 2 Diabetes: Differences between NIH and ADA Recommendations

	NIH	*ADA*
Weight loss	+ + + + + + +	+ + (but 20% of type 2 are not overweight
Lifestyle change	Ineffective	+ + (with follow-up + +)
Diet: Dietary fibre	Not convinced (? soluble if patient thinks necessary)	Soluble + +
Glycaemic index	Too variable; no mixed meal effect. Not recommended.	Principle useful; not ready for detailed exchange change yet.

Consensus Conference (Table 12) highlight the changes in thinking about the diabetic diet and the need for further research.

The diabetic diet is becoming a high carbohydrate diet. Although there is a broad measure of agreement on this issue, there still remains some debate (29). The nature of the carbohydrate in the diabetic diet is a matter of greater controversy (30), but higher fibre and low glycaemic index foods offer some hope of filling the caloric void left by the reduction of saturated fat. The fat is reduced to lower blood lipids and to minimize the risk of cardiovascular disease. At the same time, protein is held at a relatively low level to meet requirements at about 0.8 g/kg, but higher intakes are not recommended because of concerns over its possible effect in exacerbating pre-existing or incipient renal damage. It is agreed that reduction of weight is very important in those diabetic indivuduals who are overweight, since this may reverse the metabolic abnormalities of Type 2 diabetes (31). Exercise still appears a useful way to limit positive energy balance providing that energy intake is also reduced or held constant. At the same time, exercise may have possible independent benefits in terms of cardiovascular disease and bone and calcium metabolism. The use of omega-3 fatty acids in diabetes remains to be clarified as does the use of fructose to replace sucrose.

REFERENCES

1 Garcia M, Namara P, Gordon T, Kannel WB. Morbidity and mortality in diabetics in the Framingham population: sixteen year follow-up study. *Diabetes* 1974;23:105–111.

2 American Diabetes Association Position Statement. Nutritional recommendations and principles for individuals with diabetes mellitus: 1986. *Diabetes Care* 1987;10:126–132.

3 *Guidelines for the nutritional management of diabetes mellitus: a special report from the Canadian Diabetes Association*. Toronto, Ont.: Canadian Diabetes Association, revised, 1984.

4 The Nutrition Sub-Committee of the British Diabetic Association's Medical Advisory Committee. Dietary recommendations for diabetics for the 1980's – a policy statement by the British Diabetic Association. *Hum Nutr App Nutr* 1982;36A:378–394.

5 National Institutes of Health Consensus Development Conference Statement. Diet and exercise in noninsulin-dependent diabetes mellitus. *Diabetes Care* 1987;10:639–44.

6 Donahue RP, Abbott RD, Bloom E, Reed DM, Yano K. Central obesity and coronary heart disease in men. *Lancet* 1987;1:821–824.

7 Jenkins DJA. Lente carbohydrate: a newer approach to the dietary management of diabetes. *Diabetes Care* 1982;5:634–641.

8 Wolever TMS, Jenkins DJA. The effect of fiber and foods on carbohydrate metabolism. In: Spiller G, ed. *Handbook of dietary fiber*. Boca Raton, FL: CRC Press, 1986:87–119.

9 Hollenbeck CB, Coulston AM, Reaven GM. To what extent does increased dietary fiber improve glucose and lipid metabolism in patients with noninsulin-dependent diabetes mellitus (NIDDM)? *Am J Clin Nutr* 1986;43:16–24.

10 Simpson HRC, Simpson RW, Lousley S, et al. A high carbohydrate leguminous fibre diet improves all aspects of diabetic control. *Lancet* 1981;1:1–5.

11 Kelsay JL. Update on fiber and mineral availability. In: Vahouny GV, Kritchevsky D, eds. *Dietary fiber: basic and clinical aspects*. New York: Plenum Press, 1986:361–372.

12 Jenkins DJA, Wolever TMS, Jenkins AL, Josse RG, Wong GS. The glycaemic response to carbohydrate foods. *Lancet* 1984;2:388–391.

13 Jenkins DJA, Wolever TMS, Jenkins AL. Starchy foods and the glycemic index. *Diabetes Care* 1988;11:149–159.

14 Jellish WS, Emanuele MA, Abraira C. Graded sucrose/carbohydrate diets in overtly hypertriglyceridemic diabetic patients. *Am J Med* 1984;77:1015–1022.

15 Bantle JP, Laine DC, Castle GW, Thomas JW, Hoogwerf BJ, Goetz FC. Postprandial glucose and insulin responses to meals containing different carbohydrates in normal and diabetic subjects. *New Eng J Med* 1983;309:7–12.

16 Antar MA, Little JA, Lucas C, Buckley GC, Csima A. Interrelationships between dietary carbohydrate and fat in hyperlipidemic patients. Part 3: Synergistic effect of sucrose and animal fat on serum lipids. *Atherosclerosis* 1970;11:191–201.
17 Brunzell JD. Use of fructose, xylitol, or sorbitol as a sweetener in diabetes mellitus. *Diabetes Care* 1978;1:223–230.
18 Crapo PA, Kolterman OG, Henry RR. Metabolic consequences of two-week fructose feeding in diabetic subjects. *Diabetes Care* 1986;9:111–119.
19 Nehrling JK, Kobe P, McLane MP, Olson RE, Kamath S, Horwitz DL. Aspartame use by persons with diabetes. *Diabetes Care* 1985;8:415–417.
20 Nuttall FQ, Mooradian AD, Gannon MC, Billington C, Krezowski P. Effect of protein ingestion on the glucose and insulin response to a standardized oral glucose load. *Diabetes Care* 1984;7:465–470.
21 Brenner BM, Meyer TW, Hostetter TH. Dietary protein intake and the progressive nature of kidney disease: the role of hemodynamically mediated glomerular injury in the pathogenesis of progressive glomerular sclerosis in aging, renal ablation, and intrinsic renal disease. *New Eng J Med* 1982;307:652–659.
22 Roseman JB, Ter Wee PM, Meiger S, Piers-Becht TPM, Sluiter WJ, Donker AJM. Prospective randomized trial of early protein restriction in chronic renal failure. *Lancet* 1984;2:1291–1296.
23 Kupin WL, Cortes P, Dumler F, Feldkamp CS, Kilates MC, Levin NW. Effect on renal function of change from high to moderate protein intake in type I diabetic patients. *Diabetes* 1987;36:73–79.
24 Phillipson BE, Rothrock, DW, Connor WE, Harris WS, Illingworth DR. Reduction of plasma lipids, lipoproteins and apoproteins by dietary fish oils in patients with hypertriglyceridemia. *New Eng J Med* 1985;312:1210–1216.
25 Lee TH, Hoover RL, Williams JD, et al. Effect of dietary enrichment with eicosapentaenoic and docosahexaenoic acids on in vitro neutrophil and monocyte leukotriene generation and neutrophil function. *New Eng J Med* 1985;312:1217–1223.
26 Caron D, Poussier P, Marliss EB, Zinman B. The effect of postprandial exercise on meal-related glucose intolerance in insulin-dependent diabetic individuals. *Diabetes Care* 1982;5:364–369.
27 Trovati M, Carta Q, Cavalot F, et al. Influence of physical training on blood glucose control, glucose tolerance, insulin secretion, and insulin action in non-insulin-dependent diabetic patients. *Diabetes Care* 1984;7:416–420.
28 Martin AD, Houston CS. Osteoporosis, calcium and physical activity. *Can Med Assoc J* 1987;136:587–593.

29 Reaven GM. How much carbohydrate? *Diabetologia* 1981;20:508–509.
30 Hollenbeck CB, Coulston AM, Reaven GM. Glycemic effects of carbohydrates: a different perspective. *Diabetes Care* 1986;9:641–647.
31 Olefsky JM, Kolterman OG. Mechanisms of insulin resistance in obesity and noninsulin-dependent (type II) diabetes. *Am J Med* 1981;70:151–168.

DANIEL A.K. RONCARI

Individual Susceptibility to Obesity in Response to Dietary Factors

By no means is there a simple relationship between nutrient energy intake and body fat content. Indeed, wide interindividual variations exist as to the quantity of nutrient energy that contributes to the development of obesity (1–6). Variability persists even after relating intake to estimates of energy expenditure in the form of physical activity. While studies of monozygotic twins, including those reared by adoptive parents, indicate strong genetic factors for the development of adiposity (including the thermic response to food, even after physical training) (7–9), some dissimilarity might still occur because of unequal distribution of cytoskeletal elements during cleavage of the zygote.

The first part of this paper will describe meal patterns and composition which may facilitate the development of obesity. Then functional and proliferative abnormalities of adipocytes and their precursors, which may also contribute to adiposity, will be discussed. Then the issue of facultative diet-induced thermogenesis will be addressed, and whether its depression might predispose to the development of obesity. Finally, I shall present a new hypothesis, based on energy transductions, whose interindividual disparities would explain differing susceptibility to adiposity. This hypothesis does not include dissimilarities in thermogenic responses.

Influence of Meal Pattern

For the same quantity of nutrient energy, certain patterns of eating result in disproportionate deposition of triglyceride in fat tissue. A few large meals are more adipogenic than frequent small ones (nibbling) (4,5,10). The most unhealthy, but common pattern, involves scanty or no breakfast and lunch, in the face of a large supper (followed by very limited physical activity). Such a "fasting-refeeding" cycle is associated with particularly high activity of lipogenic enzymes during the refeeding phase, and a shift in the circadian rhythm of hormones regulating triglyceride storage, e.g. insulin (10). These facts have therapeutic implications, as well as the indication that programs of physical activity lead to eating patterns more appropriate for the prevailing energy requirements (4,5). Of course, exercise imparts multiple beneficial metabolic effects including attenuation of the insulin resistance in the obese, an effect that may bear significance to the subsequent discussion on facultative thermogenesis.

Influence of Dietary Composition

For the same quantity of nutrient energy, moreover, the composition of the food determines partly how much triglyceride is stored. In particular, high-fat diets lead to disproportionately high deposition (4–6,11). First of all, the energy cost, i.e. the number of kjoules, required to process dietary fatty acids to adipocyte triglyceride is low (3% compared to 23% when dietary carbohydrate is converted to lipid by *de novo* synthesis) (5,6). Relatedly, dietary fatty acids (mainly as components of triglycerides) can be incorporated rather efficiently into adipocyte triglycerides through the key action of lipoprotein lipase on plasma chylomicrons (4). Adipocyte lipoprotein lipase activity is especially high in response to a high-fat diet, partly as a result of stimulation by the responsive intestinal hormone, "glucose-dependent insulinotropic polypeptide" (GIP) (12).

Lipoprotein Lipase

In addition to physiological responses involving lipoprotein lipase activity, genetic abnormalities of its regulation may be pathogenic in some types of obesity. Not only is basal adipocyte lipoprotein lipase activity increased, but it is elevated further after weight loss, even when it is maintained (13). Assuming that it is correct that this lipase is rate-controlling for triglyceride accretion, such augmented assimilative power, which may have contributed to the development of obesity originally, would also favour weight regain. Regional *varia-*

tions of lipoprotein lipase function might also contribute to more localized forms of adiposity such as "abdominal obesity."

Exaggerated Preadipocyte Growth in Massive Obesity

The possible "constitutive" expression of lipoprotein lipase may reflect the existence of abnormal clones of adipose cells in obesity. We have found that adipose tissue from the massively obese contains clones of preadipocytes that in culture proliferate and differentiate excessively (4,14–16). This phenomenon persists through subcultures, when there is no direct influence by *in vivo* factors. Such inordinately high growth and maturation might explain the adipocyte hyperplasia characteristic of massive obesity. We have also adduced evidence for the production of paracrine/autocrine trophic proteins by preadipocytes from the massively obese (4,17,18). These growth factors, which are partially estrogen-dependent, may be responsible for the vast expansion of fat tissue in morbid adiposity, allowing it to enlarge progressively with some autonomy, i.e. independent from circulating principles.

Mature fat cells cannot replicate. We have reported, however, that such cells are able to revert to replicative forms similar to preadipocytes (4,19). Further, mature cells from the massively corpulent have retained the "memory" of their origin because, upon reversion, they proliferate excessively (16). We have thus discussed that while sustained compliance to appropriate eating and regular exercise may lead to a decrease in the total number of mature adipocytes, cycles of adherence and relapse might be worse than stable adiposity (4,16). Indeed, reversion would lead to cells which are genetically susceptible to exaggerated replication and differentiation, under appropriate environmental triggers. Then each cycle of compliance and relapse would lead to a progressive increment of mature adipocytes accommodating the immense triglyceride storage of massive corpulence.

The described cellular and biochemical hyperfunction has almost certainly a genetic basis (4). Individual variations in the complement of rapidly developing and metabolically overactive preadipocytes might explain differing susceptibility to obesity in the presence of similar nutrient energy availability. Differences in clonal composition could then account for varying vulnerability without necessarily having to invoke disparities between the lean and the obese in such possible adaptive responses as diet-induced thermogenesis.

It should be emphasized that, under conditions of sustained energy overload, relative to a particular subject, only a small fraction of the population develops massive corpulence (> 170% of reference body weight or body mass index > 37 kg/sq m). (While genetic factors are almost certainly operative, it is not known whether the cellular response is primary, or an epiphenomenon related to a more proximate abnormality.) The majority develops moderate obesity (body weight 120–170% of reference or body mass index 25–37), which features enlarged fat cells, but a normal number. It has been suggested that adaptive thermogenesis might be related inversely to the capacity of adipose tissue to store triglyceride (20). Thus, the least would occur in those massively obese persons with the greatest excess of (enlarged) adipocytes. Towards the other extreme would be the small fraction of the population remaining lean despite sustained energy overload. According to this proposal, these individuals would have rather high degrees of adaptive thermogenesis. At the pathologic extreme, generalized lipoatrophy, even small nutrient intake beyond maintenance, results in pronounced hypermetabolism, a finding consistent with, but not proving the limiting role of triglyceride storage for facultative energy dissipation (5,6).

Important Questions in Bioenergetics

In the field of nutritional bioenergetics, critical issues still requiring resolution include:

1 In addition to the formal energy cost of nutrient absorption, metabolism, and storage, are there mechanisms for energy utilization and dissipation in response to eating, e.g. Luxuskonsumption or the facultative component of diet-induced thermogenesis? This process could also be described as heat release not accounted for by obligatory functions, beyond the efficiency of the systems, and in the absence of net chemical synthesis, or biomechanical work.
2 Should such facultative mechanisms exist, where and how do they operate?
3 Are there individual differences in facultative thermogenesis, and are these responsible for the development of at least some types of obesity?

I would also postulate a novel mechanism for energy utilization, and propose that individual variations in this response, which does not depend on external losses of energy, account for differing susceptibility to the development of obesity. This hypothesis will be discussed later.

The Question of Facultative Diet-Induced Thermogenesis

A number of studies have suggested the existence of facultative diet-induced thermogenesis in human subjects, while a number of investigations have not revealed this process (5,6,21). Most investigators observing it have suggested that its main site is brown adipose tissue (5,6,22). The question whether brown adipose tissue is of any significance in humans after infancy is still unresolved (5,6,23). The uncoupling protein ("thermogenin") has recently been found in certain human adipose depots (24). It is considered to be unique to brown adipose tissue, but is it? There is also renewed interest in substrate ("futile") cycles in skeletal muscle, which according to recent work could account for an appreciable portion of facultative diet-induced thermogenesis (5,6,25,26).

Hypothalamic stimulation of sympathetic nervous system pathways plays a major role (5,6,22). Indeed, catecholamines acting through beta-1 receptors appear to be the major positive hormonal effectors in brown adipose tissue (5,6,22). It is probably relevant that high glucose diets or highly palatable diets containing sufficient quantities of sugars, augment appreciably facultative thermogenesis (in the presence of appropriate insulin action), probably through stimulation of sympathetic nervous system activity (5,6,22). The latter is promoted much less by high-fat diets, which also result in much less facultative thermogenesis. L-triiodothyronine (T_3), the biologically most potent thyroid hormone, is of course required for optimal beta-catecholamine action, and in brown adipose tissue it may have a synergistic effect on facultative thermogenesis (5,6,22). T_3, moreover, appears to be particularly important in accelerating substrate cycles (5,6,26).

A number of studies have suggested that facultative diet-induced thermogenesis is depressed in obese subjects, while a number of investigators did not observe a difference from the lean (5,6,21,22,23). Studies suggesting a depression have included influences of specific diets and catecholamine infusion. In addition, the accentuation of the thermogenic effect of exercise by a meal was dampened or abolished (5,6). Obese subjects with insulin resistance sufficient to contribute to the development of non-insulin-dependent diabetes apparently provide the best example of depressed facultative diet-induced thermogenesis (5,6,27,28). Thus, effective insulin action is also required for this thermogenic response. The interpretation of all these studies is made more difficult because the obese actually have a higher resting metabolic rate per lean body mass, and the *total* energy expenditure during eating is also augmented, partly because of the energy cost associated with this mass and the overall enlargement of the body (21).

It should be emphasized that, for any mechanism of impaired energy expenditure, only a small (i.e. 3–10% inequality at a given energy load), but sustained difference between two subjects can lead to obesity in one, but not the other.

Hypothesis Based on Interactions Between Cytoskeletal Function and Triglyceride Accretion

My novel hypothesis has been reported recently (4,29). It is based on the concept that individuals vary in the degree of their cellular biomechanical functions (e.g. cell movements, membrane ruffling, ciliary lashes), which are mediated by microfilaments, microtubules, and other components of the cytoskeletal matrix. This individual variability would have a strong genetic basis, but other factors, including neural and endocrine influences, would have a modulating role. The second main feature of the postulate is that a substantial portion of the energy that is not used for the biomechanical processes is transduced to chemical storage, predominantly as adipocyte triglyceride (4,29).

At one extreme of the variations is massive (morbid) obesity. According to the hypothesis, cellular biomechanical activity would be least in this state, leaving the most energy for eventual storage as adipocyte triglyceride (4,29). The excessive complement of adipocytes characteristic of massive corpulence accommodates the vast lipid stores. These would be the subjects most vulnerable to the development of pronounced adiposity. At the other extreme are individuals who are inordinately thin, in the absence of illness. Their cells would have the highest degree of biomechanical activity, and the least energy left over for chemical storage, with the lowest propensity to obesity. Between the two extremes would be an almost infinite variation, with a reciprocal relationship between level of biomechanical activity and deposition of adipocyte triglyceride, with corresponding susceptibilities to varying body fat contents at the same energy load. While the extremes might be due to specific mutations of genes encoding for proteins involved in cytoskeletal functions, the intervening variation may be caused, at least partly, by genetic polymorphism (4,29).

The unique aspect of the hypothesis is the *individual variation* in energy utilization for cellular *biomechanical* functions, its *genetic* basis, and the *secondary* nature of triglyceride deposition. Since all these processes and interactions (including lipid processing and accretion) proceed at a certain efficiency, any measured thermogenesis would represent a composite, and would not necessarily distinguish between utilization for biomechanical processes from anabolic functions. A fundamental feature of the hypothesis is the *internal energy transduction*.

Acknowledgment

Research described in this article was supported by grants from the Medical Research Council of Canada, the Canadian (Alberta) Heart Foundation, and the Alberta Heritage Foundation for Medical Research.

REFERENCES

1 Widdowson EM. Nutritional individuality. *Proc Nutr Soc* 1962;21:121–128.

2 Durnin JVGA, Edholm OG, Miller DS, Waterlow JC. How much food does one require? *Nature* 1973;242:418.

3 James WPT. Energy requirements and obesity. *Lancet* 1983;2:386–389.

4 Roncari DAK. Obesity and lipid metabolism. In: Spittell JA Jr, Volpé R, eds. *Clinical medicine*. Philadelphia, PA: Harper and Row, 1986; Vol. 9, Ch. 14:1–57.

5 Sims EAH. Energy balance in human beings: the problems of plenitude. In: Auerbach GD, McCormick DB, eds. *Vitamins and hormones.* Vol. 43. New York, NY: Academic Press, 1987:1–101.

6 Sims EAH, Danforth E Jr. Expenditure and storage of energy in man. *J Clin Invest* 1987;79:1019–1025.

7 Fontaine E, Savard R, Tremblay AC, Despres JP, Poehlman ET, Bouchard C. Resting metabolic rate in monozygotic and dizygotic twins. *Acta Genet Med Gemmellol* 1985;34:41–47.

8 Poehlman ET, Tremblay A, Fontaine E, et al. Genotype dependency of the thermic effect of a meal and associated hormonal changes following short-term overfeeding. *Metabolism* 1986;35:30–36.

9 Stunkard AJ, Sorensen TI, Hanis AC, et al. An adoption study of human obesity. *N Engl J Med* 1986;314:193–198.
10 Bray GA. Lipogenesis in human adipose tissue: some effects of nibbling and gorging. *J Clin Invest* 1972;51:537–548.
11 Danforth E Jr. Diet and obesity. *Am J Clin Nutr* 1985;41:1132–1145.
12 Eckel RH, Fujimoto WY, Brunzell JD. Gastric inhibitory polypeptide enhanced lipoprotein lipase activity in cultured preadipocytes. *Diabetes* 1979;28:1141–1142.
13 Schwartz RS, Brunzell JD. Increase of adipose tissue lipoprotein lipase activity with weight loss. *J Clin Invest* 1981;67:1425–1430.
14 Roncari DAK, Lau DCW, Kindler S. Exaggerated replication in culture of adipocyte precursors from massively obese persons. *Metabolism* 1981;30:245–247.
15 Roncari DAK, Lau DCW, Djian P, Kindler S, Yip DK. Culture and cloning of adipocyte precursors from lean and obese subjects: effects of growth factors. In: Angel A, Hollenberg CH, Roncari DAK, eds. *The adipocyte and obesity: cellular and molecular mechanisms*. New York, NY: Raven Press, 1983:65–73.
16 Roncari DAK, Kindler S, Hollenberg CH. Excessive proliferation in culture of reverted adipocytes from massively obese persons. *Metabolism* 1986;35:1–4.
17 Roncari DAK. Pre-adipose cell replication and differentiation. *Trends Biochem Sci* 1984;9:486–489.
18 Lau DCW, Roncari DAK, Hollenberg CH. Release of mitogenic factors by cultured preadipocytes from massively obese subjects. *J Clin Invest* 1987;79:632–636.
19 Van RLR, Bayliss CE, Roncari DAK. Cytological and enzymological characterization of adult human adipocyte precursors in culture. *J Clin Invest* 1976;58:699–704.
20 Dallosso H, James WPT. Whole-body calorimetry studies in adult men. 2. The interaction of exercise and overfeeding on the thermic effect of a meal. *Br J Nutr* 1984;52:65–72.
21 Garrow JS. *Energy balance and obesity in man*. Amsterdam: Elsevier/North-Holland Biomedical Press, 1974 and 1978.
22 Rothwell NJ, Stock MJ. Luxuskonsumption, diet-induced thermogenesis and brown fat: the case in favour. *Clin Sci* 1983;64:19–23.
23 Hervey GR, Tobin G. Luxuskonsumption, diet-induced thermogenesis and brown fat: a critical review. *Clin Sci* 1983;64:7–18.
24 Lean ME, James WPT, Jennings G, Trayhurn P. Brown adipose tissue uncoupling protein content in human infants, children and adults. *Clin Sci* 1986;71:291–297.

25 Newsholme EA. A possible metabolic basis for the control of body weight. *N Engl J Med* 1980;302:400–405.
26 Shulman GI, Ladenson PW, Wolfe MH, Ridgeway EC, Wolfe RR. Substrate cycling between gluconeogenesis and glycolysis in euthyroid, hypothyroid, and hyperthyroid man. *J Clin Invest* 1985;76:757–764.
27 Nair KS, Webster J, Garrow JS. Effect of impaired glucose tolerance and Type II diabetes on resting metabolic rate and thermic response to a glucose meal in obese women. *Metabolism* 1986;35:640–644.
28 Golay A, Schutz Y, Felber J-P, De Fronzo RA, Jequier E. Lack of thermogenic response to glucose/insulin infusion in diabetic obese subjects. *Int J Obesity* 1986;10:107–116.
29 Roncari DAK. Individual variations in energy utilized for biomechanical processes and molecular mobility account for diverse susceptibility to obesity. *Medical Hypotheses* 1987;23:11–18.

WILLIAM E. MITCH

Diet and Kidney Disease

The goals of therapy of chronic renal failure before the patient must be treated by dialysis or transplantation are: first, to minimize mineral and electrolyte disturbances; second, to lower or reduce the pool of accumulated waste products; third, to maintain adequate protein nutrition; and, fourth, to retard or, in some cases, halt the progression of renal insufficiency. The three latter goals will be discussed in this article.

Principles of nutritional biochemistry led us to use low-protein diets, and our results indicate that this type of therapy can be used safely and can have a major impact on the course of disease, at least for some kidney failure patients. When normal subjects or patients with kidney disease eat foods containing protein, the protein is broken down into essential and non-essential amino acids. Essential amino acids are those amino acids which must be provided in the diet. It they are not provided then protein synthesis cannot proceed normally, resulting in negative nitrogen balance and ultimately wasting of lean body mass. In contrast, the eleven non-essential amino acids can be synthesized by humans and it is not necessary to provide them in the diet.

Amino Acid Metabolism

Amino acids derived from dietary protein have two fates. First, they are catabolized to waste products as follows: the alpha-amino group is removed by transamination, leaving the ketoacid and ammonia, which is converted to urea; the carbon skeleton or ketoacid of the amino acid is metabolized to carbon dioxide and water or reutilized to form the amino acid. Urea must be excreted by the kidney. Metabolism of foods containing protein also yields phosphorus, hydrogen, potassium, sodium, sulphate, plus other nitrogenous waste products. Likewise, if negative nitrogen balance is present, breakdown of body protein gives rise to these same waste products, which must be excreted by the kidney. Therefore, impaired kidney function and failure to excrete urea and other waste products will lead to a build-up of waste products in body fluids and cause symptoms of uremia.

Low-Protein Dietary Therapy

To limit the accumulation of waste products and reduce symptoms of uremia, Giordano gave patients with severe kidney failure a diet containing only about 2 g of essential amino acids (1). With this very low level of dietary protein, the production of all waste products, including urea, was sharply reduced, but the patients remained in negative nitrogen balance for many weeks. Giordano proposed that uremic patients, like starved individuals, would be able to utilize protein more efficiently and achieve nitrogen balance after 6–7 weeks. He showed that when dietary protein is reduced to very low levels, the accumulation of waste products decreases and uremic symptoms improve, but overly severe restriction can lead to wasting of lean body mass.

With these very low protein regimens, wasting was so serious that most investigators disregarded low-protein dietary therapy, and this field of investigation was somewhat neglected. About ten years later, Kopple and Coburn re-examined dietary requirements in a study of eight patients with only about 10% of residual kidney function (2). In the first period, they gave patients about 40 g of protein per day, which represents the average daily protein requirement of normal subjects. Patients with kidney disease, like normal subjects, were in neutral or mildly positive nitrogen balance with this amount of protein. Patients were then switched to a modified Giordano diet; protein intake was about one-half of the daily requirement or about 20 g protein per day. In every case, nitrogen balance was worse and one-half of the patients experienced negative nitrogen balance. Over prolonged periods this would lead to wasting of body proteins. Thus, patients with kidney disease seem to have the same protein requirements as normal subjects and if they are given an adequate amount of protein they should be able to maintain lean body mass. Occasionally, this quantity of dietary protein produces excessive accumulation of nitrogen waste products.

We attempted to design a diet containing less than the normal required amount of protein because some patients with severe kidney disease will develop uremic symptoms at 0.6 g protein/kg/day. We decided to take advantage of the normal metabolism of amino acids. Since the initial step in amino acid breakdown is to remove the alpha amino group (i.e. transamination) to form ketoacids, we administered ketoacids to reverse the reaction and augment essential amino acid production. The chemical formulae of the ketoacids show that they are simply the carbon skeletons of essential amino acids without the amino group. They are not given as free acids, but as neutral salts. L-lysine and L-threonine are not used because they do not undergo transamination reactions, and must be supplied as amino acids. In the conversion of exogenous ketoacids to amino acids, nitrogen from non-essential amino acids is used, resulting in the formation of non-essential ketoacids. The latter compounds are converted into carbon dioxide and water but not nitrogen waste products. Fortunately, the transaminase reaction can occur in virtually every tissue, including muscle, heart, gut, liver, and brain (3,4).

Keto Acid Therapy of Uremia

Initially, we gave uremic patients ketoacid mixtures that were based on the essential amino acid requirements of normal subjects. However, plasma levels of amino acids in kidney patients are abnormal; histidine, alanine, phenylalanine are in the normal range, but certain amino acids, especially those containing sulphur, are very high. On the other hand, most of the essential amino acids are subnormal. Unfortunately, the cause of these abnormalities is not completely understood. The conversion of phenylalanine to tyrosine is inhibited in patients with kidney disease, and this could explain why phenylalanine is normal and tyrosine is low. Regardless, we decided to give tyrosine as if it were an essential amino acid, and eliminated phenylalanine or its ketoacid from the more recently designed supplement. Branched-chain amino acids are invariably low in patients with kidney disease; in experimental animals these amino acids are oxidized at an accelerated rate in muscle, presumably because acidosis activates the enzyme that causes their degradation (5,6). Finally, serine is synthesized predominantly in the kidney, so if kidneys are damaged, serine could be subnormal. The new ketoacid supplement was designed to correct abnormalities in amino acid pools. Tyrosine was provided, the amount of methionine was reduced sharply, and the amounts of branched-chain ketoacids and threonine amounts were increased.

An imbalanced mixture of essential amino acids such as in this supplement could cause negative nitrogen balance. To test for this effect, patients were admitted to hospital and given the same amount of protein as they were eating at home, an average of 66 g, well above their minimum daily protein requirement. Nitrogen balance was neutral on these nutrients and did not change significantly when they were given only 0.3 g protein/kg/day plus the new supplement (7). Maintenance of nitrogen balance while in the hospital satisfied two goals. First, the accumulation of waste products was reduced, since dietary protein was halved; second, nitrogen balance indicated that the regimen was nutritionally adequate, at least for a brief period. It also appears to be adequate for long-term therapy. In a group of patients treated with long-term therapy, the average values of serum albumin and serum transferrin were within the normal range before therapy. After four to six weeks, there was a small, but statistically significant, improvement in both albumin and transferrin, and this improvement was maintained over one year of therapy. There also was no loss of weight (8). Thus, we had both short-term evidence that this therapy could maintain nitrogen balance and long-term evidence that patients maintained their weight and normal values of serum albumin and transferrin.

To assess compliance, we measured the products of ketoacids in blood in random blood samples to determine if patients were taking the supplement.

To measure dietary protein, we took advantage of the nitrogen balance equation: nitrogen balance is equal to nitrogen intake minus the urea nitrogen produced each day, minus the amount of non-urea nitrogen excreted each day. Urea production is emphasized because of its linear relationship with protein intake (9,10). Patients were studied at protein intakes from as low as 12 g per day to 94 g of protein per day. As protein intake was increased, nitrogen balance did not improve, but there was a linear and predictable increase in the amount of urea produced. What about excretion of non-urea nitrogen? The components of non-urea nitrogen, fecal nitrogen and the nitrogen contained in urinary creatinine, uric acid, and unmeasured nitrogen and their sum was measured by Maroni et al. (10). Values for renal patients eating either the ketoacid regimen or different amounts of protein (up to 90 g per day) had scarcely any difference in non-urea nitrogen excretion. In the literature as well, patients studied at different levels of dietary protein from almost 200 g to 12 g per day had little variation in non-urea nitrogen excretion. The average value we found was 31 mg N/kg/day. In practical terms, we knew how much the patient should be eating because it is prescribed. A 24-hour urine is collected and its urea nitrogen content, the patient's blood urea nitrogen and weight are measured (the latter two to assure a steady-state condition). The prescribed and estimated nitrogen intake are compared and if there is a substantial difference, the patient is sent to the dietitian to find why there is a discrepancy. Fortunately, compliance is not a great problem, and in many cases nitrogen intake was found to be less than prescribed; it is critical to monitor what the patient is actually eating to ensure an adequate but not excessive intake. In summary, dietary protein can be limited to decrease the accumulated waste products while maintaining adequate protein nutrition. Simple methods can be used to monitor compliance to therapy.

Progression of Renal Insufficiency

The fourth goal, to change the course of renal insufficiency in kidney disease, is in many ways the most exciting. Survival to endstage renal failure requiring dialysis or transplantation varies widely (11). In a study from Scandinavia, about 50% of 143 patients with an initial serum creatinine of 5 mg/dL (about 15 to 20% of residual kidney function) required dialysis therapy after 10 to 12 months. Data from 132 Mayo Clinic patients with an initial serum creatinine concentration of 10 mg/dL (less than 10% of residual kidney function) indicated that half would require dialysis after 6 to 8 months. Finally, three patients from Missouri, with an initial serum creatinine of 10 mg/dL, had a poorer prognosis; 50% required dialysis after only a few months. Unfortunately, such data are of limited value for an individual patient; the patient wants to know whether he or she is moving rapidly or slowly towards dialysis. To devise a simple method of determining how fast a patient is progressing towards dialysis, we found that a plot of the reciprocal of serum creatinine concentration versus time for an individual patient is remarkably linear (12). When the relationship is linear, the effects of therapy can be observed by determining if the slope of the line changes. This finding also gives insight into the nature of kidney disease (11). After initial damage, glomerular filtration or creatinine clearance declines linearly, i.e. is lost at a constant rate until dialysis (11). The loss of renal function can be approximated by plotting the reciprocal of serum creatinine versus time.

It is important to follow the course of individual patients. Even patients with the same type of kidney disease have enormous variability in the rate at which they lose kidney function (11). This probably explains the apparently poorer outlook of the smaller group of patients in Missouri; with small numbers of patients, it is possible that the average value is skewed by patients progressing rapidly.

What has been done to change the progressive nature of kidney disease and how does it impact on nutrition? There have been three dietary regimens used to delay the progression of kidney failure (13). The first limits protein intake to 0.6 g protein/kg/day, and a high caloric intake is used to increase efficiency of protein utilization. The diet also will decrease phosphorus intake because phosphorus is associated with proteinaceous foods. A supplement of B vitamins is given to prevent water-soluble vitamin deficiency. The other two diets are similar; they limit protein intake to about 0.3 g/kg/day, or half of the minimum daily requirement. With these two regimens, the types of protein eaten are unimportant, because essential amino acid requirements are met either by an essential amino acid supplement or a ketoacid supplement. Caloric intake is high while phosphorus intake is reduced further and a B vitamin supplement is given. With all three regimens, a creative dietitian must work with the patient closely to vary the diets.

What are the results? Recall that 50% of patients with an initial serum creatinine of 5 mg/dL progress to dialysis over 10 to 12 months. In contrast, 27 patients identified as having a serum creatinine of about 5 mg/dL were treated with 0.6 g protein/kg/day to reduce phosphorus intake and combat secondary hyperparathyroidism. Over almost 27 months there was no significant change, on the average, in serum creatinine. This would be entirely unexpected, based on the data of patients eating unrestricted diets in Scandinavia (11). More recently, Maschio et al. fed a low-protein diet containing the minimum daily requirement to 20 patients for 30 months. There was no change on the average in their serum creatinine concentration of 4 mg/dL, although individual patients did progress. They also studied a control group who had a statistically poorer outcome while eating unrestricted diets.

What about the more stringent, supplemented regimens? There have been few studies of the essential amino acid supplement, but Alvestand et al. treated patients with a predictable loss of renal function, plotted as the reciprocal of serum creatinine versus time. When the patients reached an average serum creatinine of about 9 mg/dL, therapy was begun and some patients had marked slowing of progression.

Regarding the ketoacid regimen, we and others have had considerable success (13). To summarize our experience, we found that if patients began therapy before serum creatinine had reached 8 mg/dL, virtually all had stabilization of kidney function (8). If therapy began after serum creatinine was at that level, then stabilization of function occurred rarely.

These results leave the following questions: first, which patients will respond to dietary manipulation? Are there specific diseases that will respond better than other diseases? Is there a degree of renal insufficiency beyond which diet therapy is of no use? Secondly, are there differences between the dietary regimens in terms of achieving long-term compliance? We have treated some patients for five years, so therapy must be acceptable for long periods of time. Are there differences in the dietary regimens in terms of maintaining adequate protein nutrition? Finally, are there differences among the regimens in achieving stabilization of kidney function? Future studies involving large numbers of patients in carefully controlled studies will provide answers to these important questions relating to the nutrition of patients with progressive renal failure.

REFERENCES

1 Giordano C. Use of exogenous and endogenous urea for protein synthesis in normal and uremic subjects. *J Lab Clin Med* 1963;62:231–246.

2 Kopple JD, Coburn JW. Metabolic studies of low protein diets in uremia. *Medicine* 1973;52:583–595.

3 May RC, Mitch WE. Metabolism and metabolic effects of ketoacids. *Diabetes and Metabolism* 1989;5:71–80.

4 Mitch WE, Walser M. Utilization of calcium L-phenyllactate as a substitute for phenylalanine by uremic patients. *Metabolism* 1977;26:1041–1046.

5 May RC, Hara Y, Kelly RA, Block KP, Buse MG, Mitch WE. Branched-chain amino acid metabolism in rat muscle: abnormal regulation in acidosis. *Am J Physiol* 1987;15:E712-E718.

6 Hara Y, May RC, Kelly RA, Mitch WE. The influence of acidosis on branched-chain amino acid metabolism in uremic rats. *Kidney Int* 1987;32:808–814.

7 Mitch WE, Abras E, Walser M. Long-term effects of a new ketoacid-amino acid supplement in patients with chronic renal failure. *Kidney Int* 1982;22:48–53.
8 Mitch WE, Walser M, Steinman TI, Hill S, Zeger S, Tungsanga K. The effect of a keto acid-amino acid supplement to a restricted diet on the progression of chronic renal failure. *New Engl J Med* 1984;311:623–629.
9 Cottini EP, Gallina DL, Dominguez JM. Urea excretion in adult humans with varying degrees of kidney malfuncton fed milk, egg or amino acid mixture: assessment of nitrogen balance. *J Nutr* 1973;103:11–19.
10 Maroni BJ, Steinman TI, Mitch WE. A method for estimating nitrogen intake of patients with chronic renal failure. *Kidney Int* 1985;27:58–65.
11 Mitch WE. Measuring the progression of renal insufficiency. In: Mitch WE, ed. *Contemporary issues in nephrology*, vol 14: *The progressive nature of renal disease*. New York: Churchill-Livingstone, 1986:167–187.
12 Mitch WE, Lemann J, Buffington GA, Walser M. A simple method of estimating progression of chronic renal failure. *Lancet* 1976;2:1326–1328.
13 Mitch WE. Nutritional therapy and the progression of renal insufficiency. In: Mitch WE, Klahr S, eds. *Nutrition and renal disease*. Boston: Little, Brown, 1988:159–179.

Diet and Health Maintenance

ERNST L. WYNDER, J. BARONE, AND
JAMES R. HEBERT

The Role of Diet in the Maintenance of Health throughout Life

"You are what you eat" is a popular saying. Perhaps it has greater relevance than many modern health professionals are prepared to accept. As early as 1799, Easton wrote a volume, *Longevity*, in which he presented biographical data on individuals who lived to the age of 100 years or more (1). What these centenarians appeared to have in common was that they tended to eat rather sparingly and were physically active.

Modern man in the developed countries of the post-industrial age is probably more sedentary in his lifestyle than any of his forebears. In addition to his levels of activity, the composition of modern man's diet is much different from what it must have been throughout most of his history as a species. Depending on his habitat, prehistoric man may have been predominantly a hunter or a gatherer. In environments conducive to hunting, meat consumption was relatively high. Despite the varying proportions of meats and plants in his diet, prehistoric man was not a consumer of a high-fat diet. At least half of the diet of early *Homo sapiens* is believed to have consisted of plant sources, including fruits, nuts, grains, and greens.

Unlike domesticated animals, the wild game consumed by Palaeolithic man, such as deer, bison, and horses, was lower in fat than modern meat (3.9% vs 25–30%). Per unit weight, the meat of Palaeolithic range animals was lower in total calories, but five times higher in polyunsaturated fat (2). Late Palaeolithic man probably ate a diet with only about 20% of calories from fat, but one that was relatively rich in polyunsaturated fats.

Eating habits emphasizing a low-fat diet can be seen even among the hunter-gatherers of today. The Hadza of Tanzania or San of the Kalahari generally have a diet in which 50–80% of the food (by weight) comes from plants (2,3). Estimates from the Food and Agriculture Organization of the United Nations indicate that half of the people in the world eat diets from which less than 25% of the calories come from fat (4).

The Tarahumara Indians of Mexico live on a simple diet of corn and beans that is low in fat and cholesterol and high in complex carbohydrates, yet it is nutritionally adequate. When cholesterol absorption and sterol balances were studied in this population by feeding eight men a cholesterol-free diet for three weeks followed by a high-cholesterol diet for three weeks, their mean plasma cholesterol levels increased about 30%, from 113 mg/dl to 147 mg/dl. Cholesterol biosynthesis decreased during consumption of the high-cholesterol diet. Compared with other people, the Tarahumaras have a reduced ability to absorb dietary cholesterol. They have a higher total sterol turnover, probably because of an increased bile acid output (5).

To see the effects of low-fat diets, we are not limited to studies of prehistoric man or populations in distant lands. Right in our midst we have a subset of vegetarians called vegans who eat no animal products – no meat, dairy products, eggs, or fish. Unfortunately, we do not have sufficient knowledge of their morbidity or mortality. We might assume, however, that their "improved" diet could produce even greater health benefits than those we see among non-vegan, Seventh-Day Adventists who, by not eating meat, have slightly lower blood lipid levels despite their relatively high consumption of dairy products (6). Seventh-Day Adventists also live an average of six years longer than other Americans. Their longevity may also be explained by their alcohol- and tobacco-free lifestyle (7).

In our current study of a vegan Seventh-Day Adventist community in New Jersey, preliminary findings of 30 members, aged 8–38 years, show that they consume a relatively low-fat diet with a high proportion of polyunsaturated and monounsaturated fatty acids. Blood lipid analyses indicate very high HDL (average = 50 mg%) and low total serum cholesterol levels (average = 131.6 mg%). Three children aged 8, 11, and 12 who were born into the community had cholesterol levels of 102, 108, and 110 mg%, probably close to the optimal levels of serum cholesterol in children (American Health Foundation, studies in progress, 1987).

The question we need to ask is what is the optimal diet that is conducive to the avoidance of illness and permits youthfulness throughout a long life.

Heart Disease

The effect of diet on heart disease is particularly well-documented (8). Even for this relatively strong relationship, we still hear debates on the significance of diet in determining serum cholesterol levels and how these levels affect heart disease.

Currently, heart attacks are not among the ten leading causes of death in China, where the average cholesterol level in urban and rural populations in cities is about 160 mg% and 150 mg% respectively (personal communication, Haozhu Chen, Shanghai Institute for Cardiovascular Diseases). There is no doubt that a high level of serum cholesterol (especially in the form of LDL), as shown in the Framingham Study, is the key risk factor for cardiovascular disease. It is the optimum level of total cholesterol, as contrasted with the average found in Western populations, that we need to attain (Figure 1).

Cardiovascular disease risk appears especially high if the dietary P/S ratio is low. For instance, in Finland, the country with the highest rates of myocardial infarction, the P/S ratio is about 0.15 (4) versus about 0.45 in the United States.

As shown for the Tarahumara Indians, there is an interaction between genetic predisposition to respond to lipid intakes and actual dietary lipid consumption. Among people with no genetic defects in lipid metabolism, only a small proportion of blood lipid levels is determined primarily by genetic factors (9). In the majority of cases, the level depends on the amount of fat in the diet, particularly the amount of saturated fat and cholesterol.

Figure 1 shows the optimal levels of cholesterol for both youth and adult populations. These values are different from those recommended by the NIH Consensus Conference (10), which suggested that individuals aged 20–29 are at moderate risk above 200 mg%, from 30–39 at 220, and from 40–49 at 240. Recommendations of a recent European conference on atherosclerosis (11) dealing with the same issue defined adults at risk if they were over 200 mg%. In establishing public health policy, the roles of LDL and HDL cholesterol or of other blood lipids are secondary to that of total blood cholesterol. If our

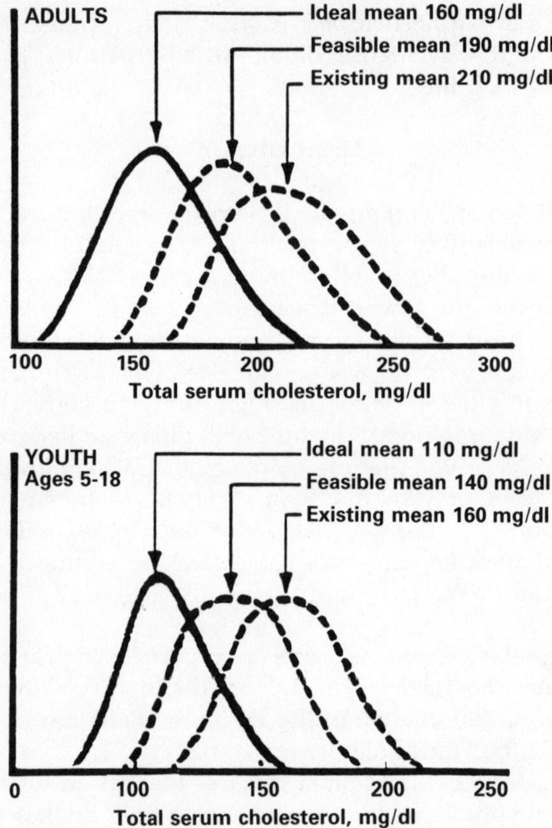

Figure 1. Ideal, feasible, and existing total serum cholesterol levels in adults (top) and in youths, age 5–18 (bottom). These idealized, smoothed curves portray, on the right hand, the present distributions of total serum cholesterol found in sampled U.S. populations. The middle curves represent distributions believed feasibly obtainable by a continuation of current changes in U.S. eating patterns over the next ten years. The left-hand curves are those thought ideal with respect to freedom from a large population burden of atherosclerotic diseases. These curves also display the phenomena that skewness and the relative excess of individuals having high values tend to diminish as the population mean is lowered. (Reprinted with permission from *Prev Med* 1979;8:612–678.)

entire population had serum cholesterol levels below 120 mg% as children and 160 mg% as adults, coronary heart disease would probably be as rare as it was in this country early in this century or currently is in China.

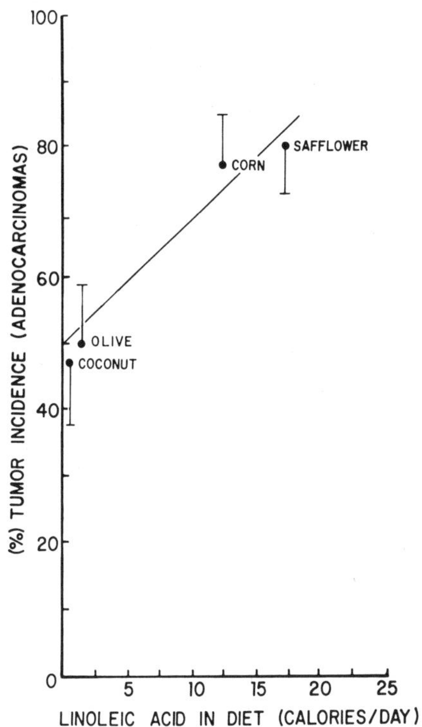

Figure 2. Animal studies: tumor enhancement as a function of % of linoleic acid in a type of fat.

Diet and Cancer

High-fat diets are also associated with several major types of human cancer. Dietary lipids, other than cholesterol, appear to be the main culprits (12,13). Animal studies show that dietary fats play an important role as tumor enhancers – an enhancement that seems to depend on the percentage of linoleic acid contained in the diet (14,15) (Figure 2). Judged on the basis of animal work, the major risk seems to be associated with polyunsaturated fats within the context of a certain minimal level of total fat. There is a lower risk associated with saturated fats, and no increase in risk noted for monounsaturated fats (13–16).

In addition to evidence from laboratory animal experiments, several sources of evidence indicate that cancers of various sites, notably

Table 1
Methods of Study in the Etiology of Cancer

1 Epidemiology
  a. Geographic pathology
  b. Special populations
  c. Time trends
2 Laboratory studies
  a. Metabolic and biochemical epidemiology-population studies
  b. Model studies in animals
  c. Model studies in cell and organ cultures
  d. Definition of mechanisms
3 Development of hypotheses
  a. Established risk factors and their mode of action
  b. Suspected risk factors and their possible role

breast, colon, and prostate, may relate to nutritional excesses, particularly high dietary fat intake. The types of evidence are summarized in Table 1. Correlations based upon geographic distribution relating dietary fat to breast cancer are striking, although we recognize that, by themselves, correlations do not prove association. These correlations, however, are supported by migrant studies showing that rates of breast cancer among Japanese living in the United States are greater after migration (17). This is also true for cancers of the prostate, colon, ovary, and endometrium, as well as for cardiovascular disease and diabetes (18,19). These findings are consistent with those from metabolic studies on risk for colon cancer that show that the pattern of bile acid metabolites (compounds proposed to affect colon cancer risk) found in stool is strikingly different in high-fat and low-fat diets as well as low- or high-fibre diets, which also affect the stool bulk as a diluent of colon carcinogens and promoters (20).

Many studies depend on dietary records to assess the role of diet on disease status. The epidemiologic method entailing the most difficulty in using dietary assessment tools is case-control studies that attempt to relate retrospective assessment of diet with current disease. In both prospective and retrospective settings, dietary assessments, including multiple dietary records, 24-hour dietary recalls, and food frequency questionnaires are, at the very least, very imprecise. Within homogenous populations, such imprecision poses severe obstacles to detecting diet/cancer relationships (21). Despite difficulties in assessing true dietary exposure, many conclusions are drawn on the basis of such data.

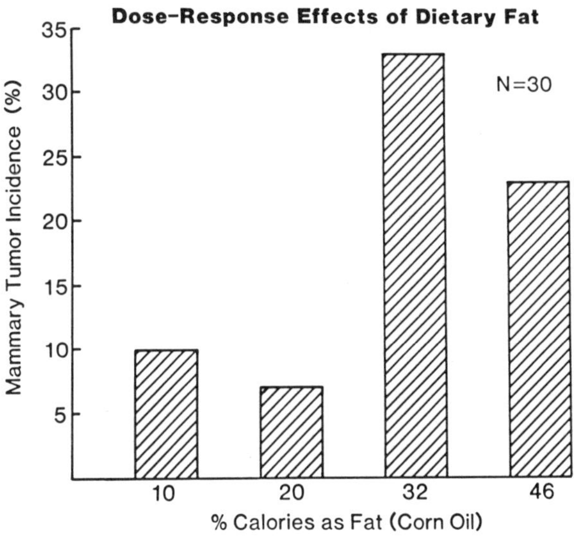

Figure 3. Dose-response effects of dietary fat.

In a recent report from a large-scale prospective study, Willett et al. (22) concluded that among nurses, 80% of whom had a dietary fat intake between 32 and 44% of calories as fat, no differences were noted in breast cancer risk. Diet was assessed by a semi-quantitative food frequency questionnaire. This assessment technique, even if it includes everything eaten, would be sufficiently imprecise in terms of type of food, quantity of food, and methods of food preparation to call for considerable caution in interpreting study results. Furthermore, the questionnaire might not accurately reflect patterns of food consumption early in life, e.g. 10 or 20 years prior to recalling diet, a time that may be of greater importance for the etiology of breast cancer than the more recent past.

Interpreting the results of this or any study requires extreme caution when extrapolating beyond the range of available data (i.e. below 30% of calories as fat). On the basis of animal studies (23), the results for intakes of 10% and 20% of calories as fat are the same, as are those for 30% compared with 40%, indicating a plateau effect between 20% to 30% of calories as fat (Figure 3). As for the animal experiments, ecological evidence relies on the use of a wide range of calories-as-fat values. The Willett et al. study (22), however, included very few individuals consuming less than 30% of total calories as fat. As the authors readily admit, their study could not draw conclusions concerning the effects of a very low (20%-of-calories-as-fat) fat diet on breast cancer risk.

Micronutrients

Deficiencies in micronutrients have been implicated in the etiology of various cancers. The key issue is to determine the optimal intake of each nutrient for each age group within a largely sedentary population.

The effect of micronutrients on cancer risk is more uncertain than for macronutrients. Most of the early work in nutrition was conducted on deficiency diseases. Therefore, decisions regarding micronutrient intake for prevention of diseases are relatively straightforward. Uncertainty about making recommendations at pharmacologic levels arises from the difficulty in determining optimal intake to prevent chronic diseases (i.e. cancer) and the problems of toxicity in moderate to high doses of certain micronutrients.

Some information on the effect of pharmacologic doses of micronutrients is known. Increased metabolic requirements under unique physiologic conditions, such as those for iron, folate, and calcium during pregnancy, are known. We do, however, need to evaluate further suggestions of "megadoses" of certain vitamins and minerals to prevent cancer, such as those proposed by Pauling (24). We project that in years to come, as several ongoing chemoprevention studies are completed, we will have learned more about the preventive qualities of certain micronutrients in the development of cancer and other diseases. Currently, emphasis is being given to such micronutrients as beta carotene, vitamins E and C, selenium, and zinc.

Application of Dietary Recommendations

Those convinced that the standard Western diet is not necessarily conducive to optimal health have asked how best to modify both the diet and the dietary habits of the population *per se*. The following decribes some relevant activities of our Institute.

THE KNOW YOUR BODY SCHOOL HEALTH EDUCATION PROGRAM (KYB)

Health habits are primarily initiated early in life. Our taste in foods is, to a large extent, dependent on what we were fed in our earliest

Table 2
First Year Cholesterol Values at Baseline, Ages 8–10

School location	*<120*	*121–149*	*150–169*	*170–184*	*185–200*	*>200*
Bronx, N.Y.C.	1.28%	17.79%	28.28%	21.72%	16.15%	13.69%
N = 1084	14	195	310	238	177	150
Westchester, N.Y.	1.71%	22.11%	33.24%	17.69%	12.13%	12.84%
N = 699	12	155	233	124	85	90

Data from Walter et al. (25)

years. The American youngster learns to like peanut butter, whereas his counterpart in Japan (perhaps more in the past) appreciates a bowl of rice.

Since it is more difficult to reach children at home, we have developed a school health education program that ranges from kindergarten through high school (25). The program attempts to teach good health habits to children.

Young children already have high cholesterol levels that can be tracked into adulthood (25) (Table 2). Studies with six-year-olds have shown that we can modify at least their intention to eat low-fat foods. The question remains whether we can translate these intentions into actual changes in behaviour. That this is possible, Walter et al. (25) have shown in a study indicating that consumption of fatty foods and actual blood cholesterol levels in ten-year-olds can be reduced over a six-year period. These results might be improved if we could use an entire school and start the program in the first grade. Aside from benefiting from the full force of group dynamics, by doing the program in an entire school we could influence school-wide environments such as the menu in the cafeteria.

The KYB program screens children for cholesterol, blood pressure, and weight each year. It teaches them for 30 hours a year through workbooks and teachers' guides to change their health behaviour, improve their self-esteem, and express assertiveness in a way that will be helpful in making and carrying out appropriate health-related decisions. Furthermore, the children receive an annual health test for attitude, knowledge, and behaviour. School health education, including nutrition education, should be a mandatory part of every school curriculum. If well done, and of sufficient intensity and duration, it could make a major impact on nutritional health and other aspects of lifestyle.

MASS SCREENING FOR CHOLESTEROL

Together with local hospitals and with the assistance of CBS-TV affiliates, we have undertaken a large-scale screening of blood cholesterol levels in major cities in the United States that has led to 120,000 screenings to date (26). As to be expected, participants are relatively well-educated, smoke less than the average population (17% are current smokers), and are, therefore, probably more health conscious than the general population. Even among this group, we are finding that about one-third of screenees have levels above the optimal cholesterol levels suggested by the NIH Consensus Conference (10), levels that we consider are still too high.

At the screening, participants receive a Health Passport, a document that, in addition to providing a Framingham-based coronary risk score, gives succinct information on how to reduce one's cholesterol and fat intake. A key issue of this exercise is the potential of changing the diet of the population. Given the tremendous burden of cardiovascular diseases to our society, physicians should give considerably more attention to dealing with elevated cholesterol levels among their patients. In our initial study in New York City, some 70% of 300 people with high cholesterol levels who responded to a follow-up telephone interview said that their physicians did not provide intervention advice (26). Thus, physician education in nutrition and behavioural modification must be an important component of the overall strategy to lower cholesterol levels in a population, preferably by dietary changes or, failing that, through prescription drugs.

Mass screening for cholesterol should also be conducted at the worksite. This practice would provide an opportunity to examine the general workforce. In a recent screening at a worksite in New Jersey, 11 out of 208 employees had cholesterol levels above 300 mg% (personal communication, N. Haley, American Health Foundation). This proportion is high compared with the self-selected sample found in our city-wide screenings.

CHANGING FOOD PRODUCTS

A long-range public health strategy is required to reduce the fat and cholesterol content of food products, particularly those we tend to consume most often. From this point of view, we are less concerned about shellfish than we are about whole milk, eggs, butter, and hamburgers. As part of this effort, we need to work towards educating

American Health Foundation Food Plan

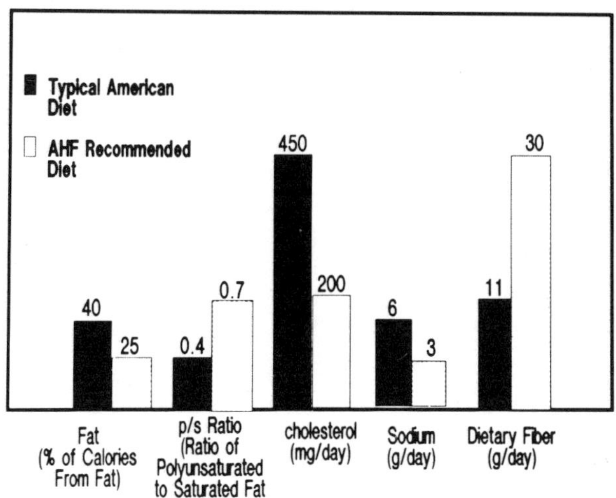

Figure 4. American Health Foundation food plan.* Salt = 40% sodium; 1 tsp salt = 2 g sodium.

consumers to know the difference in the fat content between whole and skim milk, cheddar cheese and low-fat cottage cheese, a porterhouse steak and a pot roast, and ice cream and sherbet. The consumer also needs to know that frying food adds considerable fat to the meal. We also need to encourage the food industry to reduce, wherever possible, the fat content of their products.

The American Health Foundation food plan (Figure 4) suggests eating more vegetables and fruits and reducing the consumption of beef and whole-milk dairy products. In food preparation, we should choose to broil, steam, or microwave our food instead of frying it. If we are going to change our diet from the current 40% of calories as fat to 20–25%, it is not only just what we do not eat that is critical but also the extent to which we replace high-fat, low-fibre foods and high-fat food preparation techniques with lower fat and higher fibre foods and low-fat food preparation methods. This is a long-range process that would lead to a society that has adopted a new taste for low-fat, less salty, and less sugary foods. Those who have eaten a typical Mediterranean diet on the shores of Portafino will recognize that there are Western diets that can be nutritious as well as delicious.

Concluding Thoughts

In the developed world, deficiency diseases are virtually non-existent. Nutrition-related diseases in the West are now largely a consequence of nutritional excesses. It appears that most of our dietary problems relate to a general problem of metabolic overload. Physiologic systems of detoxification, packaging, and regulation cannot handle the onslaught of tobacco smoke to the respiratory organs, the deluge of a heavy alcohol intake on the liver, and our excessive intake of macronutrients such as fat and cholesterol.

While we are interested in the mechanisms whereby nutritional overloads induce disease, the history of medicine teaches us that we do not have to understand fully the pathogenesis of a disease to prevent it. For this reason, we must proceed to modify the diets of our largely sedentary population to the extent that they become tuned to their metabolic capacities.

Our slogan is that "medicine should help us to die young as late in life as possible." What we do about our nutritional intake and other aspects of lifestyle will determine, to a large extent, if we can make this saying become a reality. Our goal is medically feasible and fiscally imperative. Perhaps man need not die from disease but simply pass from life when the genetic time clock of biological existence has run its predetermined course.

ACKNOWLEDGMENT

This paper was supported by grants from the Medical Research Council of Canada, the Canadian (Alberta) Heart Foundation, and the Alberta Heritage Foundation for Medical Research.

REFERENCES

1 Easton J. *Human longevity, Salisbury*. London: James Easton, 1799.
2 Eaton SB, Konner M. Paleolithic nutrition. *N Engl J Med* 1985;312:283–289.
3 Gaulin SJC, Konner M. On the natural diet of primates, including humans. In: Wurtman RJ, Wurtman JJ, eds. *Nutrition and the brain*. Vol. 1. New York: Raven Press, 1977:1–86.
4 FAO. *Food balance sheets*, 1979–1981. Rome: Food and Agriculture Organization of the United Nations, 1984.

5 McMurry MP, Connor WE, Lin DS, Cerqueira MT, Connor SL. The absorption of cholesterol and the sterol balance in the Tarahumara Indians of Mexico fed cholesterol-free and high cholesterol diets. *Am J Clin Nutr* 1985;41:1289–1298.
6 Sacks FM, Ornish D, Rosner B, McLanahan S, Castelli WP, Kass EH. Plasma lipoprotein levels in vegetarians: the effect of ingestion of fats from dairy products. *JAMA* 1985;254:1337–1341.
7 Philips RL. Role of life-style and dietary habits in risk of cancer among Seventh-Day Adventists. *Cancer Res* 1975;35:3513–3522.
8 Castelli WP. Epidemiology of coronary heart disease: The Framingham Study. *Am J Med* 1984;76(suppl 2A):4–12.
9 Katan MB, Beynen AC. Characteristics of human hypo- and hyper-responders to dietary cholesterol. *Am J Epidemiol* 1987;125:378–399.
10 NIH Consensus Development Conference. Lowering blood cholesterol to prevent heart disease. *JAMA* 1985;253:2080–2086.
11 Schettler G. *European Congress on Atherosclerosis*, 1986.
12 Doll R, Peto R. The causes of cancer: qualitative estimate of avoidable risks of cancer in the United States today. *JNCI* 1981;66:1191–1340.
13 Reddy BS, Cohen LA, eds. *Diet, nutrition, and cancer: a critical evaluation*, Vol. 1. Boca Raton, FL: CRC Press, 1986.
14 Braden LM, Carroll KK. Dietary polyunsaturated fat in relation to mammary carcinogenesis in rats. *Lipids* 1986;21:285–288.
15 Cohen LA, Thompson DO, Maeura Y, Choi K, Blank ME, Rose DP. Dietary fat and mammary cancer. I. Promoting effects of different dietary fats on N-nitrosomethylurea-induced rat mammary tumorigenesis. *JNCI* 1986;77:33–42.
16 Reddy BS. Amount and type of dietary fat and colon cancer: animal model studies. *Prog Clin Biol Res* 1986;222:295–309.
17 Buell P. Changing incidence of breast cancer in Japanese-American women. *JNCI* 1973;51:1479–1483.
18 Haenszel W, Kurihara M. Studies of Japanese migrants. 1. Mortality from cancer and other diseases among Japanese in the United States. *JNCI* 1968;40:43–68.
19 Locke FB, King H. Cancer mortality risk among Japanese in the United States. *JNCI* 1980;65:1149–1156.
20 Reddy BS. Diet and excretion of bile acids. *Cancer Res* 1981;41:3766–3768.
21 Hebert JR, Wynder EL. Dietary fat and the risk of breast cancer. *N Engl J Med* 1987;317:165–166.
22 Willett WC, Stampfer MJ, Colditz GA, Rosner BA, Hennekens CH, Speizer FE. Dietary fat and the risk of breast cancer. *N Engl J Med* 1987;316:22–28.

23 Cohen LA, Choi K, Weisburger JH, Rose DP. Effect of varying proportions of dietary fat on the development of N-nitrosomethylurea-induced rat mammary tumors. *Anticancer Res* 1986;6:215–218.

24 Pauling L, Cameron E. *Cancer and Vitamin C*, 2nd ed. New York: Warner Books, 1981.

25 Walter HJ, Hofman A, Connelly PA, Barrett LT, Kost KL. Primary prevention of chronic disease in childhood: changes in risk factors after one year of intervention. *Am J Epidemiol* 1985;122:772–781.

26 Wynder EL, Field F, Haley NJ. Population screening for cholesterol determination. *JAMA* 1986;256:2839–2842.

PHILIP J. GARRY AND ROBERT L. RHYNE

Nutritional Problems of the Elderly

It is by now widely recognized that the average age of Americans is increasing. The percentage of Americans over age 65, 75, or 85 has been increasing dramatically in this century, and these percentages are projected to continue to increase over the next four decades. This increase in the aging population has stimulated attention to the special health problems of elderly adults. One confusing aspect of discussions dealing with the elderly is our lack of a satisfactory definition of aging. What is old? Who is old? When does one become old? Clearly, physiological age is not the same as chronological age. On the other hand, numerous attempts to arrive at a simple and accurate indicator of physiological age have not as yet yielded a satisfactory instrument. In general terms "elderly" and "old" usually refer to all those over age 65.

The nutritional status of old people has received increasing attention from the scientific community in the past two decades. In the Western world, the elderly are the largest population at risk for protein-calorie malnutrition. Although there now exists documentation of specific nutritonal problems in the elderly, the relationship of altered nutrition to subsequent morbidity and mortality is not clear.

Age-Related Changes that Influence Nutrition

Todhunter (1) reported that 70% of a sample population of elderly subjects had made some change in food habits in recent years for reasons of health, aloneness, beliefs, or finances. The Ten State Nutrition Survey (2) found that two-thirds of the elderly had changed their diets in the four years prior to the study. Elahi et al. (3) reported a marked secular change in the diets, especially cholesterol intake, of the Baltimore Longitudinal Study of Aging male participants during the period 1961–1975. One hypothesis given for this observed secular change was that the public health advice from health professionals and the lay press about the danger of cholesterol and saturated fats in the diet was having an effect. Therefore, in order to separate true aging effects from possible time and cohort effects on nutrient intakes that can subsequently influence nutritional status, both cross-sectional and longitudinal studies are required in elderly populations. Unfortunately, most of the recent studies on nutrition and aging have been cross-sectional in nature.

PHYSIOLOGICAL CHANGES

The sensations for taste and smell decrease with age (4,5), resulting in a decreased appetite (6). Dental problems, common in old age, decrease the ability to chew certain foods (7). Diminution of visual and auditory senses makes it less pleasant for some elderly persons to eat in public places or at social gatherings (8). Decreases in basal metabolic rate and physical activity noted with increasing age result in overall lower caloric intake, which can lead to lowered intakes of essential nutrients (9,10). If total caloric intake is reduced without a change in dietary patterns, then intake of specific nutrients decreases proportionally. However, it should be pointed out that requirements for some nutrients, like riboflavin, are thought to decrease with age because of the decline in basal metabolic rate and physical activity.

Physiological changes, such as osteoarthritis, that affect mobility can decrease an old person's ability to purchase and prepare food (11). Another hindrance to adequate nutrition in the aged is malabsorption brought about by a decrease or absence in acid secretion by the stomach and by interactions with medications commonly prescribed for the elderly (12–14). It is not clear whether changes in the absorption of specific nutrients with age contributes to nutritional problems in the elderly.

PSYCHOLOGICAL CHANGES

The most common psychological variable affecting nutrition is depression (11). Of all psychiatric diagnoses, depression is most strongly correlated with increased morbidity and mortality, regardless of the age of the subjects (15,16). In the elderly, simple loneliness can contribute to poor nutrition. At least 30% of non-institutionalized men and women over the age of 65 live alone (1,17). Eating patterns are learned social behaviour, and changes in the living situation, such as loss of a spouse, can lead to significant changes in eating patterns. If the deceased partner was the caretaker of the couple, the surviving partner may be ignorant of even the basics of shopping, menu planning, and food preparation.

ECONOMIC AND SOCIAL CHANGES

Elderly individuals usually experience a net loss of income (18). However, the percentage of older individuals living below the poverty level (12.4% in 1984) has decreased substantially over the past two decades, and is now less than the percentage of those under 65 living in poverty (14.7% in 1984) (17). A major determinant of "life satisfaction" in the elderly would appear to be income, with health status also very important (19). Low income has been shown to be a major risk factor for inadequate nutrition in the elderly (20,21).

Elderly individuals are at high risk for institutionalization on either a temporary or permanent basis (22). While institutional food is likely to meet minimal standards for nutrient content, several aspects of institutional food discourage consumption. A lack of choice, a limited day-to-day variety, and the general unattractiveness of mass-prepared food increase the risk of inadequate consumption. In addition, because long-term care facilities such as nursing homes are conceived on a medical model, the admitting physician specifies the diet. This means that most residents of nursing homes are on some sort of therapeutic diet (low salt, diabetic, etc.) (23), which further discourages adequate intake. The situation is different for free-living individuals, who frequently ignore or "cheat on" their prescribed diets. In many cases, the potential benefits of therapeutic diets in elderly nursing home residents are outweighed by the detriment of possible inadequate total protein and calorie intake as a consequence of the diets. Thus, the major issue in institutionalized individuals is not that the diet is inadequate; it is that the food is often not consumed (24).

Nutritional Assessment of the Elderly

To define the nutritional status of a population, three basic methods are employed: clinical studies, dietary studies, and laboratory investigations. In general, clinical studies evaluate the physical signs of nutritional health or disease. Dietary studies compare nutrient intake with accepted standards. Laboratory investigations provide data about quantities of particular nutrients in the body or evaluate certain biochemical functions that are dependent on an adequate supply of a particular nutrient.

NUTRITION IN THE ELDERLY – CLINICAL ASSESSMENT

Anthropometric results show an increase in percent body fat for both sexes as age increases, although females possess a greater percent of body fat than males at all ages (25). The first National Health and Nutritional Examination Survey (NHANES-1) (20), Ten State Nutrition Survey (2), and Nutrition Canada National Survey (26) found obesity to be a substantial problem in the aged, especially in women. It is clear that obesity can aggravate other medical conditions such as diabetes, degenerative joint disease, and pulmonary disease (27,28).

Clinical signs of undernutrition in the elderly are less common. McClean's study of vitamin C and thiamine status in elderly men found few clinical signs of deficiencies in these vitamins (29). This is not surprising, as many of the changes in skin, subcutaneous tissue, and mucous membranes in the elderly would make it difficult to pick up relatively subtle signs such as petechiae.

NUTRITION IN THE ELDERLY – CALORIE AND PROTEIN INTAKE DETERMINED IN NUTRITIONAL SURVEYS

Calories

Over the past 20 years, several comprehensive nutritional surveys that included subjects over age 60 have been performed in the United States (2,30–32). In addition, other nutritional surveys have focused solely on the elderly. All of these studies identified a substantial proportion of elderly men and women who fell below established dietary intake recommendations for calories, protein, vitamins, calcium, and iron (33,34).

Dietary intakes in older persons have been estimated by several different methodologies. These include dietary histories, food records, and 24-hour dietary recalls. Dietary history methods are primarily designed to estimate the habitual intake for a period of one week to several months. As pointed out by Mahalko et al. (35), the subjectivity involved in describing usual eating patterns makes the dietary history method vulnerable to memory lapses, and psychological tendencies to exaggerate or minimize self-described behaviour. Food record methodology requires an individual to record all foods eaten over a specified period of time, generally from a few days to one week. Unlike dietary history methodology, which requires a trained interviewer, the burden is placed on the subject to provide accurate intake information. This requires that the individual be highly motivated, especially if required to keep records for several days. The 24-hour dietary recall methodology also requires a trained interviewer; however, the main advantage of this methodology is the minimal amount of interviewer and subject time required to complete the intake recall.

Several studies conducted in the U.S. have shown that energy intake decreases with age. In a cross-sectional study of male executives ranging in age from 20 to 93 years, McGandy et al. (9) found that there was a steady decline in energy intake from 2700 kcal/day at 30 years to 2100 kcal/day at 80 years of age. Most of the decline in energy intake was attributed to reduced physical activity (400 kcal) while 200 kcal was accounted for by a decline in basal energy metabolism as a result of a reduction in lean body mass with age. In 180 male participants (35 to 74 years) in the Baltimore Longitudinal Study of Aging, Elahi et al. (3) also found that aging had a negative effect on energy intake. A four-year longitudinal study of free-living healthy elderly men (n=91) and women (n=116) also showed a decline in energy intake with age (36). The mean age and standard deviation of men as well as women at the beginning of this study was approximately 71 ± 4.5 years. The average energy intake over the four-year period was 1545 kcal/day for women and 2118 kcal/day for men. These values were determined from three-day diet records and are substantially higher than recorded for elderly subjects between 65 and 74 years of age in NHANES-1 and 2 (20,32) studies in which 24-hour dietary recall was employed to calculate energy intake. Of the 3500 elderly examined in the NHANES-1 sample, which is representative of the U.S. civilian non-institutionalized elderly population between 65 and 74 years of age, approximately 82% were white and 18% were black. The mean energy intake for the white and black males was 1828 and 1571 kcal/day respectively. For white and black females, the mean energy intake was 1319 and 1186 kcal/day. Energy intake for those with income below the poverty level was less than the population mean regardless of sex and race. The energy intake as percent of standard Recommended Dietary Allowance (RDA), based on weight for age, sex, and height, was 77 for white and 69 for black females. The percent of standard was 75 and 64 for white and black males, respectively. Even when a conservative estimate of the standard is used, i.e., two-thirds of the RDA, only about 50% of the individuals 65 years and older met this level of intake. Because of an increased prevalence of dementia in the elderly, surveys using recall methods are biased towards decreased total nutrient intake with age (37,38). Surveys of institutionalized individuals, where actual food consumption is measured, avoid this bias. Nevertheless, most surveys have found that total energy intake of institutionalized elderly individuals is less than that of individuals living at home (39–41).

While it is difficult to compare studies of the elderly because of differences in dietary intake methodology, they usually point to decreases in energy intake with age, with possible influences of income and race on energy intake. It is not known for certain how reduced energy intakes affect the ability of elderly individuals to meet their specific nutrient requirements, but it may be difficult to meet nutrient requirements on low calorie diets (10).

Protein

The current RDA for protein intake in the elderly is 0.8 g of mixed protein per kg of body weight (42). A recent study of elderly men and women based on the RDA of 0.8 g protein/kg and energy intakes appropriate for their age and needs led to the finding that about half of the elderly are unable to maintain nitrogen balance on this level of protein, even at the end of a month (43). Munro (44) reviewed the limited number of studies designed to examine protein requirements of the elderly, including the study mentioned above, and concluded that the elderly do not need less protein than the young and that they possibly may even need more. Mean protein intakes were above the RDA for both men and women in the majority of studies (41,45–49). Yet in the studies by Jansen and Harrill (50) and Justice et al. (51), at least 24% of the women in nursing homes and 29% of the women living in private homes had diets that provided less than 0.8 g of protein/kg of body weight. In Jordan's study (41), 12% of the men and 40% of the women living at home failed to meet this criterion. Because the RDA for protein is substantially above the estimated average requirement, it is not possible to conclude from these data that persons with intake below the RDA are protein deficient or that they would benefit from additional protein intake.

NUTRITION IN THE ELDERLY – DATA ON SPECIFIC NUTRIENTS FROM DIETARY AND BIOCHEMICAL STUDIES

Calcium

Elderly people, especially postmenopausal Caucasian women, show an increased loss of bone mineral, which is reflected in their higher incidence of fractures (52). The mechanism behind the age-related loss of bone quantity is multifactorial and not understood clearly; however, chronic negative calcium balance appears to be a major contributory factor (53–55). The chronic net loss of calcium is predicated in part upon lowered efficiency for intestinal calcium absorption (56–60) and inadequate dietary calcium intakes (48,61–64). Recent reports show that increased protein intake may have a profound and sustained effect on increasing urinary calcium excretion (56). It has also been shown that high phosphorus intake reduces calcium excretion by increasing renal tubular reabsorption of calcium (56).

The RDA (1980) for calcium is currently 800 mg/day (42). It is becoming increasingly clear that this level may not be sufficient to maintain calcium balance in populations consuming Western-type diets at risk for osteopenia, particularly elderly women (53,65,66).

Stiedemann et al. (39) and Brown et al. (45) found that calcium was the nutrient that was most often marginal in the diet, with 43% of the women in nursing homes failing to get two-thirds of the 1980 RDA for calcium. In comparing two populations, Brown et al. (45) found that women living at home consumed less calcium than those in nursing homes. Grotkowski and Sims (47) found a population mean among women that was equal to only two-thirds of the RDA. Brown et al. (45) and McClean et al. (46) found similar low calcium intakes among men (660 mg/day), while Stiedemann et al. (39) and Grotkowski and Sims (47) found that the intakes among elderly males equaled or exceeded the RDA of 800 mg/day. Older people tend to avoid dairy products rich in calcium, possibly because of a fear of cholesterol or because of an intolerance to milk for a variety of reasons (67,68).

Iron

Clinicians confronted with detecting and determining the cause of anemia in the elderly are dependent on laboratory results such as hemoglobin level, hematocrit, red blood cell indices (erythrocyte count, mean corpuscular volume (MCV), mean corpuscular hemoglobin (MCH), mean corpuscular hemoglobin concentration (MCHC)), serum iron levels, total iron binding capacity (TIBC), percent transferrin saturation (PSAT), and plasma ferritin, folate, and vitamin B levels for their final diagnosis. Thus, the frequency with which anemia is encountered in the elderly and determination of its etiology depend on the criteria used for diagnosis.

In a recent review of the iron status of elderly persons in the United States, Lynch et al. (69) pointed out that very few data are available to describe the iron status of the elderly and that the conclusions in reported studies are based on hemoglobin and hematocrit values with, at most, one other index of iron nutrition. They further state that any discriminant value may lead to a large number of false-negative and false-positive results, especially when hemoglobin is the measure, as there is a marked overlap in the frequency distribution curves for anemic and normal people. Also, it has been suggested that the definitions of low and deficient hemoglobin levels need to be redefined for blacks, as Garn et al. (70) have shown that in 3321 age-matched pairs of black and white participants in NHANES-1, the difference in hemoglobin levels approximates 0.73 g/dl (i.e., blacks have lower hemoglobin levels than whites). This difference was statistically significant even after adjusting for transferrin saturation, and income, education, and other socioeconomic variables.

One national study (71) and three regional studies (72–74) showed that more than 10% of elderly white men were found to be anemic when hemoglobin levels less than 14 g/dl were used as the cut-off point to identify anemia. Using a hemoglobin level less than 12 g/dl to identify anemia in women, these same studies showed that elderly white women have a lower incidence of anemia than elderly white men. However, it should be pointed out that these studies included unselected or natural populations of elderly men who were not screened for disease states such as chronic infections, renal disease, neoplasms, and chronic blood loss, which can have a dramatic effect on erythrocyte production. It has been suggested that the increased incidence of anemia in elderly males compared to females may indicate that the cut-off point for low hemoglobin levels for males is too high. Also, decreased testosterone levels in the elderly men has been suggested as the possible cause for their high incidence of anemia, as testosterone has been shown to have a direct effect on hematopoiesis and is thought to account for the difference in hemoglobin levels between adult males and females (75).

In a study of 280 free-living and healthy elderly men (n = 131) and women (n = 149), Garry et al. (76) assessed iron status by examining dietary and supplemental iron intake as well as ten biochemical measures of iron nutriture (hemoglobin, hematocrit, erythrocyte count, MCV, MCH, MCHC, plasma iron, TIBC, PSAT, and plasma ferritin). This was a cross-sectional study of elderly individuals ranging in age from 61 to 93 years. This population was examined in 1980 when the median age for men was 71, and for women, 72 years. In this study, the association of biochemical measures of iron status with age was examined. The only significant negative correlations found were between TIBC and age for both men and women. For comparison purposes, iron status measures in an unselected group of younger men (n = 107) and women (n = 164) between the ages of 20 and 39 years were also obtained. The conclusion from this study was that anemia or iron deficiency was no more prevalent in this healthy elderly population than in younger adults when using identical criteria to assess iron nutriture. Subsequent to this report, Garry et al. (77) repeated all the previously mentioned iron status measurements in 221 of these same elderly subjects on a yearly basis over a period of five years. This longitudinal study revealed significant year-to-year variability in the population mean values for all biochemical measures of iron nutriture except plasma iron, but there were no trends for any of the changes that would suggest an increased risk of anemia. Comparison of those elderly subjects consistently taking an iron supplement to non- or infrequent supplement users showed no significant differences in the biochemical measures of iron status except for a slight but significant trend toward higher ferritin values in those taking an iron supplement.

Studies that only examine dietary intakes of iron in the elderly need to be viewed with caution, because iron stores or reserves, as determined by plasma ferritin measurements, have been shown to increase with age (78). Therefore, poor dietary intakes of iron at one point may or may not indicate an immediate risk factor. Also, the critical issue, as Monsen and Balintfy (79) point out, is not the total amount of iron ingested, but rather the amount of iron available for absorption. They point out that nonheme iron is absorbed at a 3% rate unless enhancing factors such as cellular animal protein (meat/fish/poultry) and ascorbic acid are ingested along with routine dietary iron sources. Marked improvement in nonheme iron absorption of as much as 8% is possible if these enhancing factors are present. Thus, in order to determine whether iron deficiency occurs at increased frequency among the elderly, the entire diet needs to be examined and, more importantly, biochemical parameters in additon to hemoglobin and hematocrit levels are helpful to determine the extent and cause of the deficiency.

Other Minerals

It is difficult to assess adequately trace metal intake in a population because trace metal content of many foods has not been exactly determined. The one possible exception is zinc (80).

Vitamins

While dietary intakes have been a primary source of vitamin information on elderly populations, precautions must be taken when interpreting dietary survey information. Difficulty in obtaining accurate estimates and inability of intake data to account for variations in absorption limit the usefulness of dietary information. Also, vitamin intakes below the RDA are not sufficient evidence for assigning risk levels for deficiency states unless confirmed by biochemical testing (81). These factors must be kept in mind when reviewing reports of vitamin deficiencies based only on intake information in elderly populations.

Vitamin A

Vitamin A deficiency does not seem to be a particular problem in the elderly, even though there have been reports of poor dietary intakes. In NHANES-1, which was a cross-sectional survey of the American population, approximately one-half of those over 65 had vitamin A intakes of less than two-thirds of the RDA. Nevertheless, only 0.3% of this population had low vitamin A blood levels (82,83). Similar data have been published on other populations (84,85), suggesting that elderly individuals can maintain normal vitamin blood levels even with low dietary intakes.

Vitamin D

Studies in several countries have revealed a generally lowered vitamin D status in elderly people, especially in chronically ill individuals (86,87), those living in institutions (87–89), and those with little or no sunlight exposure (90–92). Because the vitamin D endocrine system is the major regulator of intestinal calcium absorption (93), and lowered vitamin D status would promote the observed negative calcium balance in elderly people, deficiencies in this vitamin would be particularly damaging in elderly subjects. Two recent studies in the United States have found vitamin D intake to be approximately 50% of the RDA for elderly subjects (48,49). There was a good correlation between inadequate intake and low blood levels of 25-OH vitamin D (63). Fifteen percent of a healthy free-living elderly group had 25-OH vitamin D levels considered to be at least borderline deficient (< 8.0 mg/ml). Since sunlight exposure regulates the amount of provitamin D that is produced by the skin, it has been recommended that the elderly obtain minimal sunlight exposure (10–15 minutes) two or three times a week (95).

Vitamin E

Vitamin E is the subject of much interest in the scientific community and the lay press because of its antioxidant properties, which have been proposed to retard the aging process as well as prevent and/or to treat diseases as disparate as atherosclerosis and cancer (96). All of these issues involve supplementation of vitamin E frequently at "mega" doses. There is no evidence that elderly individuals are deficient either in dietary intake or tissue levels of vitamin E (81,97,98). Therapeutic trials of high dose vitamin E as an antioxidant in humans have met with some success, for example, in prolonging survival of red blood cells in some inherited hemolytic anemias (99). The use of vitamin E in intermittent claudication is promising but not yet established (96). Its use to treat or prevent atherosclerosis and cancer has not been established nor has it been conclusively proven to be ineffective in those conditions (96).

B vitamins

Hypovitaminosis reflects decreased dietary intake, absorption defects, decreased hepatic avidity, decreased storage and conversion to active metabolic forms, or excessive utilization, destruction, or excretion (100). Information that has accumulated from many dietary surveys of the vitamin status of the elderly indicates a great risk for deficiencies of these substances, but this is not always confirmed by biochemical or clinical results. No single comprehensive study for all the vitamins and their related enzyme systems has been carried out, probably because, as Brin and Bauernfeind (101) suggest, laboratory facilities are not available to do all the biochemical evaluations that would be necessary. Most individual studies have concentrated on one or two vitamins.

Davidson et al. (102) examined 104 elderly people in Boston and found that 37% had inadequate blood levels of riboflavin and 21% had low thiamine levels. Vir and Love published several articles (103–105) on the thiamine, riboflavin, and pyridoxine status of 196 institutionalized (in a hospital, residential accommodation, or a sheltered dwelling) and non-institutionalized Caucasian elderly subjects (males = 51, females = 145) as assessed by combined dietary, biochemical, and clinical studies. These subjects resided in Belfast, Ireland, and were between 65 and 94 years of age, were considered free of acute illness, and were not on a modified diet. This study revealed biochemical deficiency of thiamine in 17.6% of males and 12.5% of females as determined by the transketolase activity coefficient test in the various groups not receiving multivitamins. Biochemical deficiency of riboflavin was noted in 9.8% of males and 6.2% of females as determined by the glutathione reductase activity coefficient test. Biochemical deficiency of pyridoxine was observed in 24.3% of male and 42.7% of female subjects. Also, 20% of the subjects receiving multivitamins nonetheless had deficient pyridoxine levels as measured by stimulating erythrocyte glutamic-pyruvate transaminase in vitro with pyridoxal phosphate. The high incidence of pyridoxine deficiency in the elderly has also been noted by Hoorn et al. (106) using enzyme functional tests. Vir and Love found that the highest incidence of thiamine, riboflavin, and pyridoxine deficiency was in subjects in sheltered dwellings. In 196 subjects examined by Vir and Love, only one individual had clinical signs of vitamin deficiency.

Studies in a healthy free-living population in New Mexico using three-day diet records revealed that a substantial percentage of the population was receiving less than the RDA for vitamins B_1, B_2, B_6, B_{12}, and folate from diet alone (48). However, biochemical studies designed to assess vitamin B_2, B_{12}, and folate status in this population failed to confirm that these individuals were at risk of developing clinical symptoms associated with low intakes of these vitamins (107,108). There are several reasons for the apparent discrepancy between the dietary and biochemical assessments in this population. One is that nearly 50% of these elderly were ingesting a vitamin supplement on a regular basis. Another is that the RDAS for most nutrients represent upper limits of variability for age and sex. Also, the data on the exact vitamin content in many foods are lacking and, therefore, dietary analyses using standard reference tables may underestimate their true value.

Vitamin C

Some studies have reported low vitamin C intake and blood levels in both institutionalized and free-living elderly (102,109). Vitamin C status in 270 free-living healthy elderly was determined from dietary and supplemental intakes and plasma levels of ascorbic acid (110). Mean dietary intakes of ascorbic acid for women and men were approximately two-and-one-half times the current RDA of 60 mg/day. Of interest was the finding that men not consuming a vitamin supplement had significantly lower plasma ascorbic acid levels than women – 0.91 vs 1.14 mg/dl. This difference could not be explained by the smoking habits of men and women.

Kallner et al. (111) have been able to show, using radioactively-labelled ascorbic acid, that the total body pool of ascorbic acid reaches a maximum of approximately 20 mg/kg, and that this amount can be achieved at a steady state plasma concentration of 1.0 mg/dl. A comparison between ascorbic acid intake and plasma levels in the study reported by Garry et al. (110) revealed that women require an intake of 75 mg/day and men require an intake of 125 mg/day to achieve a plasma ascorbic acid level of 1.0 mg/dl. VanderJagt et al. (112) confirmed this finding in a clinical trial in which eight healthy men and nine women over the age of 65 were placed on controlled intakes of ascorbic acid ranging from 30 to 280 mg/day. This study also showed that the majority of men on daily intakes of 60 mg had plasma ascorbic acid levels below 0.4 mg/dl, a level often used to identify individuals at risk for developing clinical hypovitaminosis symptoms. If maintaining a maximum body pool of ascorbic acid is desirable, especially for the elderly, there may be a need to consider increasing the ascorbic acid allowances above the present value of 60 mg/day, especially for elderly men.

Conclusions

The information presented is not intended to be an exhaustive review of the causes and consequences of poor nutrition in the elderly. Instead, we have presented a general review which will allow the reader to understand better the complexity of this subject and the need for continued research required to determine all etiologies and the subsequent alleviation of nutritional problems in the elderly.

Acknowledgment

This work was supported by a grant from the United States Public Health Service AG-02049.

REFERENCES

1 Todhunter EN. Lifestyle and nutrient intake in elderly. *Curr Concepts Nutr* 1976;4:119–127.
2 Department of Health, Education and Welfare. III. Clinical, Anthropometry, Dental; IV. Biochemical; V. Dietary. *Ten State Nutrition Survey 1968–1970*. Atlanta, GA: U.S. Department of Health, Education and Welfare, Center for Disease Control, 1972. [DHEW Publication No. (HSM) 72–8131, 8132, 8133.]
3 Elahi VK, Elahi D, Andres R, Tobin JD, Butler MG, Norris AH. A longitudinal study of nutritional intake in men. *J Gerontol* 1983;38:162–180.
4 Schiffman SS, Mors J, Erickson RP. Thresholds of food odors in the elderly. *Exp Aging Res* 1976;2:389–398.
5 Kamath SK. Taste acuity and aging. *Am J Clin Nutr* 1982;36:766–775.
6 Busse EW. How mind, body and environment influence nutrition in the elderly. *Postgrad Med* 1978;63(3):118–125.
7 Albanese AA. Nutrition of the elderly: introduction. *Postgrad Med* 1978;63(3):117.
8 Newman EG, Douvenmuehle RH, Busse EW. Alterations in neurologic status with age. *J Am Geriatr Soc* 1960;8:915–917.
9 McGandy RB, Barrows CH, Spanias A, Meredith A, Stone JL, Norris AH. Nutrient intakes and energy expenditure in men of different ages. *J Geront* 1966;21:581–587.
10 McGandy RB. Nutrition and the aging cardiovascular system. Bristol-Myers Nutrition Symposia. In: Hutchinson M, Munro HN, eds. *Nutrition and aging*, vol. 5. Orlando, FL: Academic Press, 1986:263–275.
11 Garetz FK. Breaking dangerous cycle of depression and faulty nutrition. *Geriatrics* 1976;31:73–75.
12 Butler RN, Lewis MI. *Aging and mental health*, 2nd ed. St Louis: Mosby, 1977.

13 Russell RM. Implications of gastric atrophy for vitamin and mineral nutriture. Bristol-Myers Nutrition Symposia. In: Hutchinson M, Munro HN, eds. *Nutrition and aging*, vol. 5. Orlando, FL: Academic Press, 1986:56–59.
14 Roe DA. Pharmacokinetics and drug-nutrient interactions. In: Chandra RK, ed. *Nutrition, immunity and illness in the elderly*. Elmsford, NY: Pergamon Press, 1985:253–265.
15 Widgor B, Morris G. A comparison of 20-year medical histories of individuals with depressive and paranoid states: a preliminary note. *J Geront* 1977;32:160–163.
16 Nielsen J, Homma A, Bjorn-Henriksen T. Followup 15 years after a gerontro-psychiatric prevalence study. *J Geront* 1977;32:554–561.
17 American Association of Retired Persons. *A profile of older Americans: 1985*. D996, Washington, DC: AARP Publication PF3049 (1085).
18 U.S. Bureau of the Census. *Statistical abstracts of the United States*. 98th ed. Washington, DC: Government Printing Office, 1977.
19 Chatfield WF. Economic and sociological factors influencing life satisfaction of the aged. *J Geront* 1977;32:593–599.
20 Department of Health, Education and Welfare. *Preliminary Findings of the First Health and Nutrition Examination Survey, United States, 1971–72. Dietary intake and biochemical findings*. Washington, DC: U.S. Government Printing Office, 1974. [DHEW Publications No. (HRA) 74–1219–1.]
21 Guthrie HA, Black K, Madden JP. Nutritional practices of elderly citizens in rural Pennsylvania. *Gerontologist* 1972;12:330–335.
22 Kane RL. Long-term care: policy and reimbursement. In: Cassel CK, Walsh JR, eds. *Geriatric medicine*, Vol. 2. New York, NY: Springer-Verlag, 1984:380–396.
23 National Center for Health Statistics, United States Public Health Service. Characteristics of nursing home residents, health status and care received: National Nursing Home Survey. Hyattsville, MD: National Center for Health Statistics, 1981. (*Vital and Health Statistics. Series 13: Data from the National Nursing Home Survey*, No. 51.) [PHS Publication No. 81–1712.]
24 Sandman P, Adlofsson R, Nygren C, Hallmans G, Winblad B. Nutritional status and dietary intake in institutionalized patients with Alzheimer's disease and multiinfarct dementia. *J Am Geriatr Soc* 1987;35:31–38.
25 Schlenker ED, Feurig JS, Stone LH, Ohlson MA, Mickelsen O. Nutrition and health of older people. *Am J Clin Nutr* 1973;26:1111–1119.
26 *Nutrition Canada National Survey*. Catalogue No. H58–36. Ottawa: Information Canada, 1973.

27 Chope HD, Breslow L. Nutritional status of the aging. *Am J Public Health* 1956;46:61–67.

28 Jeffay H. Obesity and aging. *Am J Clin Nutr* 1982;36:809–811.

29 McClean HE, Dodds PM, Stewart AW, Beaven DW, Riley CG. Nutrition of elderly men living alone. Part 2: Vitamin C and thiamine status. *NZ Med J* 1976;84:345–348.

30 Agricultural Research Service 1972. *Food and nutrient intake of individuals in the U.S. Spring, 1965*. United States Department of Agriculture Household Food Consumption Survey, 1965–1966. Department II, Washington, DC.

31 USDA. *Food and nutrient intakes of individuals in one day in the United States, Spring, 1977*. Hyattsville, MD: Nationwide Food Consumption Survey, 1977–1978. U.S. Department of Agriculture, Consumer Nutrition Center, 1980.

32 National Center for Health Statistics. *Dietary intake findings, United States 1976–1980*. Hyattsville, MD: U.S. Department Health Human Services, 1982.

33 Bidlack WR, Kirsch A, Meskin MS. Nutritional requirements of the elderly. *Food Technol* 1986;40:61–71.

34 Symposium on: Evidence relating selected vitamins and minerals to health and disease in the elderly population in the United States. Rivlin RS, Young EA, eds. *Am J Clin Nutr* 1982;36(suppl):977–1086.

35 Mahalko JR, Johnson LK, Gallagher SK, Milne DB. Comparison of dietary histories and seven-day food records in a nutritional assessment of older adults. *Am J Clin Nutr* 1985;42:542–553.

36 Garry PJ, Hunt WC, Goodwin JS. Changes in dietary patterns over a four year period in an elderly population. In: Taylor TG, Jenkins NK, eds. *Proceedings of the XIII International Congress of Nutrition*. London: John Libbey, 1986:713–715.

37 Beaton GH. Nutritional assessment of observed nutrient intake: an interpretation of recent requirement reports. In: Draper HH, ed. *Advances in nutritional research*, Vol. 7. New York: Plenum Press, 1985:101–128.

38 Hunt WC, Leonard AG, Garry PJ, Goodwin JS. Components of variance in dietary data for an elderly population. *Nutr Res* 1983;3:433–441.

39 Stiedemann M, Jansen C, Harrill I. Nutritional status of elderly men and women. *J Am Diet Assoc* 1978;73:132–139.

40 Harrill I, Cervone N. Vitamin status of older women. *Am J Clin Nutr* 1977;30:431–440.

41 Jordan VE. Protein status of the elderly as measured by dietary intake, hair tissue, and serum albumin. *Am J Clin Nutr* 1976;29:522–528.

42 National Academy of Sciences. National Research Council. *Recommended dietary allowances*. 8th rev. ed. Washington, DC: National Academy of Sciences, 1980.
43 Gersovitz M, Motil K, Munro HN, Scrimshaw NS, Young VR. Human protein requirements: assessment of the dietary adequacy of the current recommended daily allowances for dietary protein in elderly men and women. *Am J Clin Nutr* 1982;35:6–14.
44 Munro HN. Protein nutriture and requirement in elderly people. *Bibl Nutr Dieta (Basel)* 1983;33:61–74.
45 Brown PT, Bergan JG, Parsons EP, Krol I. Dietary status of elderly people. *J Am Diet Assoc* 1977;71:41–45.
46 McClean HE, Weston R, Beaven DW, Riley CG. Nutrition of elderly men living alone. Part 1: Intakes of energy and nutrients. *NZ Med J* 1976;84:305–309.
47 Grotkowski ML, Sims LS. Nutritional knowledge, attitudes, and dietary practices of the elderly. *J Am Diet Assoc* 1978;72:499–506.
48 Garry PJ, Goodwin JS, Hunt WC, Hooper EM, Leonard AG. Nutritional status in a healthy elderly population: dietary and supplemental intakes. *Am J Clin Nutr* 1982;36:319–331.
49 McGandy RB, Russel RM, Hartz SC, et al. Nutritional status survey of healthy noninstitutionalized elderly: energy and nutrient intakes from three-day diet records and nutrient supplements. *Nutr Res* 1986;6:785–798.
50 Jansen C, Harrill I. Intakes and serum levels of protein and iron for 70 elderly women. *Am J Clin Nutr* 1977;30:1414–1422.
51 Justice CL, Howe JM, Clark HE. Dietary intake and nutritional status of elderly patients. *J Am Diet Assoc* 1974;65:639–646.
52 Seeman E, Riggs BL. Dietary prevention of bone loss in the elderly. *Geriatrics* 1981;36:71–79.
53 Heaney RP, Recker RR, Saville PD. Menopausal changes in calcium balance performance. *J Lab Clin Med* 1978;92:953–963.
54 Horsman A, Marshall DH, Nordin BEC, Crilly RG, Simpson M. The relation between bone loss and calcium balance in women. *Clin Sci* 1980;59:137–142.
55 Spencer H, Kramer L, Osis D. Factors contributing to calcium loss in aging. *Am J Clin Nutr* 1982;36:776–787.
56 Avioli LV. Postmenopausal osteoporosis: prevention verses cure. *Fed Proc* 1981;40:2418–2422.
57 Gallagher JC, Riggs BL, Eisen J, Hamstra A, Arnaud SB, DeLuca HF. Intestinal calcium absorption and serum vitamin D metabolites in normal subjects of osteoporotic patients. *J Clin Invest* 1979;64:729–736.

58 Alevizaki CC, Ikkos DC, Singuelakis P. Progressive decrease of true intestinal calcium absorption with age in normal man. *J Nucl Med* 1973;14:760–762.
59 Bullamore JR, Wilkinson R, Gallagher JC, Nordin BEC, Marshall DH. Effects of age on calcium absorption. *Lancet* 1970;2:535–537.
60 Ireland P, Fordtram JS. Effects of dietary calcium and age on jejunal calcium absorption in humans studied by intestinal perfusion. *J Clin Invest* 1973;52:2672–2681.
61 Heaney RP, Recker RR, Saville PD. Calcium balance and calcium requirements in middle-aged women. *Am J Clin Nutr* 1977;30:1603–1611.
62 Vinther-Paulsen N. Calcium and phosphorus intake in senile osteoporosis: prevention versus cure. *Fed Proc* 1981;40:2418–2422.
63 Omdahl J, Garry PJ, Hunsaker LA, Hunt WC, Goodwin JS. Nutritional status in a healthy elderly population: vitamin D. *Am J Clin Nutr* 1982;36:1225–1233.
64 Koplan J, Annest JL, Layde PM, Rubin GL. Nutrient intake and supplementation in the United States (NHANES-II). *Am J Public Health* 1986;76:287–289.
65 Matkovik V, Kostial K, Simonovik I, Buzina R, Broderec A, Nordin B. Bone status and fracture rates in two regions in Yugoslavia. *Am J Clin Nutr* 1979;32:540–549.
66 Recker RR, Saville RP. Effects of estrogen and calcium carbonate on bone loss in postmenopausal women. *Ann Intern Med* 1977;87:649–655.
67 Goodwin JS, Leonard AG, Hooper EM, Garry PJ. Concern about cholesterol and its association with diet in a group of healthy elderly. *Nutr Res* 1985;5:141–148.
68 Heaney RP, Gallagher JC, Johnson CC, et al. Calcium nutrition and bone health in the elderly. *Am J Clin Nutr* 1982;36:986–1013.
69 Lynch SR, Finch CA, Monsen ER, Cook JD. Iron status of elderly Americans. *Am J Clin Nutr* 1982;36:1032–1045.
70 Garn SM, Ryan AS, Owen GM, Abraham S. Income matched black-white hemoglobin difference after correction for low transferrin saturations. *Am J Clin Nutr* 1981;34:1645–1647.
71 Department of Health, Education and Welfare. *Hemoglobin and selected iron-related findings of persons 1–74 years of age, United States 1971–1974.* Hyattsville, MD, 1979. [DHEW (PHS) Publication No. 46.]
72 O'Neal RM, Abrahams OG, Kohrs MB, Eklund DL. The incidence of anemia in residents of Missouri. *Am J Clin Nutr* 1976;29:1158–1166.
73 Fisher S, Hendricks DG, Mahoney AW. Nutritional assessment of senior rural Utahns by biochemical and physical measurements. *Am J Clin Nutr* 1978;31:667–672.

74 Htoo MS, Kofkoff RL, Freedman ML. Erythrocyte parameters in the elderly: an argument against new geriatric normal values. *J Am Geriatr Soc* 1979;27:547–551.
75 Lipschitz DA, Mitchell CO, Thompson C. The anemia of senescence. *Am J Hematol* 1981;11:47–54.
76 Garry PJ, Goodwin JS, Hunt WC. Iron status and anemia in the elderly: new findings and a review of previous studies. *J Am Geriatr Soc* 1983; 31:389–399.
77 Garry PJ, Goodwin JS, Hunt WC. Longitudinal assessment of iron status in a group of elderly. In: Chandra RK, ed. *Nutrition, immunity, and illness in the elderly*. Elmsford, NY: Pergamon Press, 1985:77–83.
78 Casale G, Bonora C, Migliavacca A, Zurita IE, DeNicola P. Serum ferritin and aging. *Age Ageing* 1981;10:119–122.
79 Monsen ER, Balintfy JL. Calculating dietary iron bioavailability: refinement and computerization. *J Am Diet Assoc* 1982;80:307–311.
80 Sandstead HH, Henriksen LK, Greger JL, Prasad AS, Good RA. Zinc nutriture in the elderly in relation to taste acuity, immune response and wound healing. *Am J Clin Nutr* 1982;36:1046–1059.
81 Garry PJ, Hunt WC. Biochemical assessment of vitamin status in the elderly: effects of dietary and supplemental intakes. Bristol-Myers Nutrition Symposia, 1986. In: Hutchinson M, Munro HN, eds. *Nutrition* and *aging*, vol. 5. Orlando, FL: Academic Press, 1986:117–136.
82 Bowman BB, Rosenberg IH. Assessment of nutritional status of the elderly. *Am J Clin Nutr* 1982;35:1142–1151.
83 Food and Drug Administration. *Assessment of the vitamin A nutritional status of the U.S. population based on data in the Health and Nutrition examination surveys, Nov. 1985*. Washington, DC: Department of Health and Human Services, 1985. Life Science Research Office, Federation of American Societies for Experimental Biology.
84 Yearick ES, Wang MS, Pisias JJ. Nutritional status of the elderly: dietary and biochemical findings. *J Gerontol* 1980;5:663–671.
85 Garry PJ, Hunt WC, Bandrofchak JL, VanderJagt DJ, Goodwin JS. Vitamin A intake and plasma retinol levels in healthy elderly. *Am J Clin Nutr* 1987;46:989–994.
86 Petersen M, Hall MRP, Briggs RS. Plasma 25-hydroxyvitamin D levels in the elderly: difficulties in interpretation. *Clin Sci* 1981;61:43–44.
87 Weisman Y, Schen RJ, Eisenberg Z, Edelstein S, Harell A. Inadequate status and impaired metabolism of vitamin D in the elderly. *Isr J Med Sci* 1981;17:19–21.
88 Corless D, Gupta SP, Sattar DA, Switaa W, Boucher BJ. Vitamin D status of residents of an old people's home and long stay patients. *Gerontology* 1979;25:350–355.

89 Vir SC, Love AHG. Vitamin D status of elderly at home and institutionalized in hospital. *Int J Vitam Nutr Res* 1978;48:123–130.
90 Lund B, Sorensen OH. Measurement of 25-hydroxy-vitamin D in serum and its relation to sunshine, age and vitamin D intake in the Danish population. *Scand J Clin Lab Invest* 1979;39:23–30.
91 Baker MR, Peacock M, Nordin BEC. The decline in vitamin D status with age. *Age Ageing* 1980;9:249–252.
92 Lawson DEM, Paul AA, Black AE, Cole TJ, Mandal AR, Davie M. Relative contributions of diet and sunlight to vitamin D state in the elderly. *Br Med J* 1979;2:303–305.
93 Christakos S, Norman AW. Interactions of the vitamin D endocrine system with other hormones. *Miner Electrolyte Metab* 1978;1:231–239.
94 Lee CJ, Lawler GS, Johnson GH. Effects of supplementation of the diets with calcium and calcium-rich foods on bone density of elderly females with osteoporosis. *Am J Clin Nutr* 1981;34:819–823.
95 Holick MD. Vitamin D synthesis by the aging skin. Bristol-Myers Symposia 1986. In: Hutchinson M, Munro HN, eds. *Nutrition and aging,* Vol. 5. Orlando, FL: Academic Press, 1986:45–58.
96 Bieri JG, Corash L, Hubbard VS. Medical uses of vitamin E. *N Engl J Med* 1983;308:1063–1071.
97 Kelleher J, Losowksy MS. Vitamin E in the elderly. In: DeDuve C, Hayasshi O, eds. *Tocopherol, oxygen and biomembranes.* Amsterdam: Elsevier/North Holland Biomedical Press, 1978:311–327.
98 Vatassery GT, Johnson GJ, Krezowski AM. Changes in vitamin E concentrations in human plasma and platelets with age. *J Am Coll Nutr* 1983;4:369–375.
99 Corash L, Spielberg S, Bartsocas C. Reduced chronic hemolysis during high-dose vitamin E administration in mediterranean type glucose-6-phosphate dehydrogenase deficiency. *N Engl J Med* 1980;251:2357–2390.
100 Cherrick GR, Baker H, Frank O, Leevy CM. Observations on hepatic avidity for folate in Laennec's cirrhosis. *J Lab Clin Med* 1965;66:446–451.
101 Brin M, Bauernfeind JC. Vitamin needs of the elderly. *Postgrad Med* 1978;63(3):155–163.
102 Davidson CS, Livermore J, Anderson P, Kaufman S. The nutrition of a group of apparently healthy aging persons. *Am J Clin Nutr* 1962;10:181–199.
103 Vir SC, Love AHG. Thiamine status of institutionalized and non-institutionalizd aged. *Int J Vitam Nutr Res* 1977;47:325–335.
104 Vir SC, Love AHG. Riboflavin status of institutionalized and non-institutionalized aged. *Int J Vitam Nutr Res* 1977;47:336–344.

105 Vir SC, Love AHG. Vitamin B status of institutionalized and non-institutionalized aged. *Int J Vitam Nutr Res* 1977;47:364–372.
106 Hoorn RKJ, Filkweert JP, Westerink D. Vitamin B, B, and B deficiency in geriatric patients, measured by coenzyme stimulation of enzyme activity. *Clin Chim Acta* 1975;61:151–162.
107 Garry PJ, Goodwin JS, Hunt WC. Nutritional status in a healthy elderly population: riboflavin. *Am J Clin Nutr* 1982;36:902–909.
108 Garry PJ, Goodwin JS, Hunt WC. Folate and vitamin B status in a healthy elderly population. *J Am Geriatr Soc* 1984;32:719–726.
109 Leevy CM, Cardi L, Frank O, Gellene R, Baker H. Incidence and significance of hypovitaminemia in a randomly selected municipal hospital population, 1965. *Am J Clin Nutr* 1965;17:259–271.
110 Garry PJ, Goodwin JS, Hunt WC, Gilbert BA. Nutritional status in a healthy elderly population: vitamin C. *Am J Clin Nutr* 1982;36:332–339.
111 Kallner A, Hartman D, Hornig D. Steady-state turnover and body pool of ascorbic acid in man. *Am J Clin Nutr* 1979;32:530–539.
112 VanderJagt DJ, Garry PJ, Bhagavan HN. Relationship between ascorbic acid intake and plasma levels in healthy elderly. *Am J Clin Nutr* 1987;46:290–294.

HAROLD KALANT

Alcohol Use and Nutrition

It is frequently stated that alcoholism is one of the principal causes of nutritional disturbance in the adult population of North America and the rest of the developed world. This assertion appears to be consistent with the commonly held concept of the alcoholic as a "skid-row" drinker, grossly undernourished, and suffering from a variety of nutritional disorders such as beri-beri, peripheral neuropathy, macrocytic anemia, and Wernicke-Korsakoff syndrome. This picture of the alcoholic is often "explained" by two assumed "facts": 1. that the alcoholic spends all day drinking and not eating and is therefore grossly undernourished, and 2. that ethanol provides "empty calories" which are of no use in nutrition. Unfortunately, this picture is only partly true and only of some alcoholics, and fails completely to describe the complexity of the interaction of alcohol and nutrition. There are many other factors that must be taken into account.

Before considering other explanations involving these factors, we must first be clear on the facts that need to be explained. The first is that most alcoholics are *not* skid-row drinkers and are not grossly undernourished. The majority are employed, married and living with their spouses, and eating relatively well. For example, one nutritional study of a group of 69 alcoholics in Santiago, Chile (1), revealed that their diet was quite adequate in calories, only slightly suboptimal with respect to protein, phosphorus, and thiamine, but quite low (less than ⅔ of the Recommended Dietary Allowance (RDA) in calcium, vitamin A, riboflavin, niacin, and vitamin C. Anthropometric measurements showed that their body weight was normal, as was their muscle mass and amount of subcutaneous fat. Some of the patients indeed were actually overweight, and one interesting observation is that the obese alcoholics appeared to be at greater risk of developing alcoholic hepatitis or cirrhosis. The important point in the present context is that these patients were not grossly undernourished, but showed quite selective malnutrition with respect to specific constituents of the diet.

The second important fact is that the term "empty calories" as applied to alcohol is a potentially misleading term. If it is intended to convey the idea that ethanol provides calories without a corresponding content of vitamins or other essential nutrients, then the term is just as correct with respect to ethanol as it is with respect to sucrose, refined fat, or various other sources of calories. If, however, it is meant to imply that the calories generated by the oxidation of ethanol are dissipated as heat and are unavailable for metabolic use in biosynthetic reactions, then it is quite incorrect. It has been known for many years that rats will show normal growth on a diet in which a substantial portion of the carbohydrate has been replaced equicalorically by ethanol (2). In human infants, complete intravenous nutrition with a mixture of hydrolyzed casein, lipids, carbohydrate, and 2.5% alcohol to provide extra calories was able to maintain positive nitrogen balance and body growth (3).

In a recent study (4), adult humans took part in a metabolic study for four weeks. During this time they received a liquid diet by continuous nasogastric infusion. The diet provided 0.8 g of protein per kg of body weight, 12% of total calories from fat, and the rest from carbohydrate. During the second week of the study enough carbohydrate was replaced equicalorically by ethanol to provide 30% of the total calories as alcohol. During the third week this was increased to 50–60% of total calories. Direct and indirect calorimetry during the period in which ethanol provided 30% of calories revealed no change in heat loss, though the respiratory quotient (RQ) fell to 0.87, as would be expected from the metabolism of ethanol. However, the urinary and fecal energy losses were unchanged, and body weight and nitrogen balance were maintained in equilibrium. During the third week, when ethanol provided 50–60% of total calories, the blood-alcohol level rose steadily because the daily dose of alcohol exceeded the alcohol metabolizing capacity of the body. During this week the RQ fell further to 0.80, and negative nitrogen balance and weight loss were seen. The authors concluded that ethanol could be metabolized and utilized as efficiently as any other calorie source, but that the weight loss and negative nitrogen balance seen on the very high dosage of alcohol were probably indicative of a toxic effect on protein metabolism. The nature of this toxic effect is one of the things which must be explained.

While most alcoholics are not grossly undernourished, it is true that many do show clinical problems which are attributable to selective inadequacies of nutrition, and the nature of the toxic effect of ethanol that is responsible for such disturbances must be explained. What causes some alcoholics, even those with seemingly good diets, to show problems of this type? Basically, the disturbances can be attributed to a combination of a marginally and selectively inadequate diet with direct toxic effects of alcohol (5,6). In greater detail we can specify a number of problems (7) in the following respects:

1 The food intake is often selectively reduced, i.e. some foods are retained while others are omitted, because of poor appetite associated with alcoholic gastritis, or possibly because of lack of availability of money if too much has been spent on alcohol.
2 Gastrointestinal upset, including vomiting and diarrhoea, may impair the person's ability to retain food in the gastrointestinal tract for long enough to derive the maximum nutritional benefit from it.
3 Various intestinal transport mechanisms may be impaired directly by alcohol, giving rise to specific deficiencies in absorption of nutrients from the diet.
4 Storage capacity may be reduced, mainly because of alcoholic liver disease, and this may reduce the metabolic availability of various vitamins.
5 The metabolic conversion of native vitamins to their active forms, by such mechanisms as phosphorylation or one-carbon group transfer, may be impaired by alcohol, and this may result in failure of the vitamins to play their necessary metabolic role.
6 Ethanol may directly impair the ability of peripheral tissues to utilize substances brought to them in the circulating blood.
7 The urinary excretion of various minerals and vitamins is known to be increased by ethanol, and this may result in a metabolic deficiency even though the intake would otherwise be adequate.
8 It has been suggested that the metabolism of alcohol may increase the metabolic requirements for some vitamins or other nutrients.

We shall examine some of these suggestions now in further detail.

Intestinal Malabsorption

A number of experimental studies in humans have confirmed the fact that alcohol, both single doses and chronic ingestion, can inhibit the absorption of a variety of nutrients, including amino acids, sugars such as xylose, thiamine, folate, vitamin B_{12}, fat, and others (8,9). In order to understand this inhibitory effect of alcohol, it is important to note that oral intake of alcoholic beverages by humans can result in alcohol concentrations of over 5% in the lumen of the jejunum (10). This is much higher than the concentrations of alcohol found in the blood and in the lumen of the ileum after the same dose. Concentrations of the order of 1% or higher are well known from in vitro studies to be enough to inhibit a variety of mucosal transport enzymes.

The importance of this local action of alcohol within the upper small intestine has been confirmed in studies of the absorption of xylose (8). Xylose is not utilized metabolically, and the amount excreted in the urine provides a direct measure of the amount absorbed from the intestine. An oral dose of alcohol produced a significant fall in the urinary excretion of xylose, whereas the same dose of alcohol given intravenously failed to do so. This indicates clearly that the higher concentration of alcohol achieved within the jejunum is necessary for the inhibition, while the lower concentration produced by dilution of the absorbed alcohol throughout the body fluids failed to inhibit the absorption of xylose. In a similar manner, the absorption of vitamin B_{12} (cyanocobalamin) can be studied by measuring the urinary excretion of ^{57}Co after oral administration of vitamin B_{12} labelled with ^{57}Co. In three out of five subjects receiving 46% of their calories as alcohol, the excretion of ^{57}Co was reduced, as it was in five out of five receiving 60–65% of their calories as alcohol (11).

Over 20 years ago it was reported (12) that ethanol in concentrations of 0.2% or higher produced a significant inhibition of the activity of Na,K-ATPase in brain, muscle, and red blood cell plasma membranes. Later, this was shown to be true also of the Na,K-ATPase in the jejunal mucosa (13). Increasing concentrations of ethanol produced progressively greater degrees of inhibition, and 1.0 M ethanol (4.6% w/v) reduced the activity to only 20% of normal. The role of the Na,K-ATPase is to utilize metabolic energy from the splitting of ATP to pump sodium out of the cell and potassium into it. This maintains the high sodium concentration gradient from the outside to the inside of the cell and thus facilitates the movement of sodium into the cell by carrier-assisted diffusion. The same carrier forms mixed complexes with sodium and thiamine, amino acids, or various sugars. Thus the continued activity of the Na,K-ATPase is necessary to promote the entry into the cell of thiamine, amino acids, and sugars in addition to sodium. Therefore, the inhibition by ethanol of the Na,K-ATPase activity results not only in decreased sodium transport but also decreased thiamine uptake into the jejunal mucosa (7,14).

The same is true of amino acid uptake, which is also inhibited by ethanol for the same reason. This was demonstrated by addition in vitro of alcohol solutions to the incubation medium in which amino acid uptake was being studied in isolated sacs of rat small intestine (15). The same investigators then showed that a dose of alcohol given in vivo to the rat by stomach tube reduced the absorption of isotopically-labelled phenylalanine that had also been given by stomach tube. The effect of alcohol was obvious with the natural L-isomer, but was not seen with the unnatural D-isomer. This supports the interpretation that the effect of alcohol was exerted upon a specific carrier mechanism. This was later confirmed in humans (16) in whom an oral dose of 40 g of ethanol, as either a 20% or 10% solution, produced alcohol concentrations in the jejunum that were high enough to inhibit significantly and markedly the absorption of isotopically-labelled methionine.

A further factor contributing to the impairment of intestinal absorption by ethanol is the inhibitory effect of alcohol on gastrointestinal motility, resulting in retention of food in the stomach. In the rat, for example, the administration of a very large dose of alcohol together with ^{131}I-triolein in corn oil, or ^{51}Cr-labelled protein, resulted in a marked retention of the radioactive label within the stomach for as long as 16–24 hours, with a corresponding decrease in the amount found in the intestine or in the carcass (17). This delay in gastric emptying would not, by itself, result in malabsorption, but merely in a delay in absorption. However, if coupled with alcohol-induced impairment of transport enzyme activity, or with alcohol-induced diarrhoea, then the delay in gastric emptying could aggravate the malabsorption produced by these other effects of alcohol.

Impaired Storage after Absorption

If the hepatic storage capacity for a vitamin is reduced by alcoholic liver disease, then even if that vitamin has been adequately absorbed, it will not be retained as well in the body and more will be eliminated in the urine. Such an effect has been demonstrated in the case of vitamin A (18). The vitamin A content of the liver was markedly reduced in patients with fatty liver, alcoholic hepatitis, or cirrhosis compared with the content of normal liver. This effect was confirmed experimentally in baboons receiving a liquid diet providing a high proportion of the total calories as alcohol. The vitamin A content of the liver was reduced progressively more, the longer the period of alcohol feeding.

Impaired Activation of Vitamins

As noted above, many vitamins must be metabolically activated in the liver or other tissues before they can play their required metabolic role. Some of these activation reactions can be inhibited by ethanol or by acetaldehyde produced by the oxidation of ethanol. For example, pyridoxine is phosphorylated by ATP and a pyridoxine kinase to yield pyridoxine phosphate, which in turn is oxidized by a pyridoxine phosphate oxidase to yield pyridoxal-5-phosphate. This latter oxidation step uses flavin mononucleotide, produced from riboflavin, as a cofactor. Thus, the activation of one vitamin may depend upon the function of another vitamin. Since alcohol can impair the absorption of riboflavin, and since acetaldehyde produced from alcohol can directly inhibit the pyridoxine kinase, the net effect of alcohol is to produce a marked reduction in the yield of pyridoxal-5-phosphate from pyridoxine (19). In addition, the pyridoxal-5-phosphate is carried in the plasma as a complex with serum albumin, which delivers it to its sites of action in the peripheral tissues. If alcoholic liver disease results in a reduction in serum albumin, this is another factor which can reduce the ultimate metabolic efficacy of the ingested pyridoxine. Finally, acetaldehyde also stimulates a phosphatase that degrades the pyridoxal-5-phosphate and yields free pyridoxal, which is oxidized and then excreted in the urine. Thus, there are at least four different mechanisms by which alcohol can impair the activation and utilization of pyridoxine (19).

Another example is that of vitamin A. The alcoholic form, retinol, is oxidized to the aldehyde form, retinal, which is the active form in the retina, and to retinoic acid, which is active in other tissues of the body. The oxidation is catalysed by alcohol dehydrogenase (ADH), which is the same enzyme that oxidizes ethanol to acetaldehyde. The affinity of ethanol for the ADH is much greater than that of retinol, so that in the presence of alcohol the activation of retinol to retinal is markedly reduced (19).

Impaired Tissue Utilization

There are numerous examples of impairment by alcohol of the uptake and utilization in peripheral tissues of essential nutrients which have been already absorbed. For example, the plasma and hepatic concentrations of α-amino-isobutyrate are increased markedly in animals consuming alcohol, compared to the levels in pair-fed controls. This is thought to be due to a decrease in the peripheral tissue uptake of this amino acid. The branched-chain amino acids leucine and isoleucine are affected in the same way. The magnitude of the increase of plasma and liver concentrations is proportional to the duration and magnitude of alcohol intake (20).

The same applies to the uptake of thiamine into the brain. This uptake, like the absorption in the jejunal mucosa, is also linked to the function of the Na,K-ATPase, and is correspondingly inhibited by alcohol. Since the alcohol inhibition applies only to the active transport of thiamine by the carrier mechanism, it does not affect the passive diffusion of thiamine through the cell membrane, which depends only upon its lipid:water partition coefficient. Inside the cell, thiamine is converted to thiamine pyrophosphate (TPP) by a phosphorylation reaction utilizing ATP. This reaction can also be inhibited by alcohol. Moreover, there can be genetic variation in enzymes that utilize TPP as a co-factor. For example, the enzyme transketolase exists in a normal form and a variant form with a very low affinity for TPP. It has been suggested that patients having this abnormal form may have a genetic predisposition towards alcohol-induced thiamine deficiency, since the impaired binding of TPP to the enzyme would aggravate any of the effects of alcohol on the intestinal absorption, brain uptake, and phosphorylation of the thiamine (7).

These various possibilities can be differentiated by an in vitro test of the transketolase activity of red blood cells, incubated in the presence and absence of TPP added in vitro. In normal red cells containing the full normal amount of TPP, the addition of extra TPP does not affect the transketolase activity. In contrast, cells from a thiamine-deficient individual will show a decrease in transketolase activity, which is restored to normal levels by the addition of TPP in vitro. If the patient has an impairment of phosphorylation of thiamine, then the low transketolase activity will not be improved by administration of thiamine hydrochloride to the patient, but will be raised to normal levels by giving the patient an injection of TPP. Finally, if the enzyme is the genetic variant which has a very low affinity for TPP, then the addition of TPP in vitro will have little effect upon the low activity level unless a very high concentration of TPP is added. It has been proposed that this test can be used as a clinical diagnostic procedure (19).

As noted above, riboflavin also shows impaired activity in many chronic alcoholics. The deficiency is a composite result, again, of impaired absorption, impaired storage, and impaired phosphorylation to the co-factor flavin adenine dinucleotide (FAD). It has also been proposed that the riboflavin deficiency may be a relative one because in the alcoholic the total metabolic need for riboflavin may be increased, and thus the consequences of a minor deficiency in the diet may be exaggerated. This suggestion is interesting, but so far there is no strong evidence to prove it, and it is not clear why the metabolic requirement for riboflavin specifically would be raised.

Increased Excretion

A major factor in ethanol-induced deficiencies of zinc, magnesium, and potassium is the impairment by alcohol of the renal tubular reabsorptive capacity for these ions (21–23). It seems probable that this represents a direct local action of alcohol on the reabsorptive mechanisms for these ions, but the picture has not been as completely worked out as it has for some of the other deficiencies noted above. The deficiency of zinc and magnesium in alcoholics may be important in some of the alcohol-related functional and pathological disturbances, such as the fetal alcohol syndrome, the severe forms of alcohol withdrawal syndrome, and other types of tissue disturbance.

Interaction between Dietary Deficiency and Direct Effects of Ethanol

There is considerable evidence that the impairment of intestinal absorption of folic acid, noted above in alcoholics, depends not only upon the direct action of alcohol but also upon the effects of dietary folate deficiency. It has been observed, for example, that alcoholics admitted to hospital after being on a poor diet for some period of time had reduced intestinal absorption of folate, while those who were admitted with comparable degrees of alcoholism but with a history of good dietary intake did not show impaired folate absorption (24). After being on a good diet in hospital, providing ample dietary folate, all patients showed normal folate uptake after a period of abstinence. When they were then permitted to resume alcohol drinking but were kept on the good diet, they did not show a return to poor absorption of folate.

This has been confirmed experimentally. Subjects who were placed on a low-folate diet and were given 200 g of ethanol daily (625 ml of distilled spirits) developed marked impairment of the intestinal absorption of folate, glucose, sodium, and water. When the diet was supplemented with high doses of folate, their absorption of all of these nutrients returned to normal despite continued intake of the same amount of alcohol (8). However, an important observation is that while these changes were true of the group of subjects as a whole, there were individual exceptions to these trends. For example, in one such study of jejunal uptake of folic acid, all the subjects in the group showed an improvement of uptake after a two-week period of abstinence from alcohol. However, when alcohol feeding was resumed together with a good hospital diet, four subjects showed continued improvement in folate absorption, but two showed a renewed decrease in absorption. Similar findings were obtained in a study of changes in the absorption of D-xylose in alcoholic patients following admission to the hospital, with institution of a normal diet but continued ingestion of alcohol in doses of 190–256 g/day (8). In that experiment, nine subjects showed continued marked improvement in xylose absorption despite the alcohol, but two failed to improve. Similarly, fecal excretion of fat, which had been elevated in alcoholic patients on admission to the hospital (presumably because of deficiency of pancreatic or intestinal lipase activity), was reduced to normal levels following the institution of a normal diet and abstinence from alcohol in the hospital. When the same diet was continued but alcohol administration was resumed at a daily dose of 256 g, the fecal fat levels nevertheless fell in seven patients but increased in one (8).

These findings are important because they indicate that while a combination of alcohol effect and poor diet may be needed to produce serious malabsorption in most patients, there are, nevertheless, some individuals with greater sensitivity to the effects of alcohol, who will show impairment of intestinal absorption of at least some nutrients by alcohol alone, even in the presence of a good diet.

The impairment of absorption of vitamin B_{12} by ethanol does not appear to require the simultaneous presence of a deficient diet. Even when patients are placed on a good diet in hospital, the reinitiation of alcohol administration almost always impairs the absorption of B_{12} (11). In the case of thiamine uptake into the brain, the interaction of diet and alcohol effect is of a somewhat different nature. As noted above, impairment of the carrier-mediated uptake of thiamine by alcohol does not apply to the thiamine uptake that occurs as a result of simple passive diffusion through the lipid membrane. While this diffusion component is normally quite small, it is proportional to the circulating concentration of thiamine because it is a first-order process. Therefore a diet rich in thiamine can offset the inhibitory effects of alcohol upon the facilitated transport mechanism by increasing markedly the uptake through passive diffusion.

Implications for the Treatment of Alcoholics

The observations noted above carry a number of implications with respect to the treatment of alcoholics showing nutritional deficiencies associated with the use of alcohol (19). The first is that the impairment of intestinal absorption by ethanol may markedly decrease the value of the water-soluble forms of vitamins which are taken up by the carrier-mediated processes. On the other hand, alcohol-induced pancreatitis, and its resultant steatorrhea, may decrease the absorption of fat-soluble vitamins. In both of these cases it may be necessary to use parenteral administration until the absorption defects have become normalized. Alcoholic liver disease, as noted above, may also decrease vitamin storage and lead to a large loss of vitamins in the urine. Therefore the patients on admission usually require considerably larger doses for the correction of their deficiency than the normal requirements for the same vitamins in the diet. Under these conditions the parenteral use of potent forms of the vitamins is best, and therapy can be changed to oral administration of lower doses later when gastrointestinal mucosal functioning has returned to normal. If activation of vitamins is impaired by alcohol, then it may be better to use the already activated forms, such as TPP instead of thiamine hydrochloride, if the activated forms are available.

Most important of all, however, is the need for the clinician to be aware of possible nutritional deficiencies even when gross nutrition, as reflected in body weight and muscle mass, appears to be normal. Finally, the alert physician should be aware of the fact that the effect of alcohol on the uptake and utilization of nutrients, like any other biological process, has a Gaussian distribution, so that some individuals are considerably more sensitive to the effects of alcohol than the norm. Therefore, an apparently normal dietary history is not necessarily a guarantee in all subjects that alcohol has not produced a significant nutritional deficiency. The clinical state of the patient, and the necessary and relevant laboratory tests, must still be assessed in each case individually in order to decide whether vigorous therapy of dietary deficiency is necessary.

REFERENCES

1 Bunout D, Gattas V, Iturriaga H, Pérez C, Pereda T, Ugarte G. Nutritional status of alcoholic patients: its possible relationship to alcoholic liver damage. *Am J Clin Nutr* 1983;38:469–473.

2 Hawkins RD, Kalant H, Khanna JM. Effects of chronic intake of ethanol on rate of ethanol metabolism. *Can J Physiol Pharmacol* 1966;44:241–257.

3 Wei P, Hamilton JR, LeBlanc AE. A clinical and metabolic study of an intravenous feeding technique using peripheral veins as the initial infusion site. *Can Med Assoc J* 1972;106:969–975.

4 Reinus JF, Heymsfeld S, Casper K, Gibbons J, Wiskind R, Galambos JT. Metabolic balance in human volunteers fed diets containing ethanol by continuous infusion through a nasogastric tube. *Hepatology* 1985;5:1033.

5 Morgan MY. Alcohol and nutrition. *Brit Med Bull* 1982;38:21–29.

6 Thomson AD, Rae SA, Majumdar SK. Malnutrition in the alcoholic. In: Clark PMS, Kricka LJ, eds. *Medical consequences of alcohol abuse*. Chichester: Ellis Horwood, 1980:103–155.

7 Thomson AD, Majumdar SK. The influence of ethanol on intestinal absorption and utilization of nutrients. In: Leevy CM, ed. *Alcohol and the GI tract*. Clinics in Gastroenterology, 1981;10:263–293.

8 Mezey E. Intestinal function in chronic alcoholism. *Ann NY Acad Sci* 1975;252:215–227.

9 Langman MJS, Bell GD. Alcohol and the gastrointestinal tract. *Brit Med Bull* 1982;38:71–75.

10 Halsted CH, Robles EA, Mezey E. Distribution of ethanol in the human gastrointestinal tract. *Am J Clin Nutr* 1973;26:831–834.

11 Lindenbaum J, Lieber CS. Effects of chronic ethanol administration on intestinal absorption in man in the absence of nutritional deficiency. *Ann NY Acad Sci* 1975;252:228–234.

12 Israel Y, Kalant H, Laufer I. Effects of ethanol on Na,K,Mg-stimulated microsomal ATPase activity. *Biochem Pharmacol* 1965;14:1803–1814.

13 Hoyumpa AM Jr, Nichols SG, Wilson FA, Schenker S. Effect of ethanol on intestinal (Na,K)ATPase and intestinal thiamine transport in rats. *J Lab Clin Med* 1977;90:1086–1095.

14 Hoyumpa AM. Alcohol and thiamine metabolism. *Alcoholism: Clin Exp Res* 1983;7:11–14.

15 Israel Y, Salazar I, Rosenmann E. Inhibitory effects of alcohol on intestinal amino acid transport in vivo and in vitro. *J Nutr* 1968;96:499–504.
16 Israel Y, Valenzuela JE, Salazar I, Ugarte G. Alcohol and amino acid transport in the human small intestine. *J Nutr* 1969;98:222–224.
17 Barboriak JJ, Meade RC. Impairment of gastrointestinal processing of fat and protein by ethanol in rats. *J Nutr* 1969;98:373–378.
18 Leo MA, Lieber CS. Interaction of ethanol with vitamin A. *Alcoholism: Clin Exp Res* 1983;7:15–21.
19 Ryle PR, Thomson AD. Nutrition and vitamins in alcoholism. In: Rosalki SB, ed. *Clinical biochemistry of alcoholism*. Edinburgh: Churchill Livingstone, 1984:188–224.
20 Shaw S, Lieber CS. Plasma amino acids in the alcoholic: nutritional aspects. *Alcoholism: Clin Exp Res* 1983;7:22–27.
21 Harris RA. Metabolism of calcium and magnesium during ethanol intoxication and withdrawal. In: Majchrowicz E, Noble EP, eds. *Biochemistry and pharmacology of ethanol*. New York: Plenum Press, 1979;2:27–41.
22 McClain CJ, Su L-C. Zinc deficiency in the alcoholic: a review. Alcoholism: *Clin Exp Res* 1983;7:5–10.
23 McIntyre N. The effects of alcohol on water, electrolytes and minerals. In: Rosalki SB, ed. *Clinical biochemistry of alcoholism*. Edinburgh: Churchill Livingstone, 1984:117–134.
24 Halsted CH, Robles EA, Mezey E. Intestinal malabsorption in folate-deficient alcoholics. *Gastroenterology* 1973;64:526–532.

ANTHONY B. HODSMAN

Diet in Relation to Osteoporosis

To understand the possible effects of nutritional status on the skeleton, it is necessary to review briefly the central features of bone physiology. Bone tissue is formed by a specialized group of cells known as osteoblasts, which synthesize and secrete an unmineralized matrix, osteoid. Shortly after its formation, osteoid is "mineralized" by the precipitation of calcium-phosphate salts (hydroxy-appatite) within the matrix. Initial or primary mineralization occurs rapidly over a few days, but the final calcified density is not achieved for several months (1). After cessation of longitudinal growth, the whole skeleton goes through a phase of "consolidation", during which gradually increasing calcification of bone takes place over the next ten years. When consolidation is complete, "peak adult bone mass" is achieved, usually by the age of 35 years. Thereafter, bone volume gradually declines throughout the rest of adult life in both men and women.

Although peak cortical bone mass may remain constant until after the menopause (2), it is likely that trabecular bone loss begins in women before the menopause, perhaps soon after the achievement of peak adult bone mass (3). In the peri-menopausal period, trabecular bone loss from the vertebrae is accelerated to 2–3 times the normal rate of loss attributed to "aging". Cortical bone loss (e.g. from the wrist or femoral neck) is only slightly accelerated. This may account for the general division of involutional osteoporosis into Type I, predominantly affecting postmenopausal women in their 60s who present with vertebral fractures, and Type II patients in their 70s who present with hip fractures as a consequence of the slower cortical

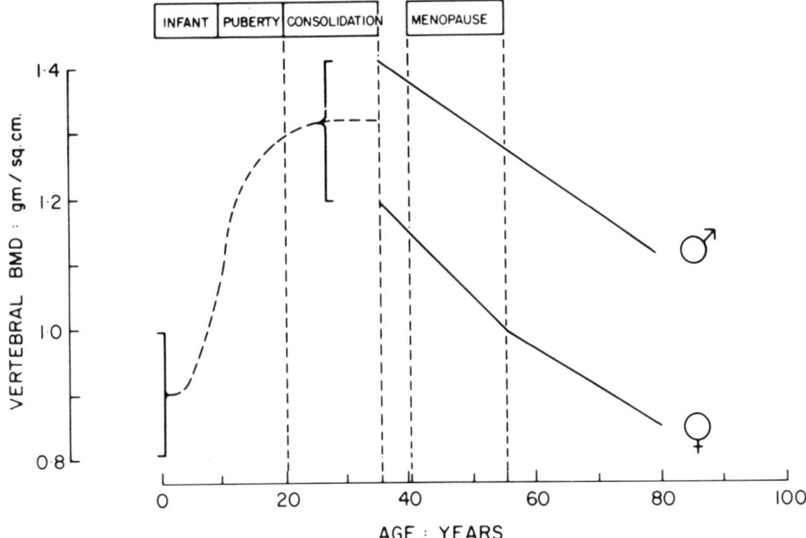

Figure 1. Diagram of "average" lumbar Bone Mineral Density (BMD); changes with age. BMD increases rapidly from birth through puberty. During "consolidation" of bone calcification Peak Adult Bone Mass is reached; this is higher for men than for women (solid lines). With age, progressive bone loss occurs, more rapidly in women during menopause (lower curve). Note that BMD for women is lower at all ages when compared to men.

bone loss. In the latter group the female:male ratio is only 2:1, compared to 3:1 in Type I patients (4).

Accompanying this age-dependent loss of bone, there is a loss of bone calcium content (commonly referred to as Bone Mineral Density, since all non-invasive measurements of bone mass depend on the detection of calcium content). For women aged 40 years or older, the steady-state decline in vertebral BMD is about 1% per year, and this accelerates with the onset of menopause, averaging 2–3% annually during the postmenopausal decade. These changes are shown diagrammatically in Figure 1.

Although these changes are thought of in terms of a skeletal calcium loss, it is important to appreciate that the mechanisms behind it are far from simple. Throughout adult life bone tissue is continually undergoing internal turnover by a process called remodelling. The process of remodelling is the same in all bone tissue, whether it be cortical bone, which is primarily found in the tubular long bones of the appendicular skeleton, or trabecular bone that surrounds marrow spaces (found at the ends of long bones, in the vertebrae and pelvis). Remodelling occurs in discreet packets by complex cellular units known as Bone Multicellular Units (BMUs). A new BMU is initiated by the differentiation of specialized marrow cells into multinucleated osteoclasts. These cells travel through cortical bone or along trabecular bone surfaces, resorbing a discreet quantity of bone tissue. This leaves a space within the bone tissue, which is later replaced by the activity of a second group of cells (osteoblasts), which synthesize new osteoid matrix. When this matrix is eventually mineralized, the original BMU has been replaced by newly formed "bone." The total cycle time of the BMU is about 90 days in young normal adults (5). However, with advancing age, the cycle time of a BMU may increase three-fold. Furthermore, while the activity of osteoclastic bone resorption appears to remain fairly constant, the efficiency of osteoblastic replacement of bone matrix is relatively diminished, leading to a net deficit in bone tissue/BMU cycle. Aggregated across the whole skeleton, this leads to a progressive net loss of bone volume, most correctly termed "osteopenia."

Osteoporosis

Osteoporosis is not a disease, but a syndrome that emerges as a consequence of the falling bone mass which occurs during aging. At a certain "threshold" of bone loss, the remaining bone (which is normally constituted in terms of its mineral and matrix components) becomes susceptible to pathological fractures. Since this bone loss occurs earlier in trabecular bone (e.g. the vertebrae) than in cortical bone (e.g. the femoral neck), vertebral fractures tend to occur at an average age of 65 years, and femoral neck fractures about a decade later.

The impact of osteoporosis in total health care terms should not be under-estimated. Twenty-five percent of women will have radiological evidence of vertebral fracturing by the age of 65, and many of them will be unable to carry out all their daily activities because of chronic back pain. Femoral neck fractures may be numerically less frequent, but their impact is more devastating. More than 10% of elderly patients with hip fractures may die within six months of such a fracture. In monetary terms, hospital health care costs directly related to osteoporosis amount to 3.8 billion dollars in the United States (6). There is no cure for osteoporosis at present, and even promising agents such as sodium fluoride probably do not benefit more than 30% of patients who enter a treatment program. Therefore, factors which might reduce the prevalence of osteoporosis, including nutritional considerations, are potentially of great importance.

FACTORS AFFECTING THE PREVALENCE OF OSTEOPOROSIS

For the purposes of this paper I have discussed only those factors which may slow or delay bone loss associated with aging.

Age

This is one of the most important factors. Osteoporotic compression fractures of the spine are very rare before the age of 45 and increase dramatically thereafter.

Peak Adult Bone Mass

Obviously, the more bone an individual has accumulated by the age of 35, the more he/she can afford to lose during subsequent decades without developing osteoporosis. In part, peak adult bone mass is geneticaly determined; one reason that very few black North Americans develop osteoporosis is their constitutionally larger skeletons. For similar reasons, small-boned Asian women living in North America have a correspondingly high prevalence of osteoporosis. Similar evidence can be seen within individual families, since height and skeletal mass are quite closely determined by the genes of the parents.

Endocrine Factors

Some endocrine factors, particularly in the calcium-vitamin D axis, may be related to nutritional status and will be discussed in detail below. However, the single most important endocrine factor leading to the development of osteoporosis relates to the menopause in women. At that time ovarian function ceases and the level of estrogen synthesis declines sharply. Thus, estrogen "lack" is the most important factor determining the development of osteoporosis in white women, who form over 90% of its sufferers; estrogen replacement therapy, at the time of menopause, prevents the accelerated bone loss that otherwise occurs (7). Replacement must start within five years of the cessation of menses and should be continued to at least the age of 65, since cessation of therapy at any time results in accelerated rates of bone loss. Fears that prolonged estrogen therapy might induce endometrial and breast carcinoma have largely proved unfounded. Although estrogens have also been linked to an increased incidence of coagulation abnormalities and thromboembolic phenomena in younger women taking oral contraceptives, this does not appear as a clinically important factor in older women taking estrogen supplements (8). Even with these considerations factored into the equation, risk-benefit analyses have confirmed that prolonged estrogen therapy is sufficiently safe to justify the benefits of a reduction in potential morbidity due to osteoporosis (9).

Exercise

It has long been known that total immobilization as experienced during prolonged hospitalization, or by paraplegic patients, is associated with a rapid, and only partially replaceable loss of skeletal mass. These findings have been accentuated in manned space flight programs because of the effects of weightlessness. Recently it has become apparent that athletic exercise in many forms leads to increased peak adult bone mass, and even graded exercise programs in older patients can be shown to increase BMD. The lack of exercise in our predominantly sedentary Western civilization may, therefore, be an important influence on the ultimate development of osteoporosis.

Nutrition

Although many nutritional factors have been linked to the development of osteoporosis, only the most important will be discussed in relation to calcium and vitamin D requirements, and dietary protein and phosphate intake.

OSTEOPOROSIS AND NUTRITIONAL FACTORS

Caveats

Before discussing nutritional factors and osteoporosis, a word of caution should be noted in the interpretation of available data.

Nutritional studies are not easy to do at the best of times. In order to detect significant impacts on a particular condition, it is often necessary to study very large numbers of subjects. Bone loss leading to osteoporosis is very slow. Typically these losses are associated with negative external calcium balances in the order of 50 mg/day. However, the nature and expense of dietary balance studies have usually allowed only small groups of subjects to be studied. For equally obvious reasons, the study of bone mass has been similarly hampered, because techniques for measuring bone mass must be extraordinarily precise to detect small differences within patient groups. Two to four years may be the minimum period needed to detect significant changes. Indeed, nutritional studies have generally been too short to even consider changes in skeletal BMD as an end-point for discussion.

Not surprisingly, the emergent data have been contradictory. Simple statistical considerations dictate that at least 40–50 subjects must be recruited to detect differences in bone mass across time between one intervention and another (10), imposing considerable problems with experimental design. For this reason many studies have used cross-sectional techniques in "at risk" populations rather than longitudinal studies of patients who subsequently develop osteoporosis.

Even studies which evaluated bone mass in osteoporotic subjects longitudinally have generally utilized a measurement of cortical bone mass (e.g. radiogrammometric measurement of metacarpal indices, or single beam photon densitometry of the distal radius). These techniques are not very sensitive when it comes to evaluating the earliest changes in bone mass within trabecular bone (e.g. vertebral bone). Although recent techniques for measuring trabecular bone mass are now more readily available (e.g. dual beam photon densitometry and quantitative computerized tomography of the lumbar spine), they have not yet addressed the issue of nutrition and the development of osteoporosis.

CALCIUM REQUIREMENTS

The daily calcium intake necessary to maintain "neutral" external calcium balance is termed the dietary calcium requirement. Nordin has postulated that middle-aged English subjects require a minimum daily calcium intake of 500–600 mg/day (11). The recommended daily allowance (RDA) of calcium is generally defined as the amount that will prevent symptoms of overt deficiency in nearly all the healthy population (theoretically 97.5%). The RDA for calcium is much higher in adolescents (1200 mg) because of the enormous requirements of the growing skeleton. In adults the RDA is set at 800 mg, slightly more than Nordin's "minimal" estimate (12).

However, calcium requirements in aging populations may greatly exceed the stated RDA. For example, by direct measurement of intestinal (jejunal) calcium transport, Ireland and Fordtram demonstrated diminishing efficiency of calcium absorption with advancing age (13). Using longitudinal and cross-sectional studies in the United States, Heaney et al. (14) have demonstrated that peri-menopausal women are in a negative external calcium balance of approximately 30 mg/day, at a self-chosen dietary calcium intake of about 660 mg/day; by regression analysis they calculated that average calcium requirements in elderly women should more realistically be set at 1200–1500 mg/day. If the usual allowance of two standard deviations is applied to the higher figure, then the RDA for post-menopausal women may be as high as 1925 mg/day – a figure almost impossible to meet through dietary habits.

From Canadian statistics, women in their 60's ingest an average intake of 600–800 mg calcium/day and thus fall well below these modified recommendations for calcium intake. In practice, the actual dietary intake available to a person consuming neither milk nor dairy products averages 400 mg/day. Most of the additional calcium intake would have to be supplied from dairy products or calcium supplements in the form of pills. Milk in its various forms supplies approximately 300 mg of elemental calcium/250 ml serving, with cheese being an equally appropriate source (15). From most dietary surveys, it is clear that elderly patients do not have a natural taste for dairy products; although the data are controversial, one possible explanation for this finding is the increasing prevalence of intestinal lactase deficiency that occurs with age, resulting in milk-intolerance (16).

Calcium deficiency, hormonal balance, and osteoporosis

While there is no dispute about the declining efficiency of calcium absorption with age, several hypotheses have been put forward to explain this. Under the first hypothesis, some authors suggest a deficiency in the renal synthesis of calcitriol brought about by age-related decreases in renal function, coupled perhaps to estrogen deficiency. Because calcitriol ($1,25(OH)_2$ vitamin D) is the most active hormone regulating dietary calcium absorption, this deficiency would lead to a tendency for hypocalcaemia stimulating a reactive increase in parathyroid hormone (PTH) secretion. The increased action of PTH on bone resorption would then lead to the eventual development of osteoporosis. Under a second hypothesis, there might be an imbalance between bone resorption and bone formation, perhaps because estrogen deficiency leads to enhanced sensitivity of bone to PTH-mediated bone resorption. As a result of enhanced bone resorption, serum calcium levels would tend to rise, leading to suppression of PTH levels, suppression of PTH-modulated renal conversion of 25-OH vitamin D to calcitriol, and resulting in a secondary reduction of dietary calcium absorption.

Both hypotheses explain the reduced intestinal absorption of dietary calcium, and increased bone loss leading to osteoporosis, but both also require the demonstration that serum levels of calcitriol are decreased in the elderly osteoporotic population. Moreover, the first hypothesis implies an increase in circulating PTH levels, and the second a decrease. Unfortunately, circulating levels of calcitriol and PTH in osteoporotic patients have been variously reported to be high, normal, or low (12,17,18), so that these biochemical hypotheses remain controversial. Schematic diagrams outlining these theories are shown in Figure 2. Furthermore, bone histomorphometric studies in patients with established osteoporosis generally show a dramatic reduction in bone turnover and bone resorption surfaces (irrespective of circulating PTH). Indeed, it is possible that bone tissue becomes resistant to the actions of circulating PTH during the aging process, leading to further difficulties in accepting either of the two hypotheses outlined above.

Dietary calcium intake and bone mass

As detailed in the foregoing arguments, suggested dietary calcium intake should approximate at least 1000 mg or more of elemental calcium/day to achieve "neutral" external calcium balance. If this condition is not met, numerous "secondary" endocrine factors might come into play to promote accelerated bone loss. Moreover, osteoporotic patients appear to have "undercalcified" bone (19), which can be improved by oral calcium supplements. Thus, it appears that there are cogent arguments to advocate dietary calcium supplementation for North American women. Have these arguments stood the test of time?

There are intriguing data about the importance of dietary calcium intake in young adults (aged 15–35 years) who are undergoing rapid skeletal growth, and subsequently "consolidation" of bone mineralization. Although often quoted as an argument to supplement calcium

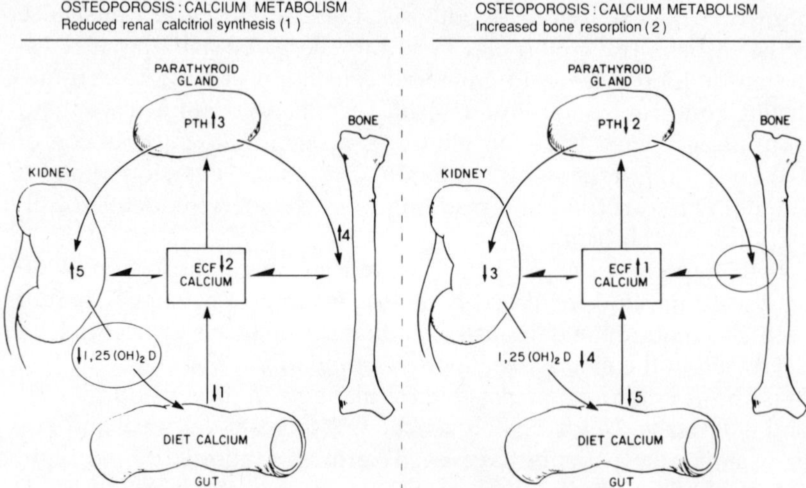

Figure 2. Theoretical endocrine mechanisms leading to Osteoporosis, based upon accepted concepts of the Calcium-Endocrine Axis.
Theory 1 (reduced renal calcitriol synthesis): There is a primary failure in renal production of calcitriol (1,25$(OH)_{2D}$). The resulting impairment of dietary calcium absorption (1) then leads to relative hypocalcemia (2), resulting in excess PTH secretion (3), increased PTH-mediated bone resorption (4), and osteoporosis. Increased PTH secretion would be a compensatory mechanism attempting to increase renal synthesis of calcitriol from circulating vitamin D stores (5).
Theory 2 (increased bone resorption): As a result of estrogen deficiency during menopause there is a primary imbalance between bone resorption and formation, such that resorption predominates; excessive release of bone calcium tends to increase serum calcium (1) which, in turn, reduces PTH secretion (2), leading to decreased renal production (3) of calcitriol (4) from circulating vitamin D stores. This results in reduced intestinal resorption of dietary calcium (5).
Both theories imply reduced dietary calcium absorption. However, the evidence for additional changes in the Calcium-Endocrine Axis in osteoporosis are controversial (see text).

intake in the elderly, the studies of Matkovik et al. (20) argue instead for an adequate calcium intake in young adults. In this widely reported study of Yugoslavians from two districts having a marked disparity between calcium intake (approximately 500 mg vs 1000 mg), the incidence of fractures in both wrists and femoral necks was much higher in the population living in a low-calcium district. The authors pointed out that the main determinant of cortical bone mass in the elderly seems to have been predicated by the prolonged early calcium deficiency seen in the low-calcium district. Other studies in North America have suggested that both cortical and trabecular bone mass in later life may be determined by the level of dietary calcium intake in the third and fourth decade (21,22) and suggest that a dietary intake in excess of one gm/day is optimal. Indeed, from dietary survey data cited by Marcus, it is apparent that North Americans have a dietary calcium intake well below the RDA from age ten onwards, *particularly* during adolescence (23). The most important impact of this would lead to a lower "peak adult" bone mass. This would predispose young adults to the earlier development of osteoporosis in later life.

However, it has become axiomatic that elderly patients with established osteoporosis benefit from large doses of calcium supplementation. The reasons behind this have been cited from a number of uncontrolled trials (6,24). In the study by Riggs et al. there was an apparent reduction in vertebral fracture rates in patients treated with calcium supplements as compared to untreated patients (24). However, the relationship between *current* dietary calcium intake and bone mass is tenuous at best (12). Although controlled prospective clinical trials have demonstrated that calcium supplements alone do not prevent bone loss in either osteoporotic or non-osteoporotic, middle-aged/elderly patients (25–28), concurrent low-dose estrogen therapy may enhance the ability of a high-dietary calcium intake to blunt post-menopausal bone loss (14).

Comment

A review of the literature shows that there are good reasons to believe that dietary calcium intake may influence bone mass, but the most important influence may occur during earlier decades before peak adult bone mass has been achieved. During middle age and later decades self-chosen dietary calcium intake may not be an important factor in the development of osteoporosis, even though there are good theoretical grounds for believing that it should. There is no sound prospective evidence that increasing dietary intake in elderly patients prevents or retards the development of osteoporosis. Although seemingly without risk (12), calcium supplements are not without cost. As a general recommendation, calcium supplementation in the middle-aged North American female population may be premature.

NUTRITIONAL VITAMIN D SOURCES AND OSTEOPOROSIS

Vitamin D is not a true "vitamin," since it can be synthesized in the skin by ultraviolet (sunlight) irradiation of 7-dehydrocholesterol leading to the formation of cholecalciferol (vitamin D_3). In North America our diet is fortified by a semisynthetic compounds, ergocalciferol (vitamin D_2), which is added to all dairy products, particularly milk, cheese, and butter. Vitamin D (either cholecalciferol or ergocalciferol) is first converted to 25-OH vitamin D by the liver, and this metabolite is further converted in the kidney to the active compound, 1,25-OH vitamin D (calcitriol). Although calcitriol is currently assumed to perform all of the major physiological actions of vitamin D, *nutritional* vitamin D status is most accurately reflected by measurement of the intermediate hepatic metabolite, 25-OH vitamin D. Vitamin D deficiency, from whatever cause, leads to impaired intestinal calcium absorption and hypocalcaemia. In its severest form, this leads to osteomalacia, whereby osteoid matrix is inadequately mineralized and leads to bone pain and fractures. Osteomalacia is very uncommon in North America and is quite distinct from osteoporosis; this form of bone disease can easily be distinguished by bone biopsy criteria.

However, mild vitamin D deficiency can be compensated for, because the resultant hypocalcaemia leads to chronic increases in parathyroid hormone secretion. Under these circumstances there may be a preferential loss of cortical bone which, in the elderly, leads to an increase in fractures primarily associated with cortical bones (e.g. femoral neck fractures) (29).

In North America, there are probably four times as many sources of dietary vitamin D as in the United Kingdom. Thus, in the elderly population, dietary vitamin D might be more important than ultraviolet irradiation of the skin, because of the frequent coexistence of chronic illness, confinement indoors, and perhaps impaired metabolism of vitamin D intermediates by the kidney (30).

The interrelationships between vitamin D and osteoporosis remain unclear, especially in North American populations where controlled clinical studies have not been performed. While patients in Europe appear to be at risk of developing overt vitamin D deficiency and osteomalacia, and may be at risk of developing osteoporotic fractures through the femoral neck, there is no existing evidence that North American patients actually suffer from vitamin D deficiency (31). Although therapy of osteoporosis patients with vitamin D supplements would theoretically enhance intestinal calcium absorption, it is significant that the study by Riggs et al. (24) showed no beneficial effects on fracture rates when osteoporotic patients were treated with vitamin D as well as a number of other therapeutic agents, including calcium, estrogens, and fluoride.

Comment

While Parfitt has suggested that the probable daily needs for vitamin D may increase in the elderly from an RDA of 400 U/day to 600–800 U/day, there is little evidence in North America to support the hypothesis that subclinical vitamin D deficiency leads to osteoporosis, and no evidence to support its use in the treatment of established osteoporosis (29,30).

DIETARY PROTEIN AND PHOSPHATE

Phosphate is primarily an intracellular mineral, found in high concentrations in protein-rich foods. Nutritional changes in phosphate intake usually parallel a corresponding change in dietary protein. There are theoretical reasons for considering that high protein diets lead to osteoporosis. The sulfur-containing amino acids contained in most natural proteins are metabolized to acidic residues essentially equivalent to a net gain of total body H_2SO_4. This potential metabolic acidosis would bring in the buffering capacity of bone calcium carbonate, liberating bone calcium, and resulting in hypercalciuria. This would lead, in turn, to osteoporosis. High phosphate diets also lead to a decrease in serum calcium and secondary increase in circulating parathyroid hormone. Secondary hyperparathyroidism might also lead to osteoporosis (see above). However, high PTH levels tend to cause a relative reduction in urinary calcium output because of a physiologic role of parathyroid hormone causing renal retention of calcium. Thus, the combined effects of high protein/high phosphate diets seem to have opposing effects on urinary calcium excretion, but similar effects upon bone loss.

The concurrence of increasing dietary phosphate as protein intake increases has led to a number of attempts to separate these two factors by dietary manipulations (for review see Marcus (17)). It seems clear that high protein diets do lead to hypercalciuria, so that roughly doubling the dietary protein intake leads to a 50% increase in urinary calcium excretion. Populations ingesting very high protein intakes (200–400 gm/day) have a lower BMD than would be expected (32). Although high phosphate diets lead to biochemical evidence of increased parathyroid hormone secretion in the short term, long-term phosphate supplementation (e.g. prescribed for patients with renal calculi) does not confirm this (33). Moreover, dietary balance studies, in which protein and phosphate intakes are increased proportionately, do not confirm that long-term urinary calcium hyper-excretion occurs, suggesting that the effects of these diets upon bone dissolution might be cancelled out (17,34). However, it is significant that all dietary studies performed to date have been of relatively short duration (less than one year), and few of them have studied skeletal BMD concurrently.

Comment

The principal objections to evaluating the effects of high dietary phosphate and protein intakes in the genesis of osteoporosis are several: 1. many of the experiments have been performed in animals, usually rodents, in which bone metabolism is considered to be very different from that leading to the osteoporotic syndrome in elderly humans; 2. studies in humans have often used non-physiological synthetic diets in order to vary the phosphate and protein intake independently; or 3. have utilized very unrealistic protein loads (in excess of 100 gm/day), that are never consumed for long periods by large sections of the population; 4. many studies have used young male volunteers, who are almost certainly not reflective of the predominantly elderly female population who go on to develop the osteoporotic syndrome in later life. It is, therefore, difficult to relate the data from experiments, however well-conducted, to the ultimate development of accelerated bone loss and the development of osteoporosis in the particular segment of the population at risk. Although studies so far conducted in humans are important, none of the theories regarding protein and phosphate intake have been put to the test in prospective, longitudinal, controlled clinical trials. Given the immense difficulties in conducting such studies, it is quite possible that they will never be done.

Conclusion

The osteoporotic syndrome is so common in the aging population that it should not be regarded as a disease. Whether it is simply a phenomenon of senescence, or whether there is a distinct subgroup of female patients who lose bone mass faster than their peers, remains to be proven. However, it is clear that the factors leading to osteoporosis are multiple, and there is no convincing evidence that nutritional factors play a predominent role in the development of this syndrome. Given that the endocrine mechanisms leading to accelerated bone loss (apart from the occurrence of estrogen "lack" during menopause) are so controversial, the role of calcium deficency in leading to osteoporosis and calcium supplementation should be viewed as an open question.

REFERENCES

1 Parfitt AM. The physiologic and clinical significance of bone histomorphometric data. In: Recker RR, ed. *Bone histomorphometry: techniques and interpretation*. Boca Raton FL: CRC Press, 1983:143–224.

2 Meema HE, Bunker ML, Meema S. Loss of compact bone due to menopause. *Obstet Gynecol* 1965;26:333–343.

3 Riggs BL, Wahner HW, Seeman E, et al. Changes in bone mineral density of the proximal femur and spine with aging: differences between the post-menopausal and senile osteoporosis syndrome. *J Clin Invest* 1982;70:716–723.

4 Peck, WA, Riggs BL, Bell NH, eds. *Physicians' resource manual on osteoporosis: a decision making guide*. National Osteoporosis Foundation, 1987.

5 Ericson EF. Normal and pathological remodelling of human trabecular bone: three dimensional reconstruction of the remodelling sequence in normal and in metabolic bone disease. *Endocrinol Rev* 1986;7:379–408.

6 NIH Consensus Conference. Osteoporosis. *JAMA*, 1984; 252:799–802.

7 Lindsay R, Aitken JM, Anderson JB, Hart DM, MacDonald EB, Clarke GC. Long-term prevention of postmenopausal osteoporosis. *Lancet* 1976;1:1038–1041.

8 Nachtigall LE, Nachtigall RH, Nachtigall RD, Beckman EM. Estrogen replacement therapy II: a prospective study in relationship to carcinoma and cardiovascular and metabolic problems. *Obstet Gynecol* 1979;54:74–79.

9 Weinstein MC. Estrogen use in postmenopausal women – costs, risks, and benefits. *N Engl J Med* 1980;303:308–316.

10 Kanis JA. Treatment of osteoporotic fracture. *Lancet* 1984;1:27–33.

11 Nordin BEC, ed. *Calcium, phosphate and magnesium metabolism*. New York, NY: Churchill Livingstone, 1976.

12 Heaney RP, Gallagher JC, Johnston CC, Neer R, Parfitt AM, Whedon GD. Calcium nutrition and bone health in the elderly. *Am J Clin Nut* 1982;36:986–1013.

13 Ireland P, Fordtram JS. Effect of dietary calcium and age on jejunal calcium absorption in humans studied by intestinal perfusion. *J Clin Invest* 1973;52:2672–2681.

14 Heaney RP, Recker RR, Saville PD. Calcium balance and calcium requirements in middle-aged women. *Am J Clin Nut* 1977;30:1603–1611.

15 *A nutrient value of some common foods*. Health and Welfare, Canada, 1979.
16 Newcomer AD, Hodgson SF, McGill DB, et al. Lactase deficiency: prevalence in osteoporosis. *Ann Int Med* 1978;89:218–220.
17 Marcus R. The relationship of dietary calcium to the maintenance of skeletal integrity in man – an interface of endocrinology and nutrition. *Metabolism* 1982;31:93–102.
18 Riggs BL. Osteoporosis – a disease of impaired homeostatic regulation? *Min Electrol Metab* 1981;5:265–272.
19 Burnell JM, Baylink DJ, Chesnut CH, et al. The role of skeletal calcium deficiency in postmenopausal osteoporosis. *Calcif Tissue Int* 1986;38:187–192.
20 Matkovik V, Kostial K, Simonovic I, et al. Bone status and fracture rates in two regions of Yugoslavia. *Am J Clin Nutr* 1979;32:540–549.
21 Sandler RB, Slemenda CW, La Porte RE, et al. Postmenopausal bone density and milk consumption in childhood and adolescence. *Am J Clin Nutr* 1985;42:270–274.
22 Picard D, Ste-Marie L-G, Carrier L, et al. Influence of calcium intake during early adulthood on bone mineral content in premenopausal women. In: *Proc. IX Int Conf on Calcium Regulating Hormones, Nice, France, 1986*. Amsterdam: Excerpta Medica, 1987, 000–000.
23 Marcus R. Calcium intake and skeletal integrity: is there a critical relationship? *J Nutr* 1987;117:631–635.
24 Riggs BL, Seeman E, Hodgson SF, et al. Effects of the fluoride/calcium regimen on vertebral fracture occurrence in postmenopausal osteoporosis. *N Engl J Med* 1982;306:446–450.
25 Martin AD, Houston CS. Osteoporosis, calcium and physical activity. *CMAJ* 1987;136:587–593.
26 Nilas L, Christiansen C, Rodbro P. Calcium supplementation and postmenopausal bone loss. *Br Med J* 1984;289:1103–1106.
27 Ettinger B, Genant HK, Cann CE. Postmenopausal bone loss is prevented by treatment with low dose estrogen with calcium. *Ann Int Med* 1987;106:40–45.
28 Riis B, Thomsen K, Christiansen C. Does calcium supplementation prevent postmenopausal bone loss? A double-blind, controlled clinical study. *N Engl J Med* 1987;316:173–177.
29 Parfitt AM. Dietary risk factors for age-related bone loss and fractures. *Lancet* 1983;2:1181–1184.
30 Parfitt AM, Gallagher JC, Heaney RP, et al. Vitamin D and bone health in the elderly. *Am J Clin Nutr* 1982;36:1014–1031.
31 Riggs BL, Melton LJ. Involutional osteoporosis. *N Engl J Med* 1986;314:1676–1686.

32 Mazess RB, Mather W. Bone mineral content of North Alaskan Eskimos. *Am J Clin Nutr* 1974;27:916–925.
33 Smith LH, Thomas WC, Arnaud CD. Orthophosphate therapy in calcium renal lithiasis. In: *Urinary calculi. Int. Symp. Renal Stone Res., Madrid, 1972*. Basel: Karger, 1973:188–197.
34 Spencer H, Kramer L, DeBartolo M, Norris C, Osis D. Further studies of the effect of a high protein diet as meat on calcium metabolism. *Am J Clin Nutr* 1983;37:924–929.

Diet and Cancer

TAKASHI SUGIMURA*, KEIJI WAKABAYASHI, MINAKO NAGAO, AND HIROKO OHGAKI

Mutagens and Carcinogens Formed during Cooking

Nutrition and diet are closely related to cancer development in human beings (1,2). For instance, intake of high levels of calories and fat is related to high incidence of cancers in the colon and breast in humans. In addition, a high intake of protein is also claimed to be related to high incidences of cancers in certain organs like the urinary bladder. Minor elements such as vitamins and selenium are also related to human carcinogenesis, and a high daily intake of salt is generally thought to enhance stomach carcinogenesis. Nitrite and nitrate intakes are closely related to in vivo production of carcinogenic nitrosamine and nitrosamide compounds. Moreover, non-nutritional components such as fibre are important factors in suppressing the incidence of colon cancer. All these relations are described in detail in this volume of the proceedings of the Symposium.

Aromatic hydrocarbons produced by heating, nitrosamines and their precursors, aflatoxin B_1 produced by mould, and other naturally occurring substances including cycasin in cycad nuts, ptaquiloside (aquilide A) in bracken fern, and pyrrolizidine alkaloids in some edible plants have been shown to be mutagens/carcinogens in food (3,4).

In this chapter, newly discovered heterocyclic amines, which are produced by cooking fish and meat, are introduced. These compounds are mutagenic to *Salmonella typhimurium* TA98 and TA100 with a metabolic activation system. They are also mutagenic and clastogenic towards cultured mammalian cells. Moreover, in long-term animal carcinogenesis experiments, all of these compounds so far tested were carcinogenic (5–7). Since this new class of mutagens and car-

Table 1
Chemical Names, Abbreviations, Sources, and References of Newly Isolated Heterocyclic Amines.

Number in Fig. 1	*Chemical name*	*Abbreviation*	*Source*	*Reference*
I	2-Amino-3-methylimidazo-[4,5-*f*]quinoline	IQ	Broiled sun-dried sardine	17
II	2-Amino-3,4-dimethyl-imidazo[4,5-*f*]quinoline	MeIQ	Broiled sun-dried sardine	18
III	2-Amino-3,8-dimethyl-imidazo[4,5-*f*]quinoxaline	MeIQx	Fried beef	19
IV	2-Amino-1-methyl-6-phenyl-imidazo[4,5-*b*]-pyridine	PhIP	Fried beef	20
V	2-Amino-3,4,8-trimethyl-imidazo[4,5-*f*]quinoxaline	4,8-DiMeIQx	Heated mixture of creatinine, threonine and glucose	21
VI	2-Amino-3,7,8-trimethyl-imidazo[4,5-*f*]quinoxaline	7,8-DiMeIQx	Heated mixture of creatinine, glycine and glucose	22
VII	3-Amino-1,4-dimethyl-5*H*-pyrido[4,3-*b*]indole	Trp-P-1	Tryptophan pyrolysate	23
VIII	3-Amino-1-methyl-5*H*-pyrido[4,3 *b*]indole	Trp-P-2	Tryptophan pyrolysate	23
IX	2-Amino-6-methyldipyrido-[1,2-*a*:3′,2′-*d*]imidazole	Glu-P-1	Glutamic acid pyrolysate	24
X	2-Aminodipyrido[1,2-*a*: 3′,2′-*d*]imidazole	Glu-P-2	Glutamic acid pyrolysate	24
XI	2-Amino-5-phenylpyridine	Phe-P-1	Phenylalanine pyrolysate	23
XII	4-Amino-6-methyl-1*H*-2,5,10,10b-tetraaza-fluoranthene	Orn-P-1	Ornithine pyrolysate	25
XIII	2-Amino-9*H*-pyrido[2,3-*b*]-indole	AαC	Soybean globulin pyrolysate	26
XIV	2-Amino-3-methyl-9*H*-pyrido[2,3-*b*]indole	MeAαC	Soybean globulin pyrolysate	26

cinogens is present in our daily food and these heterocyclic amines are produced during cooking, their formation cannot be completely prevented. Although the actual daily intakes of these compounds are much lower than the doses causing cancer in experimental animals given diets containing each compound singly, the risk of cancer development in humans by these compounds should be considered more carefully. The estimation of this risk and practical measures to control exposure of humans to these mutagens, carcinogens, and tumour promoters will be described in connection with other suitable measures for prevention of cancer.

Historical Background of Studies on Mutagenic and Carcinogenic Heterocyclic Amines in Cooked Food

In the early 1970s, the mutagenicities of typical carcinogens were first demonstrated by Ames's group in California and by us in Tokyo (8,9). Two main factors were responsible for rapid development of studies: the concept of metabolic activation, developed by Miller and Miller, Gelboin and many others (10,11); and the use of *Salmonella typhimurium* strains for mutation assay, developed mainly by Ames et al. (12). Since cigarette tar contains a variety of mutagenic and carcinogenic compounds, it is not surprising that charred parts of cooked food also contain mutagenic and carcinogenic compounds. However, curiously enough, few scientists tried to find mutagens and carcinogens in foods, although there were a limited number of reports on this subject, including a paper on the presence of aromatic hydrocarbons in broiled meat and coffee beans (13,14). Moreover, it was very difficult to find new, unknown carcinogens in cooked foods, because animal experiments for carcinogenicity may take as long as two years, and examination of many specimens in such experiments is not practically possible. In contrast with animal experiments, mutation tests on microbes take only a few days and are suitable for screening large numbers of samples obtained by fractionation of crude food stuffs. Using this test, we found high mutagenicity in the smoke produced by broiling dried fish (15,16), which we collected as a tar on a glass-fibre filter. We also detected mutagenicity in methanol extracts of charred parts of beef steak and broiled fish. By use of the mutation test for monitoring activity, we also succeeded in purifying mutagenic substances from charred parts of broiled fish, broiled beef and beef extract, and also from pyrolysates of amino acids and proteins. These compounds were identified and their organic syntheses provided sufficient amounts for use in long-term animal experiments.

Properties of Newly Isolated Heterocyclic Amines

Up to the present, 14 heterocyclic amines have been isolated and their structures determined. IQ, MeIQ, MeIQx, and PhIP were originally

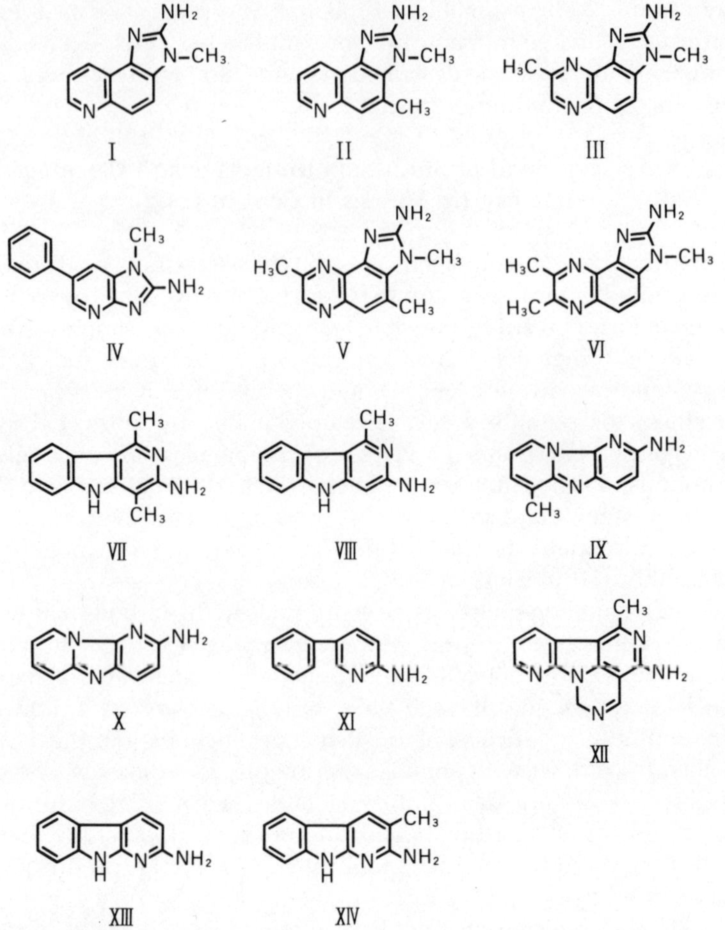

Figure 1. Structures of heterocyclic amines isolated from various pyrolysates.

isolated from cooked foods (17–20), and 4,8-DiMeIQx and 7,8-DiMeIQx were recently newly isolated together with MeIQx from a heated mixture of creatinine, amino acids, and sugars (21,22). Trp-P-1, Trp-P-2, Glu-P-1, Glu-P-2, Phe-P-1, Orn-P-1, AαC, and MeAαC were originally isolated from experimentally prepared pryolysates of amino acids or protein (23–26).

Figure 1 shows the structures of these compounds, and Table 1 lists the full chemical names, trivial abbreviations, and references to papers describing the first isolations of these compounds.

Table 2
Mutagenicities of Heterocyclic Amines and Typical Carcinogens in *Salmonella Typhimurium*

	Revertants/μg	
Compound	*TA98*	*TA100*
IQ	433,000	7,000
MeIQ	661,000	30,000
MeIQx	145,000	14,000
PhIP	1,800	120
4,8-DiMeIQx	183,000	8,000
7,8-DiMeIQx	163,000	9,900
Trp-P-1	39,000	1,700
Trp-P-2	104,200	1,800
Glu-P-1	49,000	3,200
Glu-P-2	1,900	1,200
Phe-P-1	41	23
Orn-P-1	56,800	—
AαC	300	20
MeAαC	200	120
Aflatoxin B_1	6,000	28,000
AF-2	6,500	42,000
4-Nitroquinoline 1-oxide	970	9,900
Benzo(a)pyrene	320	660
MNNG	0.00	870
N,N-Diethylnitrosamine	0.02	0.15
N,N-Dimethylnitrosamine	0.00	0.23

MNNG: *N*-Methyl-*N'*-nitro-*N*-nitrosoguanidine

These compounds are highly mutagenic towards *Salmonella typhimurium* TA98 in the presence of S9 mix (5–7). S9 mix is essential for demonstrating the mutagenicity of heterocyclic amines. Routinely, S9 mix from rats given polychlorinated biphenyls (PCB), which induces cytochrome P-450s, is used, but it can be replaced by a combination of phenobarbital and β-naphthoflavone (27). S9 mix obtained from the liver of a monkey that was not given any inducer of P-450s was effective for demonstrating the mutagenicity of heterocyclic amines (28), and S9 mix from human liver also activated heterocyclic amines efficiently (29). In Table 2, mutagenic activity is expressed as the number of revertants produced by 1 μg of substance under defined conditions. As can be seen, most of the new heterocyclic amines showed higher mutagenic activity than typical carcinogens such as aflatoxin B_1 4-nitroquinoline 1-oxide, AF-2, namely 2-(2-furyl)-3-(5-

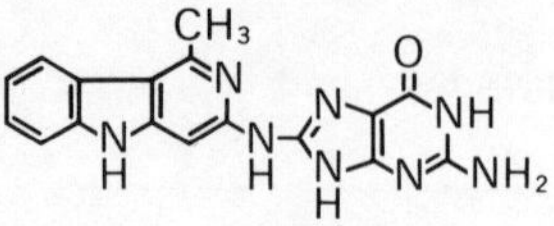

3-(C^8-guanyl)amino-1-methyl-5*H*-pyrido[4,3-*b*]indole

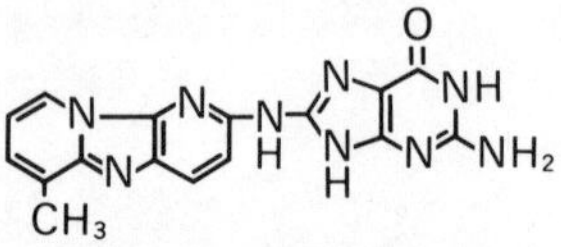

2-(C^8-guanyl)amino-6-methyldipyrido-[1,2-*a*:3′,2′-*d*]imidazole

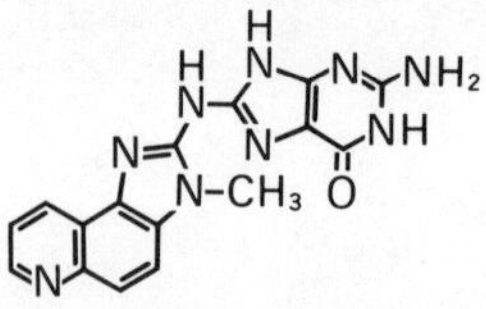

2-(C^8-guanyl)amino-3-methylimidazo-[4,5-*f*]quinoline

Figure 2. Structures of adducts of Trp-P-2, Glu-P-1, and IQ with guanine.

nitro-2-furyl)acrylamide, benzo(a)pyrene, and *N*-nitroso compounds. They showed mutagenic activity towards *Salmonella typhimurium* TA100 also, although TA98 was more susceptible.

Heterocyclic amines are converted metabolically to hydroxyamino derivatives (30). Cytochrome P-450s, and especially cytochrome P-448, induced by 3-methylcholanthrene in rat liver, are responsible for this oxidation. The hydroxyamino derivatives are further converted to their acetate or sulfate esters, yielding ultimate forms that readily react with bases of DNA. Studies by the ^{32}P-postlabeling method have revealed the presence of several modified bases in liver DNA from rats treated with these heterocyclic amines (31). The formation of adducts with DNA bases has also been demonstrated in vivo by administration of heterocyclic amines and in vitro by incubation of some heterocyclic amines with DNA in the presence of a metabolic activation system, or by incubation of the ultimate forms of heterocyclic amines with DNA (30,32). Adducts were purified and structures of major adducts were determined to be as shown in Figure 2 (33–35).

Table 3
Mutagenic Activities of Heterocyclic Amines in Chinese Hamster Lung Cells

Compound	*DT^r mutants/10^6 survivors induced by 1 μg/ml*
IQ	40
MeIQ	38
MeIQx	5.7
Trp-P-1	33
Trp-P-2	160
Glu-P-1	1.2
Glu-P-2	0.3
AαC	20

Incubation of the human c-Ha-*ras*-1 proto-oncogene with the acetoxyamino derivative of Glu-P-1 resulted in its activation (36). The sequence of this mutated c-Ha-*ras*-1 activated in vitro in transformants obtained by NIH3T3 cell transfection assay has been characterized by restriction fragment length polymorphism using restriction enzyme *Msp*1. Of fourteen transformants induced by c-Ha-*ras*-1 activated in vitro, six contained a mutation in the CCGG sequence covering two bases each of the eleventh and twelfth amino acid codons. A mutation of an amino acid at position 12, 13, 59, or 61 is known to result in the acquisition of activity to transform NIH3T3 cells. However, *ras* family oncogenes were apparently not involved in the main mechanism of activation in intestinal carcinomas and hepatocellular carcinomas of rats induced by administration of diet containing Glu-P-2 and IQ, respectively (37,38). Other mechanisms could be implicated in carcinogenesis by heterocyclic amines.

These heterocyclic amines are mutagenic towards cultured Chinese hamster lung cells with a marker of resistance to diphtheria toxin, as shown in Table 3 (39). Inclusion of a metabolic activation system enhanced their mutagenic potentials, indicating that Chinese hamster lung cells themselves do not have a sufficient capacity to activate heterocyclic amines fully. Mutagenic activities in other cultured cell lines, the production of sister-chromatide exchanges in a permanent cell line of human lymphoblastoid cells NL3, and chromosomal aberrations in a Chinese hamster cell line of lung fibroblast origin have been reported (40,41).

Table 4
Percentages of Mutagenicity due to Non-IQ and IQ Types of Heterocyclic Amines in the Basic Fractions of Various Pyrolysed Materials

Material	*Non-IQ-type*	*IQ-type*
Cigarette smoke condensate	85	6
Broiled sardine	3	88
Fried beef	24	75
Broiled horse mackerel	42	48

The metagenicities of all the heterocyclic amines were completely lost on treatment of the compounds with hypochlorite (42). Nitrite treatment (2 mM) also abolished the mutagenicities of a group of heterocyclic amines including Trp-P-1, Trp-P-2, Glu-P-1, Glu-P-2, AαC, and MeAαC by causing their deamination and conversion to hydroxy derivatives (43,44). AαC showed direct-acting mutagenicity after treatment with nitrite, yielding 2-hydroxy-3-nitroso-α-carboline which did not show mutagenicity in the presence of S9 mix (44).

On the contrary, nitrite treatment did not cause loss of the mutagenicities of IQ, MeIQ, MeIQx, and 4,8-DiMeIQx. The different sensitivities of non-IQ-type and IQ-type heterocyclic amines to nitrite and the sensitivities of both groups to hypochlorite can be used for determination of the contributions of non-IQ-type and IQ-type heterocyclic amines to the total mutagenic activity of the basic fraction of pyrolysates, including cigarette tar and charred cooked fish and meat (45). As expected, the non-IQ-type is predominant in cigarette tar, while the IQ-type accounts for almost all mutagenicity in broiled sardine and fried beef (Table 4).

The amino-group of IQ-type heterocyclic amines was found to be converted to a nitro-group by treatment with a much higher concentration of nitrite of 50 mM (46). Nitro-heterocyclic compounds do not require metabolic activation by S9 mix for mutagenicity towards *Salmonella typhimurium* TA98 and TA100, probably because they are activated by a bacterial nitroreductase. Sunlight-irradiation of IQ-type heterocyclic amines also produces nitro-derivatives.

Carcinogenesis of New Heterocyclic Amines

F344 strain rats and CDF_1 strain mice of both sexes were given diets containing each heterocyclic amine at 0.01–0.08% and water *ad libitum*

Table 5
Carcinogenicity of Heterocyclic Amines in Rats and Mice

Chemical	*Species (concentration)*	*Target Organs*	*TD_{50} (mg/kg/day)*
IQ	Rats (0.03%)	Liver, small & large intestine, Zymbal gland, clitoral gland, skin	0.7
	Mice (0.03%)	Liver, forestomach, lung	14.7
MeIQ	Rats (0.03%)	Large intestine, Zymbal gland, skin, oral cavity, mammary gland	0.1
	Mice (0.04%)	Liver, forestomach	8.4
MeIQx	Rats (0.04%)	Liver, Zymbal gland, clitoral gland, skin	0.7
	Mice (0.06%)	Liver, lung, hematopoietic system	11.0
Trp-P-1	Rats (0.015%)	Liver	0.1
	Mice (0.02%)	Liver	8.8
Trp-P-2	Mice (0.02%)	Liver	2.7
Glu-P-1	Rats (0.05%)	Liver, small & large intestines, Zymbal gland, clitoral gland	0.8
	Mice (0.05%)	Liver, blood vessels	2.7
Glu-P-2	Rats (0.05%)	Liver, small & large intestines Zymbal gland, clitoral gland	5.7
	Mice (0.05%)	Liver, blood vessels	4.9
AαC	Mice (0.08%)	Liver, blood vessels	15.8
MeAαC	Mice (0.08%)	Liver, blood vessels	5.8

continuously for 40 to 104 weeks. As shown in Table 5, tumours developed: in the liver, small and large intestines, Zymbal gland, clitoral gland, and skin of the rats (47–50,50a); and in the liver, lung, hematopoietic system, forestomach, and blood vessels of the mice (51–55).

The incidence of hepatocellular carcinomas induced by heterocyclic amines was higher in female mice than in males (51–55), but typical hepatocarcinogens, such as 7,12-dimethylbenz(a)anthracene and 1,1,1-trichloro-2,2-bis-(p-chlorophenyl)ethane, induce hepatocellular carcinomas at higher incidence in male mice than in females (56,57). In rats, the incidence of hepatocellular carcinoma induced by heterocyclic amines is significantly higher in males than in females (47,48,50) or almost the same in the two sexes (49).

On treatment with heterocyclic amines, adenocarcinomas in small and large intestines were more frequent in male rats than in females (47,48), and did not develop in mice (51–55). This interesting difference between rats and mice indicates the difficulty in estimating human risk from data on carcinogenesis in rodents, as described later. Histologically, the adenocarcinomas of the large intestine of rats were similar to those of humans (47,48).

In mice, hemangioendothelial sarcomas were found mainly in the subcutis of the interscapular region, where brown adipose tissue is present (52). These sarcomas also developed in the pleural cavity, peritoneal cavity, and axilla, but much less frequently. Histologically, hemangioendothelial sarcomas are identified by the presence of proliferating neoplastic endothelial cells and numerous erythrocytes. Hemangioendothelial sarcomas have been suspected to develop from brown adipose tissue, but they were not found in rats, although rats also have brown adipose tissue (47). Squamous cell carcinomas frequently developed in the Zymbal gland and clitoral gland of rats (47,48,50), suggesting that the carcinogens or their metabolites accumulate in sebaceous glands. Squamous cell carcinomas in the Zymbal or clitoral glands were not found with mice (51–55).

Squamous cell carcinomas developed in the forestomach of mice given a diet containing MeIQ (54). It is noteworthy that these carcinomas metastasized to the liver at an unusually high frequency in rodent experiments.

There is no correlation between the potencies of mutagenicity of these compounds towards Salmonella and their carcinogenicities in rodents. For instance, IQ, MeIQ, and MeIQx were about 1000 times more mutagenic than AαC and MeAαC, but their carcinogenecities in mice expressed as TD_{50} values were similar to those of AαC and MeAαC. Therefore, heterocyclic amines that are present in higher amounts in the environment must be more important in human carcinogenesis; for instance, PhIP (20), which shows moderate mutagenicity but is the main heterocyclic amine by weight present in many foods, may be fairly important. Experiments on the carcinogenicity of PhIP are now in progress in this laboratory. The positive data obtained in carcinogenicity experiments on newly isolated heterocyclic amines proved that use of the microbial mutation test for detecting new carcinogens in cooked food and for monitoring their purification is rational, practical, and efficient (58).

Evaluation of the Importance of Heterocyclic Amines in Development of Human Cancer

The discovery of a series of new mutagenic and carcinogenic heterocyclic amines was significant because most of these compounds were isolated from cooked fish and meat and some of those first isolated from pyrolysates of amino acids and proteins were later also found in cooked foods.

Many aromatic amines such as 2-acetylaminofluorene and β-naphthylamine have been widely used in experiments on carcinogenesis. β-Naphtylamine has been used as an intermediate in the manufacture of dyes and antioxidants (59), but most aromatic amines used in carcinogenesis experiments in the laboratory do not occur naturally and are not present in the human daily environment. On the contrary, the newly found heterocyclic amines are mainly present in ordinary cooked foods. As described earlier, primates, including humans, have a metabolic system for activating heterocyclic amines (28,29), suggesting that these compounds should be mutagenic and carcinogenic toward humans. Possible metabolites of MeIQx were recovered from the feces and urine of persons who had eaten fried ground beef (60,61), so heterocyclic amines in cooked food may be absorbed from the intestine and excreted in the urine. Moreover, since metabolites of a heterocyclic amine were found in the bile of rats given the ^{14}C-labeled heterocyclic amine by gavage (62), heterocyclic amines absorbed from the intestine are probably also excreted via the bile in the feces in humans.

There has been only one epidemiological study on broiled food, showing that a population eating much broiled fish showed a higher incidence of gastric cancer than a control population (63). When Syrian golden hamsters were given diet containing 5, 10, 20, or 40% broiled fish meal, no cancers developed in any of the organs in which tumours developed in mice and rats given pellet diet containing single heterocyclic amines at concentrations of 0.01–0.08% (64). However, in a similar experiment with Wistar rats, diets containing 25 and 50%

broiled fish meal resulted in high incidences of lesions, such as erosion, regeneration, and the appearance of hyperplastic epithelium and atypical epithelium in the glandular stomach (65). The amounts of mutagens/carcinogens in the broiled fish may not have been sufficiently high to induce malignant tumours, but the presence of a high level of sodium chloride may enhance carcinogenic processes in the glandular stomach.

Human cancer might develop with collaboration of initiation by heterocyclic amines and tumour promoters. This possibility is supported by the finding that when a limited amount of various heterocyclic amines were painted on mouse skin no tumours developed, but when a promoter, phorbol ester, was painted on the skin after the painting of heterocyclic amines, many tumours developed (66).

Ideally, all mutagens/carcinogens should be removed from our diet, but because this is not possible, we recommend that at least consumption of heavily charred parts of broiled foods should be avoided. The taste and way of cooking of food are a matter of personal choice, but just as the smoking of even a small number of cigarettes is not recommended, so the consumption of charred parts of food is not recommended, even though the amounts of heterocyclic amines in them are low compared with the amounts that cause cancers in rodents.

Some substances inhibit the mutagenicity of heterocyclic amines. These are hemin compounds, which form complexes that have planar structures with heterocyclic amines (67), and unsaturated fatty acid, whose mechanism of inhibition is unknown (68). An anticarcinogen has also been detected in fried, ground meat and was recently reported to be a derivative of linoleic acid containing a conjugated double bond system (69).

Recently a method for quantification of heterocyclic amines by their partial purification and h.p.l.c. has been developed. Results by this method on the concentrations of these compounds in various foods are listed in Table 6 (70). In addition, PhIP has been isolated from fried beef at a concentration of 15 ng/g original weight of uncooked beef (20) and from codfish at a concentration of 69.2 ng/g fried codfish (71). The heterocyclic amines identified so far constitute one-tenth to one-third of the total mutagenicity in the basic fraction from cooked food, depending on the material and the method of its cooking. This indicates the existence of as yet unknown mutagens/carcinogens.

Human beings are continuously exposed to a vast number of mutagens/carcinogens, even though each compound is usually present

Table 6
Amounts of Heterocyclic Amines in Cooked Foods

	Amount (ng/g Cooked Food)						
Sample	*IQ*	*MeIQx*	*4,8-DiMeIQx*	*Trp-P-1*	*Trp-P-2*	*AαC*	*MeAαC*
Broiled beef	0.19	2.11		0.21	0.25	1.20	
Fried ground beef		0.64	0.12	0.19	0.21		
Broiled chicken		2.33	0.81	0.12	0.18	0.21	
Broiled mutton		1.01	0.67		0.15	2.50	0.19
Food-grade beef extract		3.10					

at a very low level. Thus it seems reasonable to eliminate them from our environment as much as possible.

The ratio of actual intake of environmental mutagens/carcinogens by humans to their TD_{50} is often taken as a parameter of their risk. The TD_{50} is the dose that causes cancers in 50% of the animals tested in *ad libitum* feeding experiments for life and is expressed in mg/kg body weight/day (72). AF-2 was used as a food additive in Japan beginning in 1965 and was banned in 1974 after evidence of the compound's mutagenicity followed by carcinogenicity was discovered. During this period, the average annual production of AF-2 was 2.7 metric tons, and the levels of added AF-2 in one g of various foods, such as soy-bean cake, fish-meat cake, and fish sausages, were 5 μg, 2.5 μg, and 20 μg, respectively. Based on carcinogenesis experiments using rats, the TD_{50} value for AF-2 was calculated to be 11.4 mg/kg/day (72). If we accept the values of an average body weight of 50 kg and a total population of 100 million in Japan, then the average daily intake of AF-2 per capita calculated from its annual production is 1.48 μg/kg. Therefore, the ratio of intake of AF-2 to its TD_{50} is calculated to be 130×10^{-6}.

Rat and mouse experiments have shown that heterocyclic amines have TD_{50} values in the range of 0.1 – 15.8 mg/kg/day (Table 5), although these values are very tentative ones obtained from experiment at single-dose-level experiments. If we assume that people with an average body weight of 50 kg eat 200 g of broiled beef every day, the daily intake of heterocyclic amines is calculated to be 0.76 ng for IQ, 8.44 ng for MeIQx, 0.84 ng for Trp-P-1, 1.00 μg for Trp-P-2, and 4.80 ng for AαC per kg body weight based on the data in Table 6.

The ratio of the actual intake of five heterocyclic amines to their TD_{50} values, which are obtained from rat experiments for IQ, MeIQx, and Trp-P-1, and from mouse experiments for Trp-P-2 and AαC, are estimated to be 1×10^{-6} for IQ, 12×10^{-6} for MeIQx, 8×10^{-6} for Trp-P-1, 0.4×10^{-6} for Trp-P-2, and 0.3×10^{-6} for AαC. Regarding the sum of intake of these five heterocyclic amines, the ratio is calculated to be 21.7×10^{-6}. Therefore, the value of the ratio for AF-2 is six times larger than that for five heterocyclic amines. However, PhIP, the most abundant mutagenic heterocyclic amine by weight in cooked food, is not included in this calculation, because its carcinogenic potency is not known yet. If it is assumed that broiled beef contains 30 ng/g of PhIP, the daily intake of PhIP per capita is 6 μg. Based on the assumption that PhIP has the same carcinogenic potency as Glu-P-2, since both PhIP and Glu-P-2 show similar mutagenicity, the TD_{50} value of PhIP is estimated to be 5.7 mg/kg/day. If we take the daily intake of PhIP into consideration, the ratio for AF-2 is three times greater than the ratio for these six heterocyclic amines. Contribution of heterocyclic amines other than these six should be considered. Furthermore, cooked food contains not only heterocyclic amines but also other mutagens/carcinogens such as aromatic hydrocarbons and nitropyrenes, and nitrosable precursors. Thus, the risk from cooked food is in the same magnitude as that from AF-2.

When the mutagenicity and carcinogenicity of AF-2 were demonstrated, the general public became deeply concerned about the use of this food additive, but curiously, many people are not concerned about mutagens/carcinogens in cooked food. They feel that foods that people have eaten for many generations should be safe. But safety should be evaluated scientifically, not by feeling. Of course, simple comparison of the actual intake with the TD_{50} value does not mean very much, because the presence of tumour promoters and in vivo conditions favourable for tumour promotion may enhance the risk of mutagens/carcinogens by a factor of up to 100, while the presence of inhibitors of mutagenesis, carcinogenesis, and tumour promotion may significantly suppress the risk of carcinogenic factors. Moreover, the species differences in susceptibility to carcinogens, shown by the differences in incidences of intestinal tumours and hemangioendotheliomas in mice and rats indicate the danger of extrapolating findings in rodents to humans. Therefore, at present, the only precaution possible seems to be to avoid eating heavily charred parts of broiled fish and meat.

Gerontogenic Effects of Heterocyclic Amines besides Carcinogenicity

During carcinogenesis experiments, rats given pellet diet containing 0.08% MeAαC were found to die within nine months, while those given diet containing AαC survived. The rats given MeAαC lost weight and became severely emaciated, and at autopsy their salivary glands and pancreas were seen to have atrophied (73). Histological examination showed that the atrophy was of cells in the mucous and serous alveoli of the salivary glands, and of acinar cells and islets of Langerhans in the pancreas. This atrophy was observed in both sexes. AαC did not cause this atrophy, indicating that the presence of a methyl group in MeAαC resulted in marked pharmacological activity. Prolonged administration of a much lower level of MeAαC may produce a chronic disease resembling diabetes due to atrophy of insulin-producing cells.

Atherosclerotic plaque is thought to be a kind of benign tumour. This was proved by monoclonal growth of smooth muscle cells by showing only one band of glucose-6-phosphate dehydrogenase from female patients with heterozygosity of normal and mutated genes of this enzyme which is located in the X-chromosome (74). Intramuscular injection of 7,12-dimethylbenz(a)anthracene into chickens induced atherosclerotic lesions of the aorta (75). In a preliminary study, growth of smooth muscle cells in the wall of the aorta of chickens was also induced by injection of IQ into the pectoral muscle. Other heterocyclic amines may also induce atherosclerotic changes.

The fact that heterocyclic amines induce deteriorative changes in the pancreas and blood vessels suggests that they are related to aging phenomena. They may be called "gerontogen" or "senilogen."

Proposal of Twelve Points for Cancer Prevention

Diet, food, and nutrition are closely related to human cancer development, as described in this volume of proceedings. Our experiments reflect only one facet of this huge subject. However, since the goal of research for identification of environmental mutagens/carcinogens and tumour promoters is to establish bases for primary cancer prevention, by collecting information from many available reports of experimental, clinical, and epidemiological studies, we have proposed the 12 points for primary cancer prevention shown in Table 7 (7).

Table 7
Proposed 12 Points for Cancer Prevention

1	Eat a nutritionally balanced diet.
2	Eat a variety of types of foods.
3	Avoid excess calories, especially as fat.
4	Avoid the excessive drinking of alcohol.
5	Smoke as little as possible.
6	Take vitamins in appropriate amounts; eat fibre and green and yellow vegetables rich in carotene.
7	Avoid drinking fluids that are too hot and eating foods that are too salty.
8	Avoid the charred parts of cooked food.
9	Avoid food with possible contamination by fungal toxins.
10	Avoid over-exposure to sunlight.
11	Have an exercise program matched to your own condition.
12	Keep the body clean.

Some of these points are directly related to nutrition, food, and cancer, while others are not, but they are all recommendations for improvements in various aspects of life style. Diet and nutrition are closely related to other factors such as smoking, intake of alcoholic beverages, and exercise, so these other factors are also included. Of course, these recommendations are rather flexible and are being revised each year by a committee of scientists, journalists, essayists, and others. As demonstrated by Breslow and Enstrom, a modest life style tends to suppress cancer development (76). Consistent with this concept, our 12 recommendations are based on human wisdom.

REFERENCES

*National Institute of Nutrition Lecturer.

1 *Diet, nutrition, and cancer*. Washington, DC: National Academy Press, 1982.

2 Doll R, Peto R. The causes of cancer: quantitative estimates of avoidable risks of cancer in the United States today. *J Natl Cancer Inst* 1981;66:1191–1308.

3 Ames BN. Dietary carcinogens and anticarcinogens. *Science* 1983;221: 1256–1264.

4 Nagao M, Wakabayashi K, Sugimura T. Mutagens in food and drinks, and their carcinogenicity. In: Zimmermann FK, Taylor-Mayer RE, eds.

Mutagenicity testing in environmental pollution control. West Sussex: Ellis Horwood, 1985:69–85.
5 Sugimura T. Mutagens, carcinogens, and tumor promoters in our daily food. *Cancer* 1982;49:1970–1984.
6 Sugimura T. Carcinogenicity of mutagenic heterocyclic amines formed during the cooking process. *Mutat Res* 1985;150:33–41.
7 Sugimura T. Studies on environmental chemical carcinogenesis in Japan. *Science* 1986;233:312–318.
8 McCann J, Choi E, Yamasaki E, Ames BN. Detection of carcinogens as mutagens in the Salmonella/microsome test: assay of 300 chemicals. *Proc Natl Acad Sci USA* 1975;72:5135–5139.
9 Sugimura T, Sato S, Nagao M, et al. Overlapping of carcinogens and mutagens. In: Magee PN, Takayama S, Sugimura T, Matsushima T, eds. *Fundamentals in cancer prevention.* Tokyo: Japan Sci. Soc. Press, 1976:191–215.
10 Miller EC, Miller JA. The mutagenicity of chemical carcinogens: correlations, problems, and interpretations. In: Hollaender A, ed. *Chemical mutagens, principles and methods for their detection.* Vol. 1. New York: Plenum Press, 1971:83–119.
11 Gelboin HV. Carcinogens, enzyme induction and gene action. *Adv Cancer Res* 1967;10:1–81.
12 Ames BN, McCann J, Yamasaki E. Methods for detecting carcinogens and mutagens with the *Salmonella*/mammalian-microsome mutagenicity test. *Mutat Res* 1975;31:347–364.
13 Lijinsky W, Shubik P. Benzo[a]pyrene and other polynuclear hydrocarbons in charcoal-broiled meat. *Science* 1964;145:53–55.
14 Kuratsune M. Benzo[a]pyrene content of certain pyrogenic materials. *J Natl Cancer Inst* 1956;16:1485–1496.
15 Sugimura T, Nagao M, Kawachi T, et al. Mutagen-carcinogens in food, with special reference to highly mutagenic pyrolytic products in broiled foods. In: Hiatt HH, Watson JD, Winsten JA, eds. *Origins of human cancer.* Cold Spring Harbor, NY: Cold Spring Harbor Laboratory, 1977:1561–1577.
16 Nagao M, Honda M, Seino Y, Yahagi T, Sugimura T. Mutagenicities of smoke condensates and the charred surface of fish and meat. *Cancer Lett* 1977;2:221–226.
17 Kasai H, Yamaizumi Z, Wakabayashi K, et al. Potent novel mutagens produced by broiling fish under normal conditions. *Proc Jpn Acad* 1980; 56B:278–283.
18 Kasai H, Yamaizumi Z, Wakabayashi K, et al. Structure and chemical

synthesis of Me-IQ, a potent mutagen isolated from broiled fish. *Chem Lett* 1980:1391–1394.

19 Kasai H, Yamaizumi Z, Shiomi T, et al. Structure of a potent mutagen isolated from fried beef. *Chem Lett* 1981:485–488.

20 Felton JS, Knize MG, Shen NH, et al. The isolation and identification of a new mutagen from fried ground beef: 2-amino-1-methyl-6-phenylimidazo[4,5-*b*]pyridine (PhIP). *Carcinogenesis* 1986;7:1081–1086.

21 Negishi C, Wakabayashi K, Yamaizumi Z, et al. Identification of 4,8-DiMeIQx, a new mutagen. *Mutat Res* 1985;147:267–268.

22 Negishi C, Wakabayashi K, Tsuda M, et al. Formation of 2-amino-3,7,8-trimethylimidazo[4,5-*f*]quinoxaline, a new mutagen, by heating a mixture of creatinine, glucose and glycine. *Mutat Res* 1984;140:55–59.

23 Sugimura T, Kawachi T, Nagao M, et al. Mutagenic principle(s) in tryptophan and phenylalanine pyrolysis products. *Proc Jpn Acad* 1977;53:58–61.

24 Yamamoto T, Tsuji K, Kosuge T, et al. Isolation and structure determination of mutagenic substances in L-glumatic acid pyrolysate. *Proc Jpn Acad* 1978;54B:248–250.

25 Yokota M, Narita K, Kosuge T, et al. A potent mutagen isolated from a pyrolysate of L-ornithine. *Chem Pharm Bull* 1981;29:1473–1475.

26 Yoshida D, Matsumoto T, Yoshimura R, Matsuzaki T. Mutagenicity of amino-α-carbolines in pyrolysis products of soybean globulin. *Biochem Biophys Res Commun* 1978;83:915–920.

27 Sugimura T, Nagao M. Modification of mutagenic activity. In: de Serres FJ, Hollaender A, eds. *Chemical mutagens, principles and methods for their detection*. Vol. 6. New York: Plenum Press, 1980:41–60.

28 Ishida Y, Negishi C, Umemoto A, et al. Activation of mutagenic and carcinogenic heterocyclic amines by S-9 from the liver of a rhesus monkey. *Toxic in Vitro* 1987;1:45–48.

29 Sugimura T. Naturally occurring genotoxic carcinogens. In: Miller EC, Miller JA, Hirono I, Sugimura T, Takayama S, eds. *Naturally occurring carcinogens-mutagens and modulators of carcinogenesis*. Tokyo: Japan Sci Soc Press; Baltimore: Univ Park Press, 1979:241–261.

30 Kato R, Yamazoe Y. Metabolic activation and covalent binding to nucleic acids of carcinogenic heterocyclic amines from cooked foods and amino acid pyrolysates. *Jpn J Cancer Res (Gann)* 1987;78:297–311.

31 Yamashita K, Umemoto A, Grivas S, Kato S, Sato S, Sugimura T. Heterocyclic amine-DNA adducts analyzed by ^{32}P-postlabeling method. *Nucleic Acids Res* 1988; *Symp, Ser* 19:111–114.

32 Hashimoto Y, Shudo K, Okamoto T. Modification of nucleic acids with muta-carcinogenic heterocyclic amines *in vivo*. Identification of modified

bases in DNA extracted from rats injected with 3-amino-1-methyl-5*H*-pyrido[4,3-*b*]indole and 2-amino-6-methyldipyrido[1,2-*a*:3′,2′-*d*]imidazole. *Mutat Res* 1982;105:9–13.

33 Hashimoto Y, Shudo K, Okamoto T. Metabolic activation of a mutagen, 2-amino-6-methyldipyrido[1,2-*a*:3′,2′-*d*]imidazole. Identification of 2-hydroxyamino-6-methyldipyrido[1,2-*a*:3′,2′-*d*]imidazole and its reaction with DNA. *Biochem Biophys Res Commun* 1980;92:971–976.

34 Hashimoto Y, Shudo K, Okamoto T. Activation of a mutagen, 3-amino-1-methyl-5*H*-pyrido[4,3-*b*]indole. Identification of 3-hydroxyamino-1-methyl-5*H*-pyrido[4,3-*b*]indole and its reaction with DNA. *Biochem Biophys Res Commun* 1980;96:355–362.

35 Snyderwine EG, Roller PP, Adamson RH, Sato S, Thorgeirsson SS. Reaction of the *N*-hydroxylamine and *N*-acetoxy derivatives of 2-amino-3-methylimidazo[4,5-*f*]quinoline (IQ) with DNA. Synthesis and identification of *N*-(deoxyguanosin-8-yl)-IQ. *Carcinogenesis* 1988:1061–1065.

36 Hashimoto Y, Kawachi E, Shudo K, Sekiya T, Sugimura T. Transforming activity of human c-Ha-*ras*-1 proto-oncogene generated by the binding of 2-amino-6-methyldipyrido[1,2-*a*:3′,2′-*d*]imidazole and 4-nitroquinoline N-oxide: direct evidence of cellular transformation by chemically modified DNA. *Jpn J Cancer Res (Gann)* 1987;78:211–215.

37 Ishizaka Y, Ochiai M, Ishikawa F, et al. Activated N-*ras* oncogene in a transformant derived from a rat small intestinal adenocarcinoma induced by 2-aminodipyrido[1,2-*a*:3′,2′-*d*]imidazole. *Carcinogenesis* 1987; 8:1575–1578.

38 Nagao M, Ishikawa F, Tahira T, Ochiai M, Sugimura T. Activation of rat and human c-raf(-1) by rearrangement. In: Aaronson ST, Bishop JM, Sugimura T, Terada M, Toyoshima K, Vogt PK, eds. *Oncogenes and cancer*. Tokyo: Japan Sci Soc Press; Utrecht: VNU Sci Press, 1987:75–84.

39 Nakayasu M, Nakasato F, Sakamoto H, Terada M, Sugimura T. Mutagenic activity of heterocyclic amines in Chinese hamster lung cells with diphtheria toxin resistance as a marker. *Mutat Res* 1983;118:91–102.

40 Tohda H, Oikawa A, Kawachi T, Sugimura T. Inducton of sister-chromatid exchanges by mutagens from amino acid and protein pyrolysates. *Mutat Res* 1980;77:65–69.

41 Ishidate M Jr, Sofuni T, Yoshikawa K. Chromosomal aberration tests *in vitro* as a primary screening tool for environmental mutagens and/or carcinogens. *GANN Monograph on Cancer Res* 1981;27:95–108.

42 Tsuda M, Wakabayashi K, Hirayama T, Sugimura T. Inactivation of potent pyrolysate mutagens by chlorinated tap water. *Mutat Res* 1983;119:27–34.

43 Tsuda M, Takahashi Y, Nagao M, Hirayama T, Sugimura T. Inactivation of mutagens from pyrolysates of tryptophan and glutamic acid by nitrite in acidic solution. *Mutat Res* 1980;78:331–339.

44 Tsuda M, Nagao M, Hirayama T, Sugimura T. Nitrite converts 2-amino--carboline, an indirect mutagen, to 2-hydroxy-α-carboline, a non-mutagen and 2-hydroxy-3-nitroso-α-carboline, a direct mutagen. *Mutat Res* 1981;83:61–68.

45 Tsuda M, Negishi C, Makino R, et al. Use of nitrite and hypochlorite treatments in determination of the contributions of IQ-type and non-IQ-type heterocyclic amines to the mutagenicities in crude pyrolyzed materials. *Mutat Res* 1985;147:335–341.

46 Sasagawa C, Muramatsu M, Matsushina T. Formation of direct mutagens from amino-imidazoazaarenes by nitrite treatment. *Mutat Res* 1988;203:386.

47 Takayama S, Masuda M, Mogami M, Ohgaki H, Sato S, Sugimura T. Induction of cancers in the intestine, liver and various other organs of rats by feeding mutagens from glutamic acid pyrolyste. *Gann* 1984;75:207–213.

48 Takayama S, Nakatsuru Y, Masuda M, Ohgaki H, Sato S, Sugimura T. Demonstration of carcinogenicity in F344 rats of 2-amino-3-methylimidazo[4,5-*f*]quinoline from broiled sardine, fried beef and beef extract. *Gann* 1984;75:467–470.

49 Takayama S, Nakatsuru Y, Ohgaki H, Sato S, Sugimura T. Carcinogenicity in rats of a mutagenic compound, 3-amino-1,4-dimethyl-5*H*-pyrido[4,3-*b*]indole, from tryptophan pyrolysate. *Jpn J Cancer Res (Gann)* 1985;76:815–817.

50 Kato T, Ohgaki H, Hasegawa H, Sato S, Takayama S, Sugimura T. Carcinogenicity in rats of a mutagenic compound, 2-amino-3,8-dimethylimidazo[4,5-*f*]quinoxaline. *Carcinogenesis* 1988;9:71–73.

50a Kato T, Migita H, Ohgaki H, Sato S, Takayama S, Sugimura T. Induction of tumors in the Zymbal gland, oral cavity, colon, skin and mammary gland of F344 rats by a mutagenic compound, 2-amino-3,4-dimethylimidazo[4,5-*f*]quinoline. *Carcinogenesis* 1989;10:601–603.

51 Matsukura N, Kawachi T, Morino K, Ohgaki H, Sugimura T, Takayama S. Carcinogenicity in mice of mutagenic compounds from a tryptophan pyrolyzate. *Science* 1981;213:346–347.

52 Ohgaki H, Matsukura N, Morino K, Kawachi T, Sugimura T, Takayama S. Carcinogenicity in mice of mutagenic compounds from glutamic acid and soybean globulin pyrolysates. *Carcinogenesis* 1984;5:815–819.

53 Ohgaki H, Kusama K, Matsukura N, et al. Carcinogenicity in mice of a mutagenic compound, 2-amino-3-methylimidazo[4,5-*f*]quinoline, from

broiled sardine, cooked beef and beef extract. *Carcinogenesis* 1984;5:921–924.
54 Ohgaki H, Hasegawa H, Suenaga M, et al. Induction of hepatocellular carcinoma and highly metastatic squamous cell carcinomas in the forestomach of mice by feeding 2-amino-3,4-dimethylimidazo[4,5-*f*]quinoline. *Carcinogenesis* 1986;7:1889–1893.
55 Ohgaki H, Hasegawa H, Suenaga M, Sato S, Takayama S, Sugimura T. Carcinogenicity in mice of a mutagenic compound, 2-amino-3,8-dimethylimidazo[4,5-*f*]quinoxaline (MeIQx) from cooked foods. *Carcinogenesis* 1987;8:665–668.
56 Roe FJC, Grant GA. Inhibition by germ-free status of development of liver and lung tumors in mice exposed neonatally to 7,12-dimethylbenz(a)anthracene: implications in relation to tests for carcinogenicity. *Int J Cancer* 1970;6:133–144.
57 Tomatis L, Turusov V, Day N, Charles RT. The effect of long-term exposure to DDT on CF-1 mice. *Int J Cancer* 1972;10:489–506.
58 Sugimura T. Successful use of short-term tests for academic purposes: their use in identification of new environmental carcinogens with possible risk for humans. *Mutat Res* 1988;205:33–39.
59 2-Naphthylamine. In: *IARC monographs on the evaluation of carcinogenic risk of chemicals to man. Some aromatic amines, hydrazine and related substances, N-nitroso compounds and miscellaneous alkylating agents*. Vol. 4. Lyon: IARC, 1974: 97–111.
60 Hayatsu H, Hayatsu T, Wataya Y, Mower HF. Fecal mutagenicity arising from ingestion of fried ground beef in the human. *Mutat Res* 1985;143:207–211.
61 Hayatsu H, Hayatsu T, Ohara Y. Mutagenicity of human urine caused by ingestion of fried ground beef. *Jpn J Cancer Res (Gann)* 1985;76: 445–448.
62 Negishi C, Umemoto A, Rafter JJ, Sato S, Sugimura T. *N*-Acetyl derivative as the major active metabolite of 2-amino-6-methyldipyrido[1,2-*a*:3′,2′-*d*]imidazole in rat bile. *Mutat Res* 1986;175:23–28.
63 Ikeda M, Yoshimoto K, Yoshimura T, Kono S, Kato H, Kuratsune M. A cohort study on the possible association between broiled fish intake and cancer. *Gann* 1983;74:640–648.
64 Takahashi M, Furukawa F, Nagano K, Miyakawa Y, Kokubo T, Hayashi Y. Long-term *in vivo* carcinogenicity test of fish meat pyrolysate in Syrian golden hamsters. *Gann* 1983;74:633–639.
65 Fujii K, Nomoto K, Ishidate M, Nakamura K. Chronic toxicity of charred fish meat in Wistar rats. *Nutr Cancer* 1987;9:185–193.
66 Sato H, Takahashi M, Furukawa F, et al. Initiating activity in a two-

stage mouse skin model of nine mutagenic pyrolysates of amino acids, soybean globulin and proteinaceous food. Carcinogenesis 1987;8: 1231-1234.

67 Arimoto S, Ohara Y, Namba T, Negishi T, Hayatsu H. Inhibition of the mutagenicity of amino acid pyrolysis products by hemin and other biological pyrole pigments. *Biochem Biophys Res Commun* 1980;92:662–668.

68 Hayatsu H, Arimoto S, Togawa K, Makita M. Inhibitory effect of the ether extract of human feces on activities of mutagens: inhibition by oleic and linoleic acids. *Mutat Res* 1981;81:287–293.

69 Ha YL, Grimm NK, Pariza MW. Anticarcinogens from fried ground beef: heat-altered derivatives of linoleic acid. *Carcinogenesis* 1987;8:1881–1887.

70 Sugimura T, Sato S, Wakabayashi K. Mutagens/carcinogens in pyrolysates of amino acids and proteins and in cooked foods: heterocyclic aromatic amines. In: Woo Y-T, Lai DY, Arcos JC, Argus MF, eds. *Chemical induction of cancer, structural bases and biological mechanisms*. Vol. IIIC. New York: Academic Press, 1988:681–710.

71 Zhang X-M, Wakabayashi K, Liu Z-C, Sugimura T, Nagao M. Mutagenic and carcinogenic heterocyclic amines in Chinese cooked foods. *Mutat Res* 1988:181–188.

72 Gold LS, Sawyer CB, Magaw R, et al. A carcinogenic potency database of the standardized results of animal bioassays. *Environ Health Perspect* 1984;58:9–319.

73 Takayama S, Nakatsuru Y, Ohgaki H, Sato S, Sugimura T. Atrophy of salivary glands and pancreas of rats fed on diet with amino-methyl-α-carboline. *Proc Jpn Acad* 1985;61B:277–280.

74 Benditt EP, Benditt JM. Evidence for a monoclonal origin of human atherosclerotic plaques. *Proc Natl Acad Sci USA* 1973;70:1753–1756.

75 Albert RE, Vanderlaan M, Burns FJ, Nishizumi M. Effect of carcinogens on chicken atherosclerosis. *Cancer Res* 1977;37:2232–2235.

76 Breslow L, Enstrom E. Persistence of health habits and their relationship to mortality. *Prevent Med* 1980;9:469–483.

JOZEF V. JOOSSENS AND J. GEBOERS

Salt, Stomach Cancer, and Stroke

In 1964 one of us (JVJ) was looking at the correlation between cardiovascular disease mortality and cancer mortality using the 1958 death rates from 19 countries. Although primarily interested in the relationship between coronary mortality and lung cancer mortality, a much stronger correlation emerged by chance, i.e. that between stroke mortality and stomach cancer mortality. Only much later it appeared that the relationship had already been observed in Japan in the late '50s using mortality data of the towns, cities, and villages in the Miyagi prefecture by Hiraide, Fujisaku, and co-workers. Their paper was only published in Japanese and the authors did not pursue their investigations.

This finding was so unexpected that a series of investigations on the relationship between salt intake and blood pressure was started in 1966. It also promoted a close scrutiny of mortality data, which became available year after year since then. It became evident that, using data from many different countries, a significant correlation between stroke and stomach cancer mortality existed in each sex and for every year. Data from 1970 are shown in Figure 1 for the combined data of males and females. It was also observed that stomach cancer mortality data at middle age (e.g. age 45–64 years) were the best predictors of stroke mortality, not only in the same age group, but also in older people (age 65 years and more), thereby clearly indicating that the deaths from stomach cancer and from stroke occurred for the most part in different people.

The slope of the correlation was about 5 to 7, indicating that, under the given conditions, for each (supplementary) death from stomach

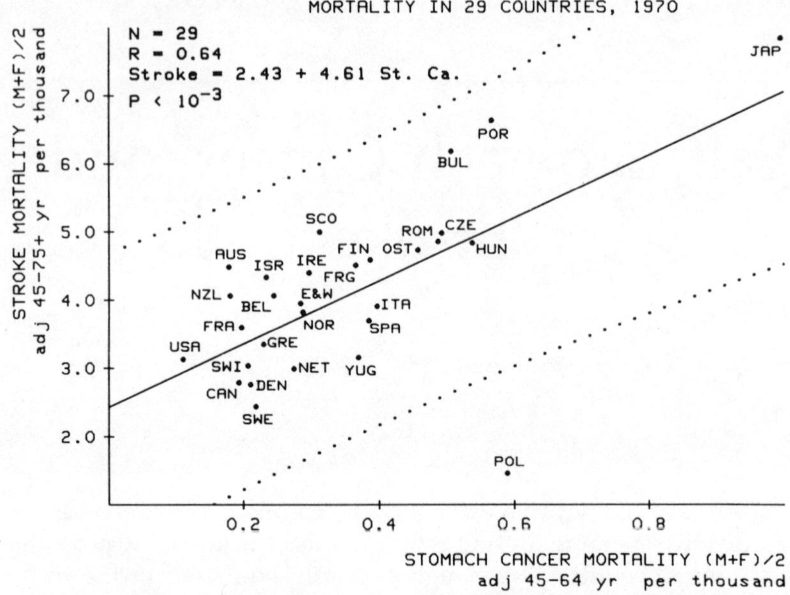

Figure 1. Relationship between stomach cancer and stroke mortality in 1970. Japan and the East European countries are on the same line as the Western countries. The very low stroke values in Poland are the result of classification errors.

cancer 5 to 7 more deaths from stroke were observed. Other important findings were that restricting the correlated data to Western countries yielded a similar regression line as in Figure 1 and that stroke mortality in Japan and East European countries could be predicted from stomach cancer in those countries using the regression line obtained for Western countries. This implied that extrapolation to more than twice the observed range still led to accurately predicted stroke mortality, suggesting that the linking factor acting in Western countries was similar to the one occurring in East European countries and Japan.

In 1980–85 the situation changed completely. The regression line obtained between the same countries as in Figure 1 no longer predicted what was happening in East European countries, nor in Japan (Figure 2). Japan had much lower stroke values than expected from stomach cancer and the reverse was true for East European countries. A possible explanation for this will be discussed later.

A second major observation was made using data from different years in a specific country. A time trend between stroke and stomach cancer

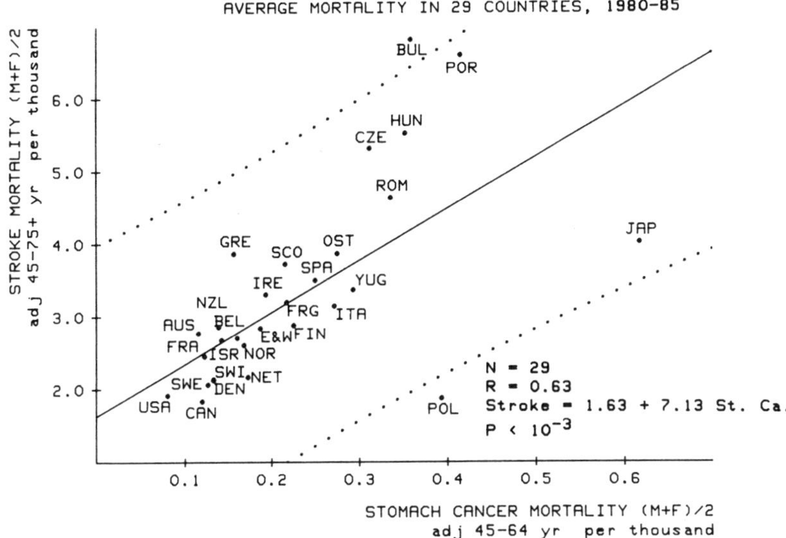

Figure 2. Same relationship as in Figure 1 but now in 1980–85. Stroke in Japan decreased markedly below the regression line, whereas the East European countries increased above it (for explanation see text).

was then obtained instead of a geographical relationship. For the time interval between 1955 and 1973 the slopes obtained in countries like England and Wales, the United States, Canada, the Netherlands, F.R. Germany, Switzerland, Denmark, Sweden, etc. were not significantly different. The relationship between stroke and stomach cancer over time is shown here for England and Wales and Canada (Figures 3 and 4). Before 1955 stroke mortality was lower than predicted from stomach cancer in many countries. In Belgium this was even true up to 1968. From an analysis of the mortality data it could be demonstrated that this was mostly due to underclassification of stroke mortality, especially in people older than 70 years. This error was gradually removed, sooner in some countries than in others. The correlation between stomach cancer and stroke mortality obtained between 1955 and 1973 was higher than 0.9 in all the countries mentioned above. The within-country regression slopes obtained in several countries over the time period 1955–73 (e.g. Figs. 3 and 4) and the between-countries regression slopes obtained for different years (1955–73 – Fig. 1) were not significantly different. This indicated that the linking factor relating stomach cancer to stroke between and

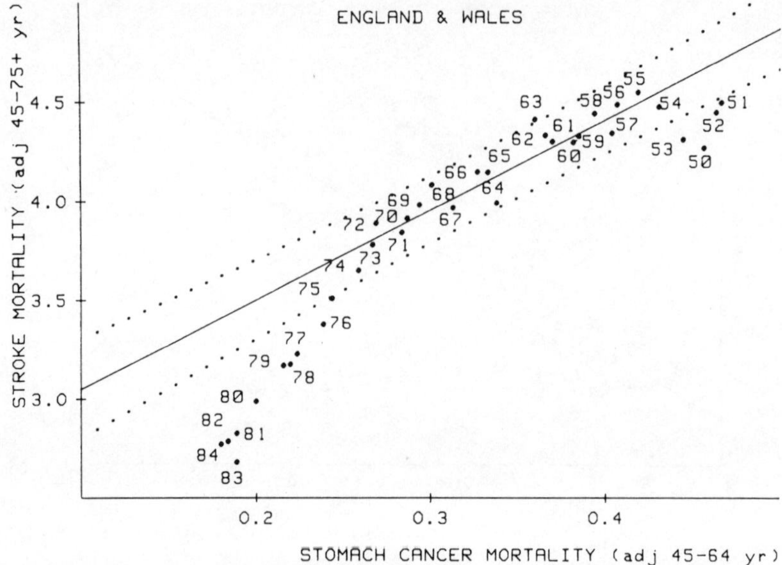

Figure 3. A within-country time trend of stomach cancer and stroke mortality, to be compared with between-country relationships (Figs. 1 and 2). The regression line was calculated between 1955 and 1973.
$n = 19$; $r = 0.95$; $p < 10^{-9}$; Stroke = 2.6 + 4.5 Stomach cancer.
Stroke decreased faster in England and Wales than stomach cancer mortality after 1973, probably because of better and more mass-oriented treatment of hypertension (*courtesy of American Journal of Clinical Nutrition* [1]).

within countries was the same and made a spurious association very unlikely. It also indicated that the linking factor between both diseases must either be unique or at least predominant. Under that condition a similar correlation between and within countries should be observed. For a complex multiple linking factor the probability of obtaining a similar distribution within and between countries becomes smaller and smaller when more factors are involved.

The relationship between stroke and stomach cancer is also present among social classes. In general, the higher the social class, the lower the mortality from stroke and from stomach cancer. This is clearly seen in England and Wales, where the richer south has much lower stroke and stomach cancer rates than the poorer north and than Wales.

All those findings suggest a simple or predominant linking factor. Since this factor also affects the stomach, it should be of nutritional

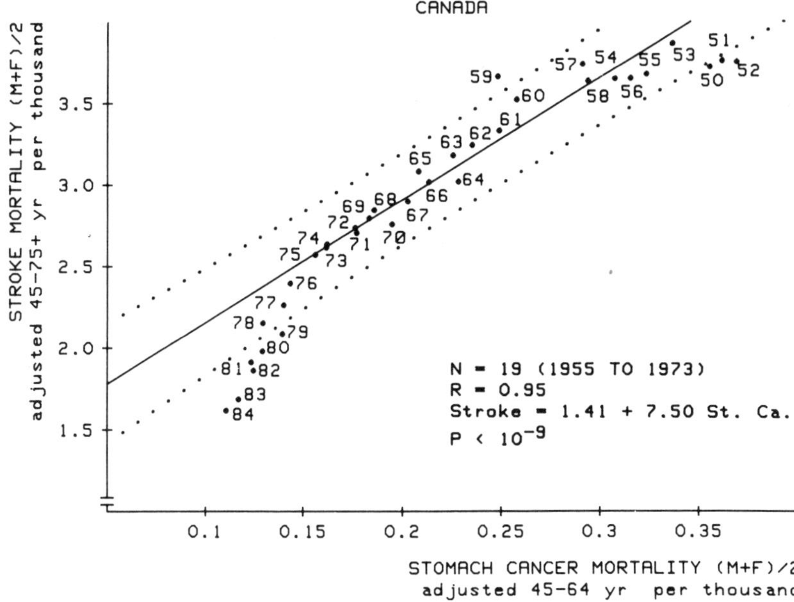

Figure 4. As in Figure 3 but for Canada.

origin. Searching the literature yielded sets of possible positive and negative etiological factors of stroke and stomach cancer which are listed in Table 1. The most important linking factor(s) should be common to the two sets of factors (the intersection of the sets). One can see from Table 1 that dietary salt is the most obvious linking factor. With the exception of vitamin C, all the factors in the intersection of sets are related to dietary salt. A high carbohydrate intake has been singled out as a possible factor promoting both stroke and stomach cancer. However, all the case-control and epidemiological studies, many of them in Japan, did not include salt as a possible confounding factor when studying the effects of a carbohydrate-rich diet. In the few areas where carbohydrates are not salted, as in the Amazon jungle or in the central part of New Guinea, hypertension and strokes are not observed. In countries like Nigeria and Uganda, with a low salt intake of only 5 g/day, cancer registries have shown very low stomach cancer rates, although the carbohydrate intake is very high.

Salt intake explains the higher prevalence of stomach cancer, stroke, and hypertension in lower social classes. Cheap foods like bread,

Table 1
Possible Risk Factors

	For Stomach Cancer Only	*For Stomach Cancer and Stroke*	*For Stroke Only*	
Positive	Nitrates/nitrites Nitroso-carcinogens Bracken fern Soil trace elements Peaty soil Talcum in rice Atrophic gastritis +	Salt + Pickled foods + Smoked foods + Lard + Soybean sauce + Carbohydrate rich foods + Low social class + Salted fish or meat +	Saturated fat − Low protein + Alcohol Lead The "Pill" Stress	Positive
Negative	Fat Selenium Milk −	Refrigeration of foods − Fresh vegetables − Vitamin C	Polyunsaturated fat − Treatment of hypertension Potassium Calcium Fiber	Negative

The column in the middle is the intersection of the sets of risk factors for stomach cancer and stroke.

\+ positively related to salt intake
− negatively related to salt intake

potatoes, cheese, sausages, dried/smoked fish or meat, canned meats and vegetables, fast food, etc. are heavily salted.

Salt intake also explains the between-countries relationship. There is a good correlation between observed salt intake and stomach cancer rates; the same applies to stroke. In general salt intake is or was very high (up to 30 g/day) in Japan, China, Korea, Portugal, Colombia, and Finland. All these countries have or had also very high stomach cancer and stroke rates. Salt intake is high in Eastern Europe (up to 20 g/day), and so are stroke and stomach cancer. Salt intake is medium in Western countries (about 8–12 g/day) with medium to low stroke and stomach cancer rates.

Salt intake can explain the within-country relationship. There is good evidence that salt intake decreased markedly over the years in Belgium, Finland, Japan, Switzerland, and France. This decrease was due to three major factors. The first is the gradual substitution of fats for carbohydrates. Since the energy density of fats is 2.4 times higher than that of carbohydrates, the intake of salt must decrease on a constant energy intake when fats are replacing carbohydrates. Secondly, the introduction of refrigerators made it possible to preserve food without salting, resulting in the gradual elimination of foods such as dried and smoked salted fish, salted meat, and salted vegetables. Unsalted frozen foods were gradually replacing the salted (canned) foods. The introduction of refrigerators varied widely all over the world. In the U.S., Australia, New Zealand, and possibly also in Canada, ice boxes and refrigerators became popular about 1925. Stroke and stomach cancer rates started to decline in the U.S. around that time. In Japan, on the contrary, refrigerators became popular only after 1960, and from that time on stomach cancer and stroke mortality started to decline simultaneously. In Western countries, except Portugal, refrigerators became widespread after 1950, with expected results on the mortality rates of both diseases. A third reason for the decreased salt intake was the mass education of the population through TV, broadcasts, the press, etc. To be effective this campaign had to be preceded by the education of the general practitioners on the value of reducing salt intake in the population. This occurred in Belgium from 1968 on, and was observed also in the U.S. and Australia. It did not occur in the United Kingdom until recently.

All this may explain why the between-countries and the within-country (between 1955 and 1973) relationships were quantitatively similar. After 1973 two major confounding factors became effective. The first was mass treatment of hypertension, resulting in a greater decrease of stroke than expected from stomach cancer (see Figs. 3 and 4, from 1973 on). If the salt hypothesis is correct, one may estimate the relative merits of reducing salt intake and of hypertension treatment in the prevention of stroke. In England and Wales about 62% of the observed decrease in stroke mortality between 1955 and 1984 is due to the stomach cancer/stroke relationship, i.e. lowering salt intake, and 38% is due to mass treatment of hypertension or to other environmental changes influencing blood pressure. In the U.S., using a similar approach as above, it follows that about 45% of the decline in stroke mortality is related to a reduction of salt intake and 55% predominantly to mass treatment of hypertension, whereas in Canada this amounts to 71% and 29% respectively (Fig. 4).

The second confounding factor started to act in the mid-seventies. Because of increasing affluence, all the East European countries increased their fat intake. Traditionally, the fat intake has been relatively low in those countries, i.e. about 20–30% of energy. The increased butter consumption (e.g. 9 kg/day/adult person in the G.D.R. in 1969, 15 kg in 1980) resulted in a marked increase of the total fat and the saturated fat intake in the East European countries. Saturated fat can increase blood pressure and enhances also the thrombotic tendency. Polyunsaturated fat has opposite properties. In general, it can be observed that not only stroke, but also coronary, total cardiovascular, rectal cancer, colon cancer, and diabetes mortality increased markedly in the East European countries. Life expectancy either remained unchanged or even decreased after 1968. The opposite change in mortality with a markedly increasing life expectancy was observed in the U.S., Canada, Finland, Belgium, etc. All this is consistent with the role of dietary fat as a disease risk factor.

The increasing P/S (polyunsaturated/saturated fat) ratio in the U.S. may also explain why after 1973 the stroke mortality decreased more, relative to stomach cancer, in the U.S. than in England and Wales (see above).

How Can Salt Intake Influence Stomach Cancer and Stroke?

Apart from the epidemiological evidence relating salt intake to *stomach cancer*, there are also several case-control studies showing that salted and pickled food increase the relative risk of stomach cancer and that fresh vegetables and fruits (which are generally low in salt) decrease the risk. Of course vitamin C may also play a protective role by blocking the nitrate-to-nitrite conversion in the stomach.

Experimental evidence for the link between salt and stomach cancer became available in the mid-seventies when it was shown by Tatematsu and co-workers that salt enhanced the influence of nitrosocarcinogens in the induction of experimental stomach cancer. More recently several investigators in Japan, the U.S., and Korea have shown that salt is a caustic substance in hypertonic solution producing atrophic gastritis in animals; that it induces DNA-synthesis in the gastric mucosa, indicating increased mitotic activity similar to the effects of gastric carcinogens; that it induces ornithine decarboxylase activity in the gastric mucosa, again similar to the action of gastric carcinogens; that it is also co-carcinogenic; and that it is a promoter of stomach cancer when given in hypertonic solution after the initiation with a carcinogen (2).

Table 2 gives the possible etiology of stomach cancer.

All this evidence is consistent with clinical and epidemiological observations. It should also be remembered that salt is caustic to the

Table 2
Possible Etiology of Stomach Cancer

High salt intake hypertonic stomach content

Delayed emptying through duodenal osmoreceptors

Longer contact with caustic salt solution, especially in lower part of the stomach

Damaged gastric mucosa, increased DNA synthesis,
ornithine decarboxylase induction
(proven in animals)

Atrophic gastritis anacidity bacterial overgrowth nitrates to nitrites

Nitroso-carcinogens (salt is cocarcinogenic and promotes stomach cancer in animals)

Stomach cancer, especially in lower part of the stomach

skin, as observed among workers in salt mines and among lobster fishermen. Salt also damages the taste buds.

Blood pressure is the major contributor to *stroke*, as shown by the Framingham study and as confirmed by many others.

The relationship between salt intake and blood pressure was observed in China more than 6000 years ago when the Yellow Emperor noticed that people who indulged in salt eating had hard pulses. He also observed a relation between hard pulses and stroke with aphasia. Since then many observations have been made in favour of the role of salt in hypertension. They are of historical, patho-physiological, pharmacological, clinical, experimental, and epidemiological origin and have been reviewed recently (1). A few of the epidemiological data will be presented here.

In populations with a high salt intake (15–30 g/day; see above) the prevalence of hypertension is also high. Consistently, the prevalence of hypertension is medium or near zero in populations on a medium salt intake (8–12 g/day) or on a no-added salt intake, respectively.

The epidemiological data linking blood pressure to salt intake in middle-aged people in Western countries are not consistent, but positive relations have been found in infants and in the elderly. In developing countries with a high salt intake (South Korea and China) significant correlations between salt and blood pressure were found in adults within the population. Blood pressure in Beijing was significantly higher than in Fuchow, and so was salt intake (3).

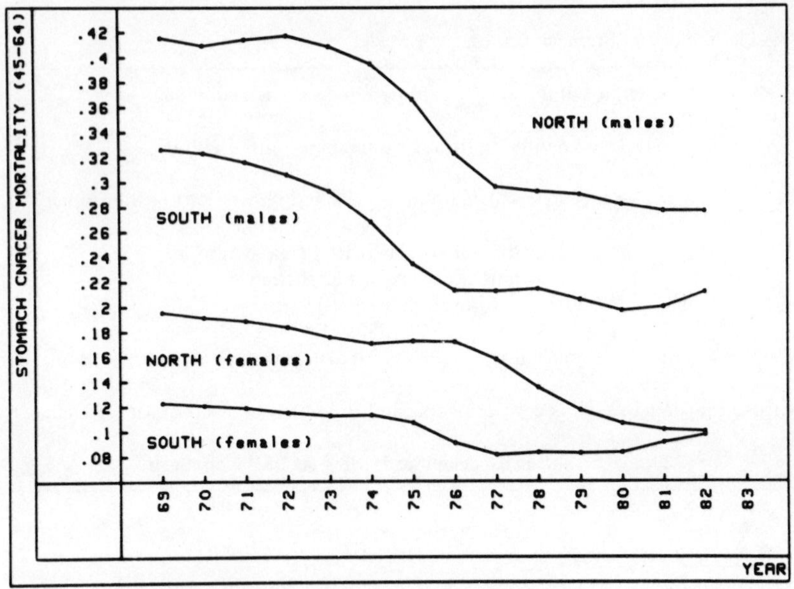

Figure 5. Recent time trends of stomach cancer mortality in males and females of the north and the south of Belgium. Traditionally the salt intake was higher in the north. Salt intake decreased by one-third from 1966 to 1975. After that it levelled off at 10 g/ day (courtesy of Royal Academy of Medicine of Belgium).

The relationships among salt, stomach cancer, and stroke are so strong that it was possible to predict that salt intake was high in Portugal and in Colombia as reflected by their mortality data. This prediction was later confirmed in those countries by measuring salt intake. Similarly it can be stated rather surely that salt intake is high in Chile, though decreasing markedly during recent years. As far as is known to the authors, salt intake has not been measured in Chile up to now.

The Belgian Natural Experiment

Salt consumption in Belgium, especially in the northern part of the country, was traditionally very high. More than 150 years ago it must have been higher than 30 g/day because of the high intake of bread and potatoes and the use of salted dried codfish (stockfish), of pork and vegetables preserved in brine, etc. Since then many changes have

Table 3
Percent Change in Belgium in Age-Adjusted (45–74 y) Mortality from 1968 to 1983, Calculated Over 10 Years

	Males	*Females*		*Males*	*Females*
All Causes	−15.1***	−20.8***	All Cancer	+5.7**	−2.9*
Total Cardiovascular	−22.6***	−29.5***	Esophagus	+16.6**	N.S.
Ischemic heart disease	−22.5***	−27.8***	Stomach	−38.8***	−45.6***
Stroke	−40.9***	−40.1***	Colon	N.S.	−14.7***
Diabetes	−33.6***	−62.3***	Rectum	−26.2***	−26.5***
			Lung	+17.1***	+30.5***
			Prostate	+12.0**	
			Breast		+15.2**

N.S.: not significant
* $p<0.05$
** $p<0.01$
*** $p<0.001$

occurred. Bread consumption is now five times and potato consumption three times lower. Stockfish, pork, and vegetables kept in brine are no longer eaten. Refrigerators are now owned by 98% of all families. Fat intake has increased tremendously, from 15–20% of energy to 42% at present. In 1968 an educational campaign was launched aiming to reduce intake of salt and saturated fat and to increase polyunsaturated fat intake. The final targets were to reduce stroke and stomach cancer mortality by decreasing salt consumption and to reduce ischaemic heart disease by changing fat consumption, thereby simultaneously reducing total cardiovascular mortality and all-causes mortality. By careful monitoring of the population, it was shown that the salt intake decreased from 15 g/day in 1966 to 10 g/day at present. Saturated fat intake in northern Belgium decreased from 20% of energy in 1960 to 17% at this time. The P/S ratio in the northern part changed from 0.2 previously to 0.5 now, whereas in the southern part it increased to only 0.35. The changes in salt and fat intake occurred mainly between 1968 and 1975, after which only minor changes were observed. With a time lag of approximately five years, stroke, ischaemic heart disease, and stomach cancer started to decline markedly (Figures 5 and 6 and Table 3). After 1980 the mortality rates levelled off.

Of course many factors may influence those changes, as, for example, the effect of treatment of hypertension on stroke, but the main arguments for the importance of nutritional factors were, first, the

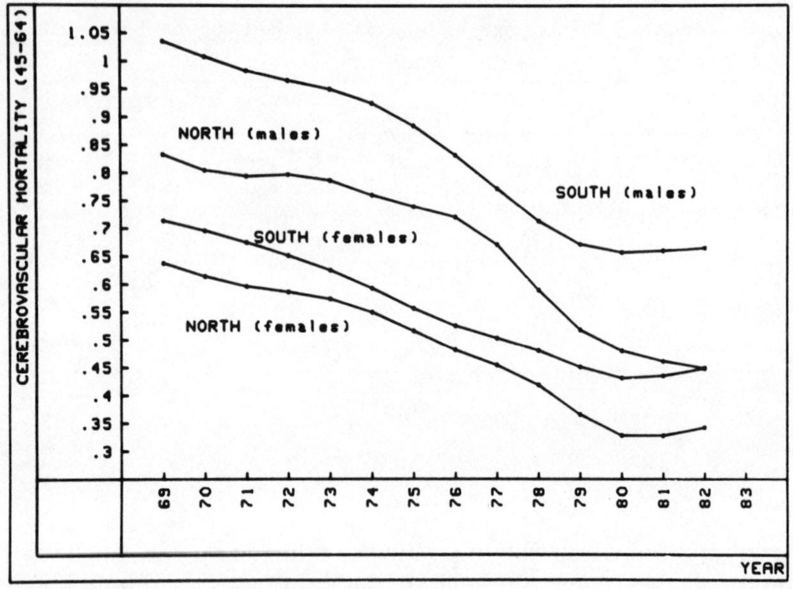

Figure 6. Similar trends as in Figure 5 but for stroke mortality. The time relationship is similar to that of stomach cancer (Fig. 5) but stroke is higher in the south, whereas from salt intake the reverse would be expected. This is probably because of differences in fat intake (see text) (courtesy of Royal Academy of Medicine of Belgium).

time-relationship of the changes (Figs. 5 and 6) and, second, the magnitude of the changes as compared to neighbouring countries (Table 3, Figures 7 and 8). Up to 1980 the declines in stomach cancer, stroke, and ischaemic heart disease in Belgium were the highest in the Common Market.

Conclusion

From the historical, patho-physiological, clinical, pharmacological, experimental, and epidemiological data it becomes more and more evident that salt is not such an innocuous substance as it appears. If salt was not used in the U.S. and one requested the FDA to authorize the addition of salt to food it would undoubtedly be refused. It can be agreed that the final proof, i.e., a controlled double-blind trial with morbidity and mortality as end points has not yet been carried out. One can wonder whether such a trial is feasible and, if so, whether

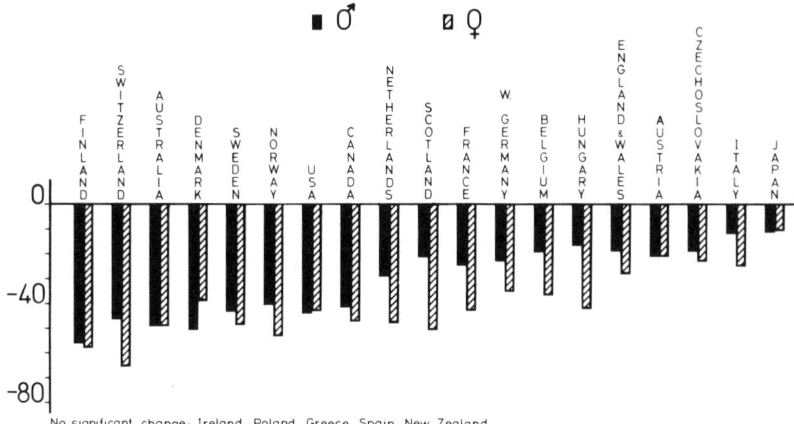

Figure 7. Significant changes of stomach cancer mortality, age adjusted 45–64 years, in % of average mortality values. The countries are ranked according to the values of both sexes averaged. Belgium ranked 13th among 24 countries.
Changes estimated over 10 years, period 1955–1965.

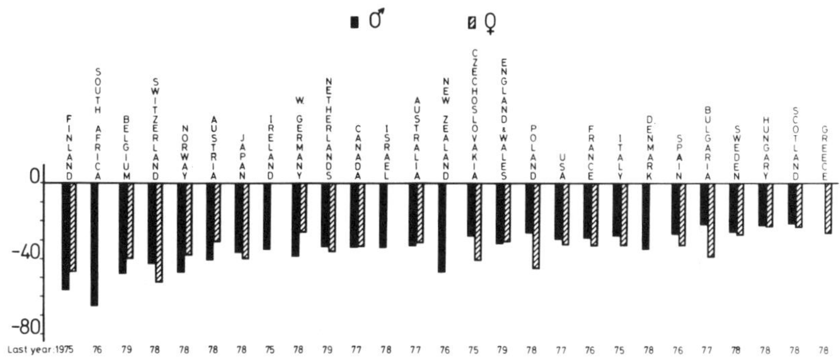

Figure 8. As in Figure 7 but for the period 1968 to 1979. Belgium now ranked third among 27 countries.

it will ever be done. A weaker alternative is doing what has been done in Belgium, i.e. lowering the salt intake at the population level, carefully monitoring the change in salt consumption, and looking for the effects on mortality. Such predicted effects occurred in Belgium. They are consistent, dose-related, and definitely encouraging.

REFERENCES

1 Joossens JV, Geboers J. Dietary salt and risks to health. *Am J Clin Nutr* 1987;45:1277–1288.
2 Takahashi M, Hasegawa R. Enhancing effects of dietary salt on both initiation and promotion stages of rat gastric carcinogenesis. In: Hayashi Y, et al., eds. *Diet, nutrition and cancer*. Tokyo: Japan Sci Soc Press; Utrecht: VNU Sci Press, 1986:169–182.
3 Kesteloot H, Huang DX, Li YL, Geboers J, Joossens JV. On the relationship between cations and blood pressure in The People's Republic of China. *Hypertension* 1987;9:654–659.
4 Kaplan NM. Diet and hypertension. In this collection.

ANTHONY B. MILLER

Epidemiology of Breast and Colon Cancer

I shall discuss the epidemiology of these two cancers from the viewpoint of the possible association between them and dietary fat consumption.

There are remarkable similarities in the epidemiology of these two cancers; both show substantial international variation, with high rates in North America and Western Europe and low rates in Japan and other parts of Asia (1). In individual cancer registries the correlation between incidence of colon cancer and breast cancer in women is high, 0.84, almost as high as the correlation between breast and rectal cancers, 0.72. In fact, the correlation is higher than that between colon and rectal cancers, 0.67. There is almost as strong correlation with the incidence of uterine corpus and ovarian cancer.

Both cancers show changes of incidence in migrant groups. This has been demonstrated in people from Eastern Europe migrating to the United States, people from Japan migrating to the United States and Canada, and people from Southern Europe migrating to Australia. In general the trend is for migrant groups to acquire the incidence pattern of the host country, the rate of change being greater for colon cancer than for breast cancer, though this is not universal; indeed, in Israel the rate of increase of both breast and colon cancer in Jews born in Africa and Asia seems very similar (2). One feature of the epidemiology of breast cancer is an apparent differing age-specific pattern in different parts of the world, with lower rates particularly in post-menopausal women in Japan, compared to North America. However, this has been demonstrated to be largely due to a birth cohort phenomenon with increasing incidence being seen in younger women in recent years (3).

Correlational Studies

A number of authors have pointed to the high correlation between dietary fat intake and the incidence of colon, rectal, and breast cancer. The strong correlations have been seen for both men and women, and, where data have been analyzed, they suggest that the correlation for animal protein intake is less than for fat intake (4). Gray et al. (5) looked also at the influence of height, weight, and age at menarche as well as estimated animal protein and total fat intake on incidence and mortality from breast cancer. They found an inverse correlation with age at menarche, a positive correlation with all other factors, with an indication of a stronger association when all factors were considered together.

There are many disadvantages in correlational studies, but one advantage is that the range of variation between countries is often much greater than is found within countries. Thus the level of the association seen internationally may more closely reflect the strength of the association between dietary fat and these two cancer sites than that seen in analytic studies.

Obesity

De Waard was one of the first to point to the association between overweight or, latterly, body mass index, and risk of breast cancer in post-menopausal women (6). Although some studies did not confirm this, the follow-up of American Cancer Society participants (7) and case-control studies in California (8) and Israel (9), as well as the earlier studies in the Netherlands (6), have demonstrated a consistent association with increasing risk of breast cancer and increasing weight or body mass index. The studies in Holland also demonstrated an association with increasing height (6), but this has not been replicated elsewhere. The association is restricted to post-menopausal women and in Israel to women age 60 or more (9). Some studies suggest the reverse effect for pre-menopausal women.

For colon cancer there has been less evaluation of the obesity issue, but for men at least there was some suggestion in the American Cancer Society that there was increasing mortality with increasing weight. Our own case-control study, however, did not show such an association.

Case-Control Studies

Much of the bulk of analytic epidemiologic evidence relating fat intake to both breast and colo-rectal cancer has come from case-control studies. These have varied in quality, from studies in which dietary information was collected by simple questionnaires, eliciting just frequency of a few standard food items, to much more complex inquiries with a detailed dietary history, quantitative estimation of intake, and calculation of nutrient intake through computerized data bases. In general, the more sophisticated the dietary methodology the stronger the association found between dietary fat and these two cancers. One of the earliest studies for breast cancer was performed by Phillips among Seventh-Day Adventists (10). He showed an association with fat-containing foods. In our own study in Canada, a relatively weak association was found, largely restricted to total fat intake (11). However, in a subsequent re-analysis incorporating two methods of dietary assessment, Howe found a dose-response relationship for saturated fat consumption which was stronger in premenopausal women (12). In another study in Canada, Lubin et al. (13) found increasing risk with increasing estimated consumption levels of beef, pork, animal fat, and animal protein. Although this study can be criticized methodologically, because a separate control group was interviewed by a completely different team at a different time period, it is not clear why this should have been a source of systematic bias, with suggestive dose-response relationships. A large study from Roswell Park, however, was entirely negative, though this study was based on a very simple questionnaire and used hospital controls (14). A more recent study from Canada found increasing risk with increasing consumption of whole milk, beef, and a protective effect from fish consumption (15). Subjects were asked about their consumption of visible fat on meat and there was a suggestion that those who consumed such fat often in childhood as well as in adult life had increased risk. Another study, which pointed to increased risk from consumption of milk – in this case, full cream milk – was performed in France (16). A large study in Israel has pointed to the importance of dietary pattern. Risk was increased in those with a high consumption of fat and protein and a low consumption of fibre, whereas risk was lowest in those with a low consumption of fat and protein, and a high consumption of fibre (17).

For colon cancer, again a series of case-control studies have been performed. One of the earliest, on Hawaiian Japanese, demonstrated increased risk for those who rarely consumed Japanese-style meals or who consumed beef frequently (18). A study in Israel showed that high consumption of food that contained fibre was protective for colon cancer, but no effect could be demonstrated for rectal cancer (19). A study on Seventh-Day Adventists showed that meat of any type, beef products, beef hamburger, and lamb, increased risk, whereas vegetarian products and green leafy vegetables were protective (10). Similarly, in a study in Roswell Park, frequent consumption of Brassica-type vegetables was protective, particularly for colon cancer but also to a lesser extent for rectal cancer (20). In a study of Bay area blacks, the highest risk was found in those with low consumption of foods containing fibre and a high consumption of 5% or more saturated fat foods (21). Those with high fibre and low fat consumption had lowest risk. In our own study, saturated fat intake seemed to increase risk to the greatest extent, with a suggestive dose-response relationship (22). We could, however, find no protective effect for dietary fibre and only a weak protective effect from cruciferous vegetables (23). A study in Adelaide, Australia, also found increased risk for fat consumption, but the most consistent finding was increased risk for protein consumption, particularly of animal origin (24). In this study there was no indication of a protective effect of fibre, indeed in females fibre appeared to increase risk. In Marseilles, however, it was demonstrated that vegetables containing low amounts of fibre produced a significant protective effect; those with medium amounts of fibre a less dramatic protective effect (25). In this study, both milk consumption and oil consumption appeared to be protective, the oil being largely olive oil. A further study in Australia found increased risk for beef consumption, fat, and high milk consumption. Other meats did not increase risk; fibre appeared to be protective (26).

Cohort Studies

An early cohort study in Norway appeared to show a protective effect of vegetables for colon cancer. Hirayama in his study has found that those with high meat consumption appeared to have increased risk of colon cancer and of breast cancer (27). He pointed out that fat intake had increased substantially in Japan and that this was associated with increase in the incidence of breast cancer. A large recent cohort study in American nurses, who were aged 34 to 59 years at the time of completion of a dietary questionnaire and have so far been followed for four years, has found no association with estimated fat intake (28). However, the difference in intake between the upper and lower quintiles of fat intake in this study could not be expected to demonstrate more than a relative risk of 1.4 if the international correlational studies are a guide. With this weak risk anticipated, and with the possibility of measurement error from a self-administered questionnaire, it is perhaps not surprising that such a study would be negative.

Conclusion

Although not all the findings are consistent, the evidence appears to be accumulating that both breast and colo-rectal cancer are associated with high fat intake. Perhaps most typically the pattern of high risk is associated with dietary consumption of high fat, possibly especially saturated fat from animal sources, and low consumption of vegetables and possibly fibre, though the relevance of fibre as distinct from other potential protective factors from vegetables containing fibre has not yet been established. Using the available data, as in our own study, it seems likely that the population attributable risk from saturated fat for colo-rectal cancer is of the order of 42%, with possibly 50% or more of cases explained by dietary variables. For breast cancer the attributable risk from total fat is of the order of 27% as estimated from our study, with an additional 12% from obesity; it seems possible that up to 40% of breast cancer may be preventable by dietary modification, although there is some concern that the effect of dietary modification for breast cancer could be delayed, as exhibited by the lack of change of breast cancer incidence in some religious groups that have adopted a low-fat diet (29). For colon cancer there seems to be less possibility for delay. One might postulate a fairly rapid impact of dietary modification on colon cancer rates, with a possible delay of 40 or 50 years for breast, especially if the full effect of dietary modification has to occur for women in their teens and twenties.

REFERENCES

1 Waterhouse J, Muir C, Shanmugaratnam K, Powell J. *Cancer incidence in five continents*. Vol. IV, IARC Scientific Publ No. 42. Lyon: International Agency for Research on Cancer, 1982.

2 Steinitz R. Cancer risks in immigrant populations in Israel. In: Aoki K, ed. *Proceedings of the first UICC conference on cancer prevention in developing countries*. Nagoya: University of Nagoya Press, 1982:363–381.

3 Stevens RG, Moolgavkar SH, Lee JH. Temporal trends in breast cancer. *Am J Epidemiol* 1982;115:759–777.
4 Armstrong B, Doll R. Environmental factors and cancer incidence and mortality in different countries, with special reference to dietary practices. *Int J Cancer* 1975; 15:617–631.
5 Gray GE, Pike MC, Henderson BE. Breast cancer incidence and mortality rates in different countries in relation to known risk factors and dietary practices. *Br J Cancer* 1979;39:1–7.
6 de Waard F, Baanders-van Halewijn EA. A prospective study in general practice on breast cancer risk in postmenopausal women. *Int J Cancer* 1974;14:153–160.
7 Lew EA, Garfinkel L. Variations in mortality by weight among 750,000 men and women. *J Chron Dis* 1979;32:563–576.
8 Paffenbarger RS, Kampert JB, Chang HG. Characteristics that predict risk of breast cancer before and after the menopause. *Am J Epidemiol* 1980;112:258–268.
9 Lubin F, Ruder AM, Wax Y, Modan B. Overweight and changes in weight throughout adult life in breast cancer etiology. *Am J Epidemiol* 1985;122:579–588.
10 Phillips RL. Role of life-style and dietary habits in risk of cancer among Seventh-Day Adventists. *Cancer Res* 1975;35:3513–3522.
11 Miller AB, Kelly A, Choi NW, et al. A study of diet and breast cancer. *Am J Epidemiol* 1978; 107:499–509.
12 Howe GR. The use of polytomous dual response data to increase power in case control studies: an application to the association between dietary fat and breast cancer. *J Chron Dis* 1985;38:663–670.
13 Lubin JH, Burns PE, Blot WJ, Zeigler RG, Lees AW, Fraumeni JF. Dietary factors and breast cancer risk. *Int J Cancer* 1981; 28:685–689.
14 Graham S, Marshall J, Mettlin C, Rzepka T. Nemoto T, Byers T. Diet in the epidemiology of breast cancer. *Am J Epidemiol* 1982;116:68–75.
15 Hislop TG, Coldman AJ, Elwood JM, Brauer G, Kan L. Childhood and recent eating patterns and risk of breast cancer. *Cancer Detect Prev* 1986;9:47–58.
16 Le MG, Moulton LH, Hill C, Kramer A. Consumption of dairy produce and alcohol in a case-control study of breast cancer. *J Natl Cancer Inst* 1986;77:633–636.
17 Lubin F, Wax Y, Modan B. Role of fat, animal protein, and dietary fiber in breast cancer etiology: a case-control study. *J Natl Cancer Inst* 1986;77:605–612.
18 Haenszel W, Berg JW, Segi M, Kurihara M, Locke FB. Large bowel cancer in Hawaiian Japanese. *J Natl Cancer Inst* 1973;51:1765–1779.

19 Modan B, Barell V, Lubin F, Modan M, Greenberg RA, Graham S. Low fiber intake as an etiological factor in cancer of the colon. *J Natl Cancer Inst* 1975;55:15–18.
20 Graham S, Dayal H, Swanson M, Mittleman A, Wilkinson G. Diet in the epidemiology of cancer of the colon and rectum. *J Natl Cancer Inst* 1978;61:709–714.
21 Dales LG, Friedman GD, Ury HK, Grossman S, Williams SR. A case-control study of relationships of diet and other traits to colo-rectal cancer in American blacks. *Am J Epidemiol* 1979;109:132–144.
22 Jain M, Cook GM, Davis FG, Grace MG, Howe GR, Miller AB. A case control study of diet and colo-rectal cancer. *Int J Cancer* 1980;26:757–768.
23 Miller AB, Howe GR, Jain M, Craib KJP, Harrison L. Food items and food groups as risk factors in a case control study of diet and colo-rectal cancer. *Int J Cancer* 1983;32:155–161.
24 Potter JD, McMichael AJ. Diet and cancer of the colon and rectum: a case control study. *J Natl Cancer Inst* 1986;76:557–569.
25 Macquart-Moulin G, Riboli E, Cornee J, Charnay B, Berthezene P, Day N. Case control study on colo-rectal cancer and diet in Marseilles. *Int J Cancer* 1986;38:183–191.
26 Kune S, Kune GA, Watson LF. Case control study of dietary etiological factors: the Melbourne colo-rectal cancer study. *Nutr Cancer* 1987;9:21–42.
27 Hirayama T. A large scale cohort study on the relationship between diet and selected cancers of digestive organs. In: *Gastrointestinal cancer, endogenous factors. Banbury report 7*. Cold Spring Harbor, NY: Cold Spring Harbor Laboratory, 1981:409–429.
28 Willett WC, Stampfer MJ, Colditz GA, Rosner BA, Hennekens CH, Speizer FE. Dietary fat and the risk of breast cancer. *N Engl J Med* 1987;316:22–28.
29 Kinlen LJ. Meat and fat consumption and cancer mortality: a study of strict religious orders in Britain. *Lancet* 1982;1:946–949.

DAVID KRITCHEVSKY

Calories and Cancer

In 1981 Doll and Peto (1) published a review and assessment of causes of cancer in the United States which further stimulated the already vigorous research on diet and cancer. In discussing the earlier studies of caloric restriction, they suggested that the direction of research might have been changed drastically had the control mice been regarded as fat instead of the calorically-restricted mice being seen as undersized. Their estimation was right on target!

The earliest study of caloric restriction (in the form of underfeeding) was reported by Moreschi (2) in 1909, who found that transplanted sarcomas grew less vigorously in mice whose daily intake of food was restricted, than in mice fed *ad libitum*. Tumour growth was inhibited as a function of dietary restriction. Other investigators confirmed Moreschi's findings. The most active work in this area was carried out by Tannenbaum in the 1940s. He investigated caloric restriction as both underfeeding (feeding less of the control diet) and true caloric restriction (in which specific sources of calories are restricted). In both cases – using several strains of mouse and spontaneous as well as experimentally induced tumours – he found caloric restriction to inhibit tumorigenesis. Some of Tannenbaum's findings (3) are summarized in Table 1.

The early investigators also examined the contribution of dietary fat. Lavik and Baumann (4) found caloric intake, rather than fat, was the principal determinant of incidence of methylcholanthrene-induced skin tumours in mice (Table 2). Boutwell et al. (5) found that the incidence of chemically-induced skin tumours in mice fed isoca-

Table 1
Inhibition of Tumorigenesis by Caloric Restriction*

Type of Tumor	*Mouse Strain*	*Percent Inhibition*
Induced epithelial	ABC	58
	Swiss	35
	DBA	66
Induced sarcoma	C57 Black	32
	Swiss	55
Spontaneous mammary	DBA	64
Spontaneous lung	ABC	48
	Swiss	83

*After Tannenbaum (3).

Table 2
Effect of Fat or Calories on Chemically-Induced Skin Tumors in Mice*

Fat	*Calories*	*Incidence (%)*
Low	Low	0
High	Low	28
Low	High	54
High	High	66

*After Lavik and Baumann (4).

loric diets containing 2 or 61% fat differed by only 28%. The entire field was reviewed by White (6) in 1961 but lay dormant until recently. We have investigated some of the different aspects of caloric restriction in an effort to assess contributions of extent of caloric restriction and type of fat. In our initial study (7) we compared effects of *ad libitum* feeding and 40% caloric restriction in rats treated with 7,12-dimethylbenz(a)anthracene (DMBA) in order to induce mammary tumours. The control rats were fed 3.9% fat (2.9% coconut oil, and 1.0% corn oil, to provide sufficient essential fatty acid). Calorically-restricted rats were fed 8.4% fat. Diets were designed to provide the same level of every nutrient except fat and carbohydrate, which was reduced in order to reduce calories. In that study (7) tumour incidence in the control group was 58% while no tumours were found (either by palpation or at necropsy) in the restricted rats. A similar experiment in rats given 1,2-dimethylhydrazine (DMH) to induce colonic tumours

Table 3
Effect of 40% Caloric Restriction and Fat Type on Chemical Carcinogenesis

Carcinogen	Rat Strain	Dietary Fat*	Tumor Incidence (%) Ad Libitum	Restricted
DMBA	Sprague-Dawley	CNO	58	0
		CO	80	20
DMH	F344	BO	85	35
		CO	100	53

* CNO – coconut oil; CO – corn oil; BO – butter oil.

showed tumour incidence of 85% and 35% in *ad libitum* or calorie restricted rats, respectively. The fat used was butter oil. Repetition of both studies using corn oil as the sole source of fat showed tumour incidences of 80% and 20% in *ad libitum* and calorically-restricted rats given DMBA and 100% and 53% in *ad libitum* and restricted rats given DMH (8) (Table 3). These experiments showed that 40% caloric restriction did indeed inhibit experimental carcinogenesis and that saturated fat was less co-carcinogenic than unsaturated fat, as Carroll and Khor (9) had shown. However, the caloric restriction was drastic and fat levels had been rather low. Experiments were then designed to examine the effects of increased fat and decreased caloric restriction.

In one experiment, rats were given DMBA and calories were restricted by either 10, 20, 30, or 40% (10). Restriction of calories by only 10% (fat intake equivalent to that of control) did not affect incidence of tumours but reduced tumour burden (total tumour weight) by 47%. At 30% caloric restriction, tumour incidence was reduced by 42% and tumour burden by 95% (Table 4). In a second study (11), also involving DMBA-induced mammary tumours, *ad libitum*-fed rats were given 5, 15, or 20% corn oil and rats whose calories were restricted by 25% were fed 20 or 26.7% corn oil, thus their daily intake of corn oil was equivalent to that of the *ad libitum*-fed rats receiving 15 or 20% corn oil. Compared to rats fed 5% corn oil *ad libitum*, the rats fed 26.7% corn oil in the 25% calorically-restricted diet exhibited a tumour incidence which was 54% lower and tumour burden which was 45% lower (Table 5). Thus, caloric restriction inhibited tumorigenesis even at high fat intake.

Could body fat play a role? In the study in which caloric intake was restricted by 10, 20, 30, or 40% (10), weight gain closely reflected caloric restriction. However, body fat content was much greater than

Table 4
Effect of Graded Caloric Restriction on DMBA-Induced Mammary Tumors in Sprague-Dawley Rats

Regimen	*Tumor Incidence (%)*	*Tumor Multiplicity*	*Tumor Burden (g)*
Ad libitum	60	4.7 ± 1.3	10.1 ± 3.3
10% restricted	60	3.0 ± 0.8	5.4 ± 3.0
20% restricted	40	2.8 ± 0.7	4.7 ± 1.9
30% restricted	35	1.3 ± 0.3	0.9 ± 0.8
40% restricted	5	1.0 ± 0	—
p	<0.005	NS	<0.05

Table 5
Effect of Fat Level and 25% Caloric Restriction on DMBA-Induced Mammary Tumors in Sprague-Dawley Rats

Regimen	*Tumor Incidence (%)*	*Tumor Multiplicity*	*Tumor Burden (g)*
Ad libitum			
5% corn oil	65	1.9 ± 0.3	4.2 ± 1.9
15% corn oil	85	3.0 ± 0.6	6.6 ± 2.7
20% corn oil	80	4.1 ± 0.6	11.8 ± 3.2
25% Restricted			
20% corn oil	60	1.9 ± 0.4	1.5 ± 0.5
26.7% corn oil	30	1.5 ± 0.3	2.3 ± 1.6
p	<0.005	<0.0001	<0.0001

would have been expected. Caloric restriction by 10, 20, 30, or 40% reduced total body fat by 16.3, 43.3, 63.3, and 72.2%, respectively. The final body weights of rats fed 15 or 20% corn oil *ad libitum* were 28 and 26% higher than those of rats fed the same amount of fat but whose calories were restricted by 25% (11). The retroperitoneal fat pads of the calorie-restricted rats weighed 70 and 62% less than those of the rats fed *ad libitum*. To test the possible effect of body fat, we used the LA/N corpulent rat, a genetically obese animal. Obese rats given DMBA and fed *ad libitum* exhibited a 100% incidence of mammary tumours. Restriction of calories by 40% reduced tumour incidence to 27% but the total body fat of the control and restricted groups was 51 and 47%, respectively (12).

Could growth factors play a role? In the experiment in which we tried stepwise caloric restriction (10), plasma insulin was 122 ± 16 μU/ml in the control rats and 42 ± 5 or 41 ± 8 μU/ml in rats whose calories were restricted by 20 or 40%, respectively. Plasma insulin levels in control and calorically-restricted obese rats were 1003 and 328, respectively.

There is ample evidence that caloric restriction inhibits experimental carcinogenesis whether spontaneous or induced by chemical carcinogens or by other means such as ultraviolet irradiation (10,13,14). Albanes (15) has reviewed data from 82 studies of caloric restriction and carcinogenesis in mice and finds reduced tumour incidence with increased restriction. Caloric restriction also enhances the activity of enzymes such as hexokinase and glucose-6-phosphate dehydrogenase (16). We must now seek to explain the mechanism(s) by which caloric restriction exerts its cancer-inhibiting effect in hopes of obtaining information which will be useful for extension to human studies.

REFERENCES

1 Doll R, Peto R. The causes of cancer: quantitative estimates of avoidable risks of cancer in the United States today. *J Natl Cancer Inst* 1981;66:1192–1308.

2 Moreschi C. Beziehungen zwischen Ernahrung und Tumorwachstum. *Z Immunitatsforsch* 1909;2:651–675.

3 Tannenbaum A. The genesis and growth of tumors. II. Effects of caloric restriction *per se*. *Cancer Res* 1942;2:460–467.

4 Lavik PS, Baumann CA. Further studies on tumor-promoting action of fat. *Cancer Res* 1943;3:749–756.

5 Boutwell RK, Brush MK, Rusch HP. The stimulating effect of dietary fat on carcinogenesis. *Cancer Res* 1949;9:741–746.

6 White FR. The relationship between underfeeding and tumor formation, transplantation and growth in rats and mice. *Cancer Res* 1961;21:281–290.

7 Kritchevsky D, Weber MM, Klurfeld DM. Dietary fat versus caloric content in initiation and promotion of 7,12-dimethylbenz(a)anthracene-induced mammary tumorigenesis in rats. *Cancer Res* 1984;44:3174–3177.

8 Klurfeld DM, Weber MM, Kritchevsky D. Inhibition of chemically induced mammary and colon tumor promotion by caloric restriction in rats fed increased dietary fat. *Cancer Res* 1987;47:2759–2762.

9 Carroll KK, Khor HT. Effect of level and type of dietary fat on incidence of mammary tumors induced in female Sprague-Dawley rats by 7,12-dimethylbenz(a)anthracene. *Lipids* 1971;6:415–420.
10 Kritchevsky D, Klurfeld DM. Caloric effects in experimental mammary tumorigenesis. *Am J Clin Nutr* 1987;45:236–242.
11 Kritchevsky D, Weber MM, Buck CL, Klurfeld DM. Calories, fat and cancer. *Lipids* 1986;21:272–274.
12 Klurfeld DM, Lloyd LM, Buck CL, Davis ML, Tulp DL, Kritchevsky D. Inhibition of mammary tumorigenesis in LA/N-cp (corpulent) rats. *Fed Proc* 1987;46:436.
13 Kritchevsky D, Klurfeld DM. Influence of caloric intakes on experimental carcinogenesis: a review. In: Poirier LA, Newberne PM, Pariza MW, eds. *Essential nutrients in carcinogenesis.* New York: Plenum Publishing, 1986;55–68.
14 Kritchevsky D. Fat, calories and cancer. In: Ip C, Birt DF, Rogers AE, Mettlin C, eds. *Dietary fat and cancer.* New York: Alan R. Liss, 1986:495–515.
15 Albanes D. Total calories, body weight and tumor incidence in mice. *Cancer Res* 1987;47:1987–1992.
16 Ruggieri BA, Klurfeld DM, Kritchevsky D. Biochemical alterations in 7,12-dimethylbenz(a)anthracene-induced mammary tumors from rats subjected to caloric restriction. *Biochim Biophys Acta* 1987;929:239–246.

Dietary Guidelines

C. WAYNE CALLAWAY*

Development and Use of Dietary Guidelines for Whole Populations versus Populations at High Risk

There are two points to be considered in this presentation. These are the development and use of dietary guidelines, including goals and recommendations; and the question of guidelines for whole populations as opposed to groups or individuals at high risk.*

Collection and Analysis of Data

The development of dietary guidelines on which to base a rational public policy is dependent first of all on the collection and analysis of data. Opinions are of little value, and it is important to have a sound base of factual information. Where there is wide disparity in the data that are being reported, the methodology needs to be examined and the differences resolved if possible.

It is also important to have independent confirmation of data. One study is not a sufficient basis for drawing conclusions, and confirmation by a different group of investigators is desirable. To give some examples from Dr. Kaplan's excellent summary of hypertension (1), one could conclude that there is now sufficient evidence on sodium, obesity, alcohol, and perhaps potassium, for an expert analysis of the data base, but evidence on calcium is still evolving, and evidence on trace elements and fibre is practically non-existent. Thus, there is no point in having an expert panel review the evidence on fibre and hypertension until more information is available.

* This chapter is an edited version of the tapescript of the talk presented by Dr. Callaway at the Symposium on Diet, Nutrition and Health.

In assembling an expert panel to review the evidence, care should be taken to ensure that the full spectrum of legitimate scientific opinion is represented. Otherwise, the credibility of the report will be undermined. This does not mean that every constituency must be represented, but that panels in which most of the members share more or less the same point of view should be avoided.

In analyzing the data, it is helpful to divide them into categories such as epidemiologic studies, animal studies, and human intervention trials. There is also the question of consistency among and within populations. For example, if you look cross-culturally, there is no doubt that sodium intake is related to blood pressure, but if you study people living in a specific location, such as Rochester, MN, it is more difficult to show this relationship. Reducing sodium intake may still lower blood pressure in a substantial number of individuals, but in a society where there is a relatively homogeneous diet, genetic factors often play a more dominant role statistically. For example, Stunkard et al. (2), in a study on genetics, environment and obesity, estimated that about 20% of the variance in body weight was environmental and about 80% was genetic. This was a population in which there was adequate food and where physical activity was relatively low. In other populations, such as farmers living in the Andes and engaging in heavy physical activity, environmental factors may be of far greater importance than genetics, and it is important to distinguish between these factors. Readers interested in further discussion of this topic should consult the December 1979 supplement to the *American Journal of Clinical Nutrition* (3).

It is critical in dealing with expert panels that the task be divided according to the types of data and that specific criteria be established for evaluating the strength and consistency of the evidence before asking the panel to make recommendations.

Public Health Policy

In dealing with public health issues, one has to integrate not only the data on a specific disease in relation to diet, but also the whole pattern of morbidity and mortality as well as the major subgroups in the country involved. The issues can also change with time, and what is effective public health policy in 1987 may be totally irrelevant in 1990. If, for example, coronary artery disease were reduced to the level of 1890, it would be anachronistic to continue to focus on issues related to this particular disease.

Thus, public health policy must change to reflect the patterns of morbidity and mortality that exist. It also has to deal with trade-offs. For example, in developing dietary guidelines in 1980, some individuals in the National Heart, Lung and Blood Institute felt strongly that there should be a recommendation to increase polyunsaturated fatty acids to approximately 10% of total calories and to make specific mention of the P/S ratio. Others within the National Cancer Institute were quite concerned about potential adverse effects of raising the level of polyunsaturated fatty acids. Another factor to be considered is whether the public health policy will be accepted and will be effective. An example of an effective public health program in Finland was presented earlier in this symposium (4). This is a critical consideration in embarking on any public health policy.

The implementation of public health policy involves a variety of different modes of intervention, including educational programs and programs designed specifically to change behaviour. These include incentives and disincentives, such as surcharges, taxes, food labelling, the provision of food and, at the other extreme, prohibition. The exact means used depend on factors such as the seriousness of the problem, the strength of the evidence, the economic implications, the political and legal systems that exist, and the attitudes of society. For example, although cigarette smoking is generally recognized as harmful, prohibition has not been considered politically feasible, although things are beginning to move in that direction. Thus, the decision may have little to do with science. In fact, the people who are most affected may be totally ignorant of the science base.

In any expert panel examining the evidence there are likely to be differences of opinion. This can be expressed in various ways, and it is very helpful for policy makers to have some idea of how strongly the experts feel about a subject and whether or not there is great divergence or fairly coherent agreement. In the task force of the American Society for Clinical Nutrition chaired by Drs. Ahrens and Connor (3), panel members were asked to evaluate the evidence on the basis of associations among population groups, associations among individuals within a given population, intervention trials, animal models, and biological explanation, and to assign arbitrary scores from 0 to 20, with 20 being an absolute rock-solid association and 0 being no association at all. Then the scores were summed and expressed as the mean score plus or minus one standard deviation. This provides a semiquantitative way of representing opinion.

This document was used quite extensively in preparing the 1980

Dietary Guidelines for Americans (6). The following are some examples: the association between alcohol and liver disease was given a very high score, indicating that most of the people on the panel felt that this was a strong association with a very small standard deviation. On the other hand, carbohydrates and atherosclerosis received a low score with a small standard deviation. The score for dietary cholesterol alone, as opposed to cholesterol and fat, was in the middle with a large standard deviation. This was interpreted to mean that this panel felt more strongly about the combination of cholesterol and fat than about cholesterol alone. This helps to give policy makers some idea of reality, and the degree of difference of opinion among experts on these issues.

Dietary Recommendations, Goals, and Guidelines

Dietary recommendatons, goals and guidelines have been considered recently by Truswell (5). In the following discussion, I will deviate somewhat from Truswell's definitions. I think we are dealing here with three major areas.

Recommended Dietary Allowances (RDAS), at least in the U.S. version, are recommendations for average intakes of essential nutrients by groups, designed to avoid nutrient deficiencies. These are used for a variety of public policy purposes, and, in essence, represent levels which, if ingested on the average over time by groups, will result in practically no one suffering from malnutrition.

In contrast, dietary goals are objectives that are future oriented. They imply some change, some direction, and should be quantitative and measurable. A minor criticism of objectives has been that some of them have dealt with issues for which baseline data were not available. It is thus difficult to measure progress, although one can measure some end point. I think that goals are a statement of public policy. For example, this is a way of saying that it is our policy to achieve a reduction in average serum cholesterol levels from 220 to 210 or 200, or some other chosen value, by 1990. By referring to a shift in the 75th percentile for adult males, the emphasis can be focussed on a higher risk group. Thus, goals have to be specific and measurable. They are not intended as a document to be read in the grocery store.

Guidelines, on the other hand, really are concerned with implementation, although this is just one aspect of implementation. They represent an information document. Guidelines, I think, should be general, and there are many advantages to making them non-quantitative and quite simple. They can still deal with the heterogeneity and multifactorial nature of chronic diseases in relation to diet. The following is an example from the 1980 Guidelines (6): "The major hazard of excessive sodium is for people who have high blood pressure. Not everyone is equally susceptible." This contains no quantitative information but makes the point that many people can eat larger amounts of sodium without developing high blood pressure. Sodium is only one factor, and obesity can also play a major role. If I were writing this today, I would probably include alcohol as well. As other information becomes established, more things can be added.

It is important to realize that there is heterogeneity. We are not dealing with a magic formula that nutrient X = disease Y; and foods cannot be arbitrarily classified as good or bad. Avoiding too much fat does not mean prohibiting the use of any food item. Eggs and liver contain cholesterol but also have other desirable nutrients. If your serum cholesterol is not elevated and your intake of cholesterol from other sources is not excessive, eggs and liver can be eaten in moderation. This kind of information can be incorporated into the overall message of dietary guidelines.

A final point about guidelines, and in fact goals and RDAs as well, is that they should have a conservative bias. This means that they should be changed only when the evidence for change is fairly strong. Any panel evaluating the evidence is likely to reach a slightly different conclusion from any other panel, and we want to avoid the situation of saying that things that were once considered bad are now good, because that causes confusion.

Whole Populations versus High Risk Groups

Now let us deal with the issue of whole populations versus high risk groups. Should we make recommendations for only one or the other? This is like asking whether four plus two equals six or three plus three equals six. The answer is obviously both. In addition, we also need to make recommendations for individuals.

For whole populations, the level of intervention is different. Dietary guidelines and other information, such as the pamphlets prepared by the U.S. Department of Agriculture based on the dietary guidelines, are helpful. Gradual changes in the nutrient content of commonly used foods, whether it is reducing the sodium content or moving to lower fat meats and dairy products over time, are things that can be done for the whole population. Fortification of foods may play a role, as it did in the mid-forties, when vitamin deficiencies were much more widespread.

Changes in regulations can help to lessen the economic impact of dietary change for whole populations. For instance, if the public perceives that high-fat diets are not healthful, sales of high-fat products will decrease; and in this situation it is better not to pay farmers on the basis of fat content of their products.

I think that on a population basis we can reinforce the idea that foods cannot be categorized as good or bad. For example, it is not fast food that is harmful, but the fat and sodium in fast food. If we can redefine that, we can encourage producers to modify the content of their foods in the direction that is consistent with good public health, without making them feel that they are the villains of the twentieth century.

With regard to groups at high risk, a great deal needs to be done. For instance, age and gender have been largely ignored in dietary goals and guidelines, although in the RDAS there has been some attention to this. For example, they need modification for premenopausal as compared to postmenopausal women. The American Dietetic Association attempted to deal with this in a set of recommendations for dietary intakes for women (7). These emphasized fat not only in terms of coronary artery disease but also in terms of cancer and obesity. They also gave prominence to calcium and iron, because for premenopausal women, many people feel that calcium and iron are at least as important as dietary cholesterol.

As discussed during this symposium, there may well need to be distinctions between infants on the one hand, growing children on the other, and different stages of maturation, including the "young old" and the "old old". I think in this targeting there is also a role for disease-specific recommendations. The recent recommendation by the American Heart Association (8) of limiting dietary cholesterol to 100 mg per 1000 calories may, as I think, have been designed for middle-aged males, and isn't really appropriate for women or for elderly people. Disease-specific recommendations such as this need to be considered in the broader, public health perspective. There is, however, a need to emphasize the diet/disease connection, as well as the cancer-related recommendations of the American Cancer Society (9), based in part on the report from the Food and Nutrition Board in 1982 (10).

Screening programs are also important, including the hypertension program (11) and the cholesterol program that is now being mounted

(12). I also think that education of physicians is a very critical activity, and the National Institutes of Health are planning to do this with their intervention program. If public recommendations are made without educating the physicians, a patient may go to his physician and say, "I was in the screening program for cholesterol and I was told to come and see you because I have a serum cholesterol level of 290 mg/dl." The physician consults reference values indicating that normal values may range from 150 to 300, and says, "Yours is normal, don't worry about it. Don't smoke so many cigars." Physician education is needed, along with multiple other interacting reinforcing mechanisms that exist in our society. How do we integrate concern for deficiency on the one hand with concern for excess on the other? A small ad hoc group has been working with Steve Kline, an evaluation psychologist in Rancorp, to devise some rules and develop a model, with the support of the Dairy Council of California, which is interested in evaluating its education programs in relation to the quality of the overall diet.

An idea that is being considered is to select leading nutrient indicators and use them in the same way as leading economic indicators are used. Certain nutrients tend to cluster together, so it may be possible to pick a leading nutrient from each of these clusters; these must be nutrients for which data are available. The range of nutrient intake is then divided arbitrarily into a level that is adequate and safe, with the beginning part of that range defined by the RDAs, below which malnutrition and deficiency are probable, and at the upper end a level where toxicity increases to the point where toxicity clearly occurs in nearly everybody. This can then be expressed mathematically in various ways by assigning relative scores, based on intake, for each of the leading nutrient indicators. Since these nutrients will not be of equal importance for all people at all ages, the scores will have to be given weighting factors depending on age, gender, etc. Thus, the percentage of calories from saturated fat and cholesterol is a much greater concern for males and would be given a higher weighting than calcium or iron. The sum of the weighted scores can then be used as an index of the nutrient quality of a diet. This would make it possible to rank order menus or diets. It would not tell you that a score of 1400 is necessarily twice as good as a score of 700, but it would indicate that a score of 1400 is better than a score of 700 to 800.

This can then be utilized in relation to national dietary goals. Suppose that we want to improve our scores in a certain fashion. They can be divided into male versus female, pre- and postmenopausal females, the very elderly versus middle-aged people, etc., and eventually considered in terms of individual risk factors. On the basis of family history, lipoprotein levels, blood pressure, etc., individuals could be told that a certain weighting seems appropriate for their dietary intake, that this is the score based on their current diet, and that these are ways the diet could be improved over time. In fact, with personal computers, the 24-hour dietary history could be entered once a week or once a month and a running score kept to see if the diet was changing with time. Although this sounds like science fiction, it is one way of trying to get at the issue of dealing with deficiencies on the one hand and chronic diseases on the other.

What is needed at this stage is not a decision about whether to look at whole populations or groups at high risk but at the virtues of a pluralistic approach of complementary and reinforcing messages. Knowledge changes with time, disease patterns change with time, and there is nothing wrong with changing recommendations so long as it is not done arbitrarily.

My message is that our task is to provide good scientific data, to improve the process of expert analysis and, when given the opportunity, to participate in the formulation of balanced public health policy. Arguments certainly help to sharpen our thinking and often provide great entertainment, but I think we have to be willing to keep our debates within some reasonable balance, so that they remain constructive and designed to meet the goal defined by Ernst Wynder as "dying young as late in life as possible."

REFERENCES

1 Kaplan NM. Diet and hypertension. This volume.
2 Stunkard AJ, Foch TT, Hrubec Z. A twin study of human obesity. *JAMA* 1986:256:51–4.
3 Ahrens EH Jr, Connor WE, Co-chairmen. Report of the task force on the evidence relating six dietary factors to the nation's health. *Am J Clin Nutr* 1979;32(suppl):2619–2748.
4 Pietinen P. A public health program for prevention of cardiovascular disease. This volume.
5 Truswell AS. Evolution of dietary recommendations, goals, and guidelines. *Am J Clin Nutr* 1987;45(suppl):1060–72.
6 U.S. Department of Agriculture and U.S. Department of Health and Human Services. *Nutrition and Your Health: Dietary Guidelines for Americans.* Home and Garden Bulletin no. 232. Washington, D.C.: U.S. Government Printing Office 1980, p. 17.

7 American Dietetic Association. Nutrition recommendations for women. *J Am Dietet Assoc* 1986;86:1663–4.
8 American Heart Association. Dietary guidelines for healthy American adults: a statement for physicians and health professionals by the Nutrition Committee. *Circulation* 1986;74:1465A-8A.
9 American Cancer Society. *Nutrition and Cancer: Cause and Prevention.* New York: American Cancer Society, 1984.
10 National Research Council. *Diet, Nutrition, and Cancer. Report of Committee on Diet, Nutrition, and Cancer.* Food and Nutrition Board, Assembly of Life Sciences, Washington, DC: National Academy Press 1982.
11 Lenfant C, Roccella EJ. Trends in hypertension control in the United States. *Chest* 1984;86:459–62.
12 Report of the National Cholesterol Education Program Expert Panel on detection, evaluation, and treatment of high blood cholesterol in adults. *Arch Int Med* 1988;148:36–69.

LEWIS E. LLOYD AND CLAIRE CRONIER

Dietary Guidelines: Implications for Agriculture

It is not that long ago that dietary guidelines were considered to be of almost exclusive interest to departments of health and to health professionals. During more recent years their significance to a wider range of interest groups has been recognized. Among these one must include the various chronic disease associations, consumer groups, and of course the agri-food industry.

In most developed countries, the interest and concern of the average consumer in a variety of nutrition issues is growing. These nutrition concerns have had, and continue to have, an impact on food consumption trends, with these trends having a direct influence upon the economic viability of specific segments of the agricultural industry. The producer, the processor, the distributor, and the retailer are all affected.

At the turn of this century, six of the ten principal causes of death in developed countries were attributed to infectious diseases. Today, with one current and notable exception, these have essentially disappeared, only to be replaced by degenerative diseases such as coronary heart disease, cancer, hypertension, etc. Diet can be one of the important factors in all of these, and is certainly one factor which individuals can control. Specific nutrient deficiency diseases can be ruled out as a main issue in developed countries. Therefore, our chief nutritional preoccupation at the present time appears to be associated with nutrition-disease relationships, and how to cope with an overwhelming choice of foods available in our markets. Dietary guidelines must attempt to deal with these issues.

Dietary Guidelines and Chronic Diseases

Let us assume that dietary guidelines can be elaborated which will serve as effective risk reduction measures against the major degenerative diseases that afflict large segments of the populations of developed countries. We know that most of these diseases are multifactorial in nature and that diet is but one, albeit an important, etiological factor. Hence, adhering to even the most effective of dietary guidelines will at best decrease the probability of the occurrence of the disease or delay its onset. It is overly optimistic to suggest that dietary guidelines will eliminate any disease.

It is not the function of this paper to enumerate and compare the relative merits of the numerous sets of dietary guidelines that have been proposed by different countries and various health-related agencies within countries. Most of these have been outlined by O'Connor and Campbell (1).

It is universally recognized that the data, upon which the relationship between diet and chronic disease is based, are far from complete. For this reason, some of the existing dietary guidelines have been criticized (2–4). However, the basic question is how much scientific proof is required prior to making general recommendations with regard to modification of diet and prevention of specific chronic diseases. There should be some "happy medium" in this respect.

Obviously, dietary modifications cannot be based upon inadequate and incomplete data. On the other hand, withholding information from the public that might require a human generation to obtain scientific confirmation could be equally disastrous. The "happy medium" could be O'Connor and Campbell's (1) suggestion that overwhelming support for dietary modification occurs when there is consistency of evidence in epidemiological studies, clinical studies, and animal studies, and where the biological plausibility of the relationship is impressive.

There is one dietary guideline which is extremely simple, does not require extensive, long-term research to confirm its validity and which, if adhered to, would go a long way towards resolving many of the current nutrition issues. It is simply "eat a wide variety of wholesome foods, each in moderation." However, it is highly unlikely to gain any degree of acceptance because it does not tell people what specific foods *to eat* and which foods *not to eat*. It does not provide a magic formula which will solve difficult food choices or provide precise recipes, percentages, and, above all, cautionary warnings – all these "deficiencies" at a time when so many people want rather detailed instructions as to how to accomplish a given dietary lifestyle.

A Stance for Agriculture

As indicated earlier, a heightened concern of the consumer with a variety of nutrition issues has had, and will continue to have, an influence on food consumption trends. Because dietary guidelines are meant to guide the consumers' attitudes towards nutrition issues, they will, if they function properly, have a significant influence upon food consumption patterns. Their influence upon the agri-food industry can be profound, and this emphasizes the obligation that dietary guidelines be devoid of any frivolous considerations.

An example of the latter might be a recommendation that the level of intake of nutrient *X* should be reduced to 1.0 gram per day, the main consideration being that a level of this low magnitude could not be harmful to the body. This could be a frivolous but harmful recommendation – frivolous in that it has no solid biological basis, and harmful in that the consumption of perhaps two agricultural commodities high in nutrient *X* content would be needlessly reduced or even avoided by the consumer.

On the other hand, agriculture must be prepared to accept and react positively to the consumption consequences on any segment(s) of the industry that happens to be negatively influenced by sound dietary guidelines. The industry must not insist on attaining the virtually impossible goal of complete scientifc confirmation of several of the nutrition-disease relationships. However, it must insist on the soundness of each dietary guideline proposed to the public, with soundness being based upon, as a minimum, "consistency of evidence in epidemiological studies, clinical studies and animal studies, and the biological plausibility of the relationship." In addition, agriculture must insist that dietary guidelines be valid for the total population rather than being applicable mainly to a selected group of "high risk" individuals.

Generally Accepted Dietary Guidelines

When the various dietary guidelines available on a world-wide basis are examined, differences are certainly found to exist, but the most striking result of such an examination is that three recommendations are made by practically every country and by almost every health-related agency within these countries. They are the following:

1 Caloric adjustments to achieve and maintain ideal body weight, i.e. avoid or eliminate obesity.
2 Reduction in the percentage of the caloric intake that originates from dietary fats, i.e. from the present level of 40–42% down to 30–35%.
3 Increased consumption of complex carbohydrates via such foods as fruits, vegetables, and cereal grains, i.e. increased intake of dietary fibre.

The same kind of unanimity is not present among the other recommendations. For example, while the kind of fat consumed appears to be of general concern, there is a lack of agreement as to the ideal distribution of saturated, monounsaturated, and polyunsaturated fatty acids in the diet; furthermore, the omega-3 fatty acid story may add another dimension. Many, but by no means all, the guidelines recommend a reduction in the present salt and sugar intake and the avoidance of excessive alcohol consumption. A reduction in the level of cholesterol intake is recommended in less than half of the dietary guidelines published to date.

The validity of all three of the generally accepted dietary guidelines cannot be disputed by the agri-food industry, even though they may have a profound effect upon it. The first guideline relating to the maintenance of ideal body weight would have an influence by decreasing the total consumption of agricultural products in general. The second and third would bring about changes in the kind of agricultural commodities consumed. To illustrate the impact on specific commodities, the latter two guidelines will be examined.

Menu Modifications Involved in Attaining Two Generally Accepted Dietary Guidelines

The starting point in this exercise was to design a one-day menu that could be considered "typical" of that consumed in 1987 by a male between the ages of 25 and 49 years and at moderate activity. This involved the provision of 2700 kcal, the inclusion of lipid sources sufficient to provide 40–42% of the caloric intake from dietary fat, and ensuring that the Recommended Nutrient Intakes (RNIs) of all major nutrients were met.

The next step was to modify this "typical" menu to the extent that the daily caloric intake from dietary fat was reduced to approximately 30%, while maintaining the total energy level at 2700 kcal and meeting the RNIs of all major nutrients. The fatty acid profile was also considered in this step. This was called the "fat-modified" menu, and accommodated the second generally accepted dietary guideline.

The final step was to alter the "fat-modified" menu to increase the dietary fibre level to 30–35 grams. All other features were maintained (i.e. total energy level at 2700 kcal, provision of approximately 30% of daily caloric intake from dietary fat, adequate levels of all major nutrients), and this was called the "fat-and-fibre-modified" menu. It accommodated the second and third generally accepted dietary guidelines.

Details of the typical menu and of the modifications required to effect the desired dietary fat and fibre changes are provided in Table 1. In order to create the fat-modified menu, the following alterations were made. At breakfast, the two fried eggs were replaced by one boiled egg, the white toast was increased from two to three slices, margarine replaced the butter, the jam portion was increased by 50% and the cream was replaced by whole milk. At lunch, the soup was changed from mushroom to tomato, the sandwich contained salmon rather than ham and low-fat rather than regular processed cheese, the serving of canned fruit cocktail was doubled, two cookies were added, and 2% milk replaced the whole milk. At dinner, the lean rump roast was replaced by roast turkey, the serving of mashed potatoes was doubled, margarine replaced the butter, plain white cake replaced the apple pie, and ice milk replaced the ice cream.

Although it is often said that reducing the dietary fat level will automatically increase the fibre content of the diet, this exercise proved otherwise. In order to create the fat-and-fibre-modified menu, the following additional alterations (i.e. to the fat-modified menu) had to be made. At breakfast, the orange juice was replaced by an orange, and the toast was changed from white to whole wheat (w/w). At lunch, split pea soup replaced the tomato soup, the sandwich bread was changed from white to whole wheat, and fresh fruit salad replaced the canned fruit cocktail. At dinner, the mashed potatoes were replaced by a baked potato with margarine, a large rather than small mixed salad was used, the dinner roll was changed from white to whole wheat, and fruit cake replaced the plain white cake.

It is recognized that the menu modifications could have been made in a variety of other ways; however, essentially the same food (or

Table 1
Example of a Typical Menu for Adult Males and of Modifications to Accommodate Two Generally Accepted Dietary Guidelines.

Typical Menu	*Fat Modified Menu*	*Fat and Fibre Modified Menu*
Breakfast	Breakfast	Breakfast
4 oz. orange juice	4 oz. orange juice	1 large orange
2 fried eggs	1 boiled egg	1 boiled egg
2 sl. toast (white)	3 sl. toast (white)	3 sl. toast (w/w)
2 tsp. butter	2 tsp. margarine	2 tsp. margarine
4 tsp. jam	6 tsp. jam	6 tsp. jam
1 coffee	1 coffee	1 coffee
1 oz. cream (10% b.f.)	1 oz. milk (whole)	1 oz. milk (whole)
1 tsp. sugar	1 tsp. sugar	1 tsp. sugar
Lunch	Lunch	Lunch
6 oz. mushroom soup	8 oz. tomato soup	8 oz. split pea soup
4 crackers	4 crackers	4 crackers
1 ham and cheese sandwich	1 salmon & cheese sandwich	1 salmon & cheese sandwich
2 sl. bread (white)	2 sl. bread (white)	2 sl. bread (w/w)
2 tsp. margarine	2 tsp. margarine	2 tsp. margarine
2 oz. chopped ham	2 oz. salmon	2 oz. salmon
1 tbsp. dressing	1 tbsp. dressing	1 tbsp. dressing
1 oz. processed cheese	1 oz. processed cheese (skim)	1 oz. processed cheese (skim)
½ c. fruit cocktail (canned)	1 c. fruit cocktail (canned)	1 c. fresh fruit salad
8 oz. milk (whole)	8 oz. milk (2% b.f.)	8 oz. milk (2% b.f.)
	2 cookies (oatmeal/raisin)	2 cookies (oatmeal/raisin)
Dinner	Dinner	Dinner
6 oz. rump roast(lean)	6 oz. roast turkey	6 oz. roast turkey
½ c. mashed potatoes	1 c. mashed potatoes	1 large baked potato with ½ tsp. margarine
½ c. peas	½ c. peas	½ c. peas
1 small mixed salad	1 small mixed salad	1 large mixed salad
1 tbsp. French dressing	1 tbsp. French dressing	1 tbsp. French dressing
1 dinner roll (white)	1 dinner roll (white)	1 dinner roll (w/w)
1 tsp. butter	1 tsp. margarine	1 tsp. margarine
⅛ apple pie	1 piece white cake (no icing)	1 piece fruit cake
½ c. ice cream	½ c. ice milk	½ c. ice milk

commodity) groups would have been involved in attaining the reduction in dietary fat and increase in dietary fibre levels.

Table 2
Certain Nutritionally Relevant Descriptors of the Typical and Modified Menus.

	Energy Content (kcal)	*Total Kilocalories from* Fat (%)	Protein (%)	Carbohydrate (%)	*Cholesterol* (mg)	*Fibre* (g)
Typical menu	2 727	43	18	39	886	14
Fat modified menu	2 706	30	19	51	520	16
Fat and fibre modified menu	2 700	28	20	52	509	33

Table 3
Fat and Fatty Acid Profiles of the Typical, Fat Modified, and Fat and Fibre Modified Menus.

	% of total kilocalories				
	Fat	*SFA*	*MUFA*	*PUFA*	*Linoleic*
Typical menu	43	17	18	6	6
Fat modified menu	30	8	12	7	6
Fat & fibre modified menu	28	7	11	7	6

Nutritional Description of Typical and Modified Menus

The three menus are described in Table 2 with respect to actual energy intake, the proportion of this energy originating with fat, protein, and carbohydrate, as well as their dietary fibre and cholesterol contents. It should be noted that each menu provides essentially the same levels of energy and protein, while the carbohydrate component was increased by approximately 30% in the modified menus. A reduction in the proportion of kilocalories originating from dietary fat was accomplished in each of the modifed menus, while an approximate doubling of the dietary fibre level was obtained in the second modified menu. The cholesterol content of the typical menu was significantly reduced with each of the modifications; however, removal of the single egg from each of the modified menus would have been required to reduce the cholesterol level below 300 mg.

The fat and fatty acid profiles of the three menus are given in Table 3. Most notable is the reduction in the saturated (SFA) and monounsaturated fatty acids (MUFA) in the two modified menus and the constant level of polyunsaturated fatty acids (PUFA) in all three menus. A precise ratio among the SFA:MUFA:PUFA of 1:1:1 was virtually impossible to attain in the modified menus.

Table 4
A Comparison of the Major Nutrients Provided by the Typical and Modified Menus to RNI's (male 25–49).

	Protein (g)	*Calcium (mg)*	*Phosphorus (mg)*	*Iron (mg)*	*Potassium (mg)*	*Sodium (mg)*
RNI	61	800	800	8	2 200	666
Typical menu	121	954	1 667	19	2 791	4 950
Fat modified menu	127	1 142	1 764	17	3 520	4 369
Fat & fibre modified menu	137	1 229	2 259	20	4 542	3 899
	Vitamin A (RE)	*Vitamin C (mg)*	*Thiamin (mg)*	*Riboflavin (mg)*	*Niacin (NE)*	*Folacin (μg)*
RNI	1 000	60	1.1	1.4	19.4	220
Typical menu	1 369	77	2.0	2.3	47	295
Fat modified menu	1 392	146	2.0	2.2	55	321
Fat & fibre modified menu	1 768	148	2.1	2.2	58	410

The comparisons provided in Table 4 illustrate that all three menus provide well in excess of an adult male's Recommended Nutrient Intakes (RNIS) for the nutrients indicated. The excess sodium in each menu is startling and could only be reduced by the elimination of the processed foods (e.g. soups, cheese, ham, salmon, dressings, etc.). The improved K/Na ratio, particularly in the fat-and-fibre-modified menu, and the significant increment in vitamin C, niacin, and folacin in both modifications, are noteworthy.

Cleveland and Pfeffer (5) examined the changes in food consumption patterns of adult men and women in the U.S.A. in order to meet dietary criteria consistent with the RDA's and/or the National Research Council's interim guidelines for reducing cancer risk. They pointed out that the RDA for zinc is one of the most difficult to meet, particularly in diets with relatively low caloric levels, such as those of adult women. Although not shown in Table 4, our three menus supplied well in excess of the 9 mg of zinc required by adult men. If each menu was to be consumed at a level to provide 2000 kcal daily, the zinc requirement for adult women would also be met.

Financial Consequences of Following These Two Dietary Guidelines

The consequences of consumption changes in food items and in commodity groups that were associated with the menu modifications are shown in Table 5. The consequences are expressed in terms of changes

Table 5
Consequences of Food Consumption Changes in Commodity Groups Associated with Menu Modification to Meet Two Generally Accepted Dietary Guidelines[1]

Commodity Group	Typical Menu					Fat Modified Menu: Net Gain (+) or Net Loss (−)					Fat & Fibre Modified Menu: Net Gain (+) or Net Loss (−)				
Food Item	*quantity*	*retail value #*	*value to producer**	*value to processor**	*value to distributor**	*quantity*	*retail value #*	*value to producer**	*value to processor**	*value to distributor**	*quantity*	*retail value #*	*value to producer**	*value to processor**	*value to distributor**
Horticulture	(g)	($000)	($000)	($000)	($000)	(g)	($000)	($000)	($000)	($000)	(g)	($000)	($000)	($000)	($000)
Fruits															
orange juice	128	505	91	265	146						−128	−505	−91	−265	−146
fresh orange											+200	+1 094	+777	—	+317
jam	27	631	114	331	183	+13	+309	+56	+162	+93					
fruit cocktail (canned)	128	1 767	318	928	512	+128	+1 767	+318	+928	+512	−256	−3 534	−636	−1 856	−1 025
apple (pie)	60	547	98	287	159	−60	−547	−98	−287	−159					
fruit (cake)											+10	+184	+33	+97	+55
fruit (cookies)						+5	+92	+17	+48	+28					
fresh fruit salad											+272	+4 509	+2 931	—	+1 578
total		3 450	622	1 811	1 001		+1 621	+292	+851	+474		+1 748	+3 014	−2 024	+779
Vegetables															
lettuce	45	295	194	—	100						+55	+360	+238	—	+122
potatoes	75	168	111	—	57	+75	+168	+111	—	+57	+56	+126	+83	—	+43
peas	85	1 052	189	552	305										
carrots	20	84	56	—	29						+20	+84	+56	—	+29
mushrooms (soup)	35	646	116	339	194	−35	−646	−116	−339	−194					
tomatoes (soup)	120					+120	+1 545	+278	+811	+464					
split peas (soup)											+100	+454	+82	+238	+136
total		2 245	667	892	685		+1 067	+173	+542	+327		+1 024	+458	+238	+330
horticulture total		5 696	1 288	2 703	1 686		+2 688	+465	+1 393	+801		+2 772	+3 472	−1 785	+1 109
Cereal															
bread (white)	60	443	173	133	142	+30	+223	+87	+67	+71	−90	−669	−261	−201	−214
bread (whole wheat)											+90	+640	+249	+192	+205
crackers	11	168	19	103	47										
rolls (white)	40	421	164	126	135						−40	−421	−164	−126	−135
rolls (whole wheat)											+40	+447	+174	+134	+143

baked goods															
apple pie	58	1 683	252	976	471	−58	−1 683	−252	−976	−471					
cake white						+60	+1 902	+285	+1 103	+533	−60	−1 902	−285	−1 103	−533
fruit cake											+50	+1 627	+244	+944	+456
cookies						+21	+700	+77	+427	+196					
total		2 715	608	1 338	795		+1 142	+197	+621	+329		+1 060	+479	+241	+350
Dairy															
butter	18	505	247	151	106	−18	−505	−247	−151	−106					
cream (10% b.f.)	28	295	144	88	62	−28	−295	−144	−88	−62					
milk (whole)	258	926	454	278	194	−230	−825	−404	−248	−173					
(2% b.f.)						+272	+809	+397	+243	+170					
cheese processed (23% b.f.)	30	884	433	265	186	−30	−884	−433	−265	−186					
cheese processed (7% b.f.)					283	+30	+1 106	+542	+332	+232					
ice cream (10% b.f.)	70	1 346	660	404		−70	−1 346	−660	−404	−283					
ice milk						+92	+960	+470	+288	+202					
total		3 925	1 938	1 187	831		−980	−480	−294	−206					
Red Meat															
pork (ham)	60	2 609	1 304	730	574	−60	−2 609	−1 304	−730	−574					
beef (rump)	180	5 554	2 777	1 555	1 222	−180	−5 554	−2 777	−1 555	−1 222					
total		8 163	4 081	2 286	1 796		−8 163	−4 081	−2 286	−1 796					
Poultry															
egg	100	631	379	177	76	−50	−316	−189	−88	−38					
turkey						+180	+5 049	+2 525	+1 338	+1 146					
total		631	379	177	76		+4 734	+2 335	+1 250	+1 108					
Fish															
salmon						+60	+360	+177	+108	+76					
total							+360	+177	+108	+76					
Fats & Oils															
margarine	10	84	22	40	22	+15	+204	+53	+98	+53					
salad dressing	15	379	98	182	98										
dressing	15	129	34	62	34										
total		592	154	284	154		+204	+53	+98	+53					

[1]Calculations based on menu changes for 1 day for total male population age 25–49 yrs according to Statistics Canada, 1981.

#Retail value calculated on the average food price of two food items chosen at random in two retail stores in the Ottawa area on April 22, 1987.

*Values calculated using shares of retail dollar to producer, processor and distributor provided by Barewal, S., Food Markets Analysis Division, Agriculture Canada.

in the quantity (g) of food items and commodity groups, as well as in the retail value resulting from these menu changes for one day for the total Canadian male population between the ages of 25 and 49 years, according to Statistics Canada, 1981. In addition, the shares of the retail dollar going to the producer, processor, and distributor are provided. (It should be noted here that the dollar values to the producer, processor, and distributor do not always add up to the retail value, because the percentage share figures and the dollar values were rounded off.)

A detailed examination of Table 5 provides the following general observations. The fat-modified menu resulted in significant increases in the consumption of fruits (canned fruit cocktail), vegetables (potatoes and tomatoes), some cereals (white bread and oatmeal cookies), 2% milk, ice milk, turkey, and salmon; these were accompanied by significant decreases in certain dairy products (butter, cream, whole milk, and ice cream), red meats (pork and beef), and eggs.

The fat-and-fibre-modified menu resulted in additional changes, but only in the horticulture and cereal groups. In the category of fruits, the increase in fresh oranges at the expense of orange juice, and in fresh fruit salad at the expense of canned fruit cocktail resulted in a particularly heavy dollar loss to the processor. The increased intake of vegetables (lettuce, potatoes, and split peas) completes the increment in food dollars to the horticulture commodity group. In terms of cereals, the notable change was to less refined flour products in the bread and rolls.

The financial consequences, in terms of retail value only, are summarized in Table 6. These data indicate that if all Canadian males between the ages of 25 and 49 years consumed the fat-modified menu for one day, the horticulture industry would benefit to the extent of about 2.7 million dollars, the cereal grain industry by 1.1 million dollars, and the poultry industry by some 4.7 million dollars, where a loss in egg consumption was more than compensated by an increase in poultry meat. On the other hand, the dairy industry would lose about one million dollars and the red meat industry 8.1 million dollars.

If these same Canadian males were to consume the fat-and-fibre-modified menu for one day, the financial consequence (relative to the fat-modified menu) would be essentially to double the gain to the horticulture and cereal grain industries, while maintaining the gains or losses to the other industries.

The financial consequences of the menu changes used in this example of attaining a fat-reduced or a fat-reduced and fibre-increased diet are staggering, especially if one projects the changes taking place

Table 6
Net Effects on Retail Values of Commodity Groups Associated with Menu Modification to Meet Two Generally Accepted Dietary Guidelines.

Commodity Group	*Typical Menu retail value ($000)*	*Fat Modified Menu retail value ($000)*	*Fat Modified Menu % change from typical menu*	*Fat & Fibre Modified Menu retail value ($000)*	*Fat & Fibre Modified Menu % change from typical menu*
Horticulture					
Fruits	3 450	+1 621	+47	+3 369	+98
Vegetables	2 245	+1 067	+48	+2 091	+93
total	5 696	+2 688	+47	+5 460	+96
Cereal	2 715	+1 142	+42	+2 202	+81
Dairy	3 925	−980	−25	−980	−25
Red meat	8 163	−8 163	−100	−8 163	−100
Poultry	631	+4 734	+750	+4 734	+750
Fish	—	+360	+360	+360	+360
Fats & oils	592	+204	+34	+204	+34

over more than one day in the year and extending beyond the young adult male population. Let us zero in on the red meat and poultry industries to illustrate the point that should be made in respect to recommended dietary changes.

The suggestion of eliminating red meats from one's diet is heard fairly widely around the world. How many of those who readily make this recommendation are aware that the removal of 6 oz. of rump roast plus 2 oz. of chopped ham from the menu of all young Canadian males for one day would cost the red meat industry over eight million dollars, with half of this loss going to the primary producer?

The egg has been the first dietary victim when attempts have been made to reduce the level of cholesterol intake. How many of those who suggest that a reduced level of cholesterol intake should not be confined to those individuals found to be at risk to cardiovascular disease are aware that the removal of one egg from the menu of all young Canadian males for one day would cost the poultry industry over 300 thousand dollars, with 60% of this loss going to the primary producer? All of this provides substantiation for the following points. While agriculture must be prepared to accept the consequences of all sound dietary guidelines, it must ensure that dietary guidelines are devoid of any frivolous considerations. Relatively few health professionals are fully aware of the economic and social implications that a "reasonable sounding" but scientifically unsubstantiated dietary guideline may have upon the agri-food industry.

Agriculture's Reaction – Past

The agri-food industry has not been totally indifferent to the nutritional considerations of the food supply. An example of this is its response to consumer concerns about the fat content of a number of animal products. Although perhaps not exclusively for nutritional reasons, different segments of the Canadian animal industry have taken steps to decrease the fat content of their products (6).

For example, Canada introduced a new beef carcass grading system in 1972 which was designed to encourage the production of leaner beef. As a result, total lean output from beef carcasses increased by 7% over a ten-year period, a change which can probably be attributed to a general reduction in the stage of maturity at slaughter and to the use of later fattening breeds in cross-breeding programs. Research done by Jones in 1985 at the University of Guelph and by Agriculture Canada (Ottawa) in 1986 confirmed that Canadian prime cuts of beef are substantially lower in fat content than their U.S.A. counterparts. Further revisions to the Federal Beef Grading Regulations were made in 1978 and 1986 to reflect this trend.

As with beef, the most significant change in pork product composition has been in the amount of fat. A new grading system was introduced in 1968 which was primarily based on carcass weight and backfat thickness. Over the following 14-year period, an increase of almost 12% in lean pork output was observed, with both increased carcass weight and reduced carcass fat content as contributory factors. There is limited information on the fat content of Canadian cooked pork products. A pilot study conducted at the University of Guelph (7) indicates that the fat content of Canadian retail cuts is lower than published American values; the results of a more detailed study by Agriculture Canada will be available during the summer of 1987.

The dairy industry, for reasons that were not originally based upon nutritional considerations, has accommodated an apparent consumer demand by making 2% milk available. The increase of almost 500% in the use of this product since 1963 indicates its strong status with the consumer. The doubling of cheese consumption in Canada over the same period of time focuses attention on this dairy product and justifies the industry's attempts to produce a consumer-acceptable, low-fat cheese.

The past decade has also been marked by the introduction of a new line of products lower in salt, sugar, fat and energy content, and higher in dietary fibre. Canadian meat processors, for example, have lowered the sodium content of processed meats – industry estimates suggest that compared to 25 years ago, bacon and hams now contain at least 25% less sodium (8). The cereal industry has introduced a variety of breakfast cereals which are higher in dietary fibre and lower in sugar. The canned food industry has brought out a line of vegetables with "no salt added" and fruit "packed in its own juice." A variety of low energy pre-prepared meals have also taken an important place on the market. These steps certainly denote a positive response on the part of the agri-food industry.

Agriculture's Reaction – Future

There is little doubt that the agri-food industry in general is becoming more conscious of its responsibilities in respect to the provision of food products of optimal nutritional value. It is not easy for certain segments of the industry to bring about rapidly meaningful improvements in the nutritional characteristics of the foods they produce. On the other hand, it is important that the industry is seen to be making a genuine effort in this direction.

Agriculture Canada is reorienting its functions, communications, and resource allocation along commodity lines. In this context, it is currently preparing a "commodity strategy framework" involving the future directions for such sectors as Red Meats, Poultry, Dairy, Grains & Oilseeds, Horticulture, and Special Crops. The final document will represent the outcome of representations from industry, provincial governments, consumer groups, other federal government departments, as well as all the participants from Agriculture Canada.

While the final document has not yet been prepared, a number of recommendations that have originated with the sector teams are of interest to the nutrition community. Examples are as follows:

1 Improve consumption statistics by using retail disappearance and consumer equivalents data and through research and surveys, determine the breakdown of actual components consumed to aid research in the relationship between coronary heart diseases, mammary and colon cancer, and red meat consumption.
2 Continue to research the composition of retail cuts and processed meats, and make a strong effort to reduce the salt content of the latter.
3 Continue to research methods to find the most economical and efficient methods of reducing the fat levels in chicken.

4 Develop methods of cooking other than deep-fat frying for the production of consumer-desired processed, poultry products.
5 Minimize or eliminate the injection of oils into turkey and roasting chicken carcasses by the industry.
6 Conduct research to determine what are adequate levels of calcium in the diets of Canadians and to develop a better understanding of the disease risks associated with sub-optimal calcium intake.
7 Investigate the development of an assortment of low-fat cheeses.

Other areas of concern which need further attention include:

1) more updated compositional data on the nutritive and non nutritive substances of Canadian food commodities; 2) data on actual food consumption by Canadians, particularly for such groups as adolescents, pregnant women, elderly persons; 3) research on the status of lipids in the diet, i.e. proportions of SFA:MUFA:PUFA, omega-3 fatty acids, cholesterol levels; 4) research on the physiological role of fibre in the diet, i.e. its role in such conditions as hypercholesterolemia, hyperglycemia, tumour development; and 5) reduction of salt levels in all processed foods.

Conclusions

Agriculture must be prepared to accept the consequences on any segment of the industry that may be negatively influenced by sound dietary guidelines. On the other hand, it must insist on scientific substantiation for all dietary guidelines.

Those directly involved in the formulation of dietary guidelines must resist making recommendations that merely sound reasonable but whose implementation might have a profound impact on some segment of the agri-food industry. This impact could be either positive or negative, involve millions of dollars (not to mention economic and social implications), and be unwarranted in either case if the scientific justification is not clearly established. However, the agri-food industry must accept the responsibility of maintaining a nutritious food supply since the nutritional status of a population depends on the quality of the food commodities available to it.

Under these conditions, the health professions and agriculture can be productive partners in ensuring optimal nutritional health for the human population.

REFERENCES

1 O'Connor TP, Campbell TC. Dietary guidelines. *Prog Clin Biol Res* 1986;222:731–772.
2 Harper AE. Dietary goals – a skeptical view. *Am J Clin Nutr* 1978;31:310–321.
3 Olson RE. The U.S. quandary: can we formulate a rational nutrition policy? In: Chou M, Harman DP, eds. *Critical foods issues of the eighties*. New York: Permagon Press, 1979:119–133.
4 Pariza MW. A perspective on diet, nutrition and cancer. *J Am Med Assoc* 1984;251:1455–1458.
5 Cleveland LE, Pfeffer AB. Planning diets to meet the National Research Council's guidelines for reducing cancer risk. *J Am Dietet Assoc* 1987;87:162–168.
6 Jones SDM. Changes in animal product composition and implications for animal production systems. Presentation given at Joint Symposium of the CSAS and CSE on Animal Products, Nutrition and Health, Charlottetown, P.E.I., June 25, 1985.
7 Jones SDM. Chemical composition of selected cooked beef steaks and roasts. *J Can Dietet Assoc* 1985;46:40–44.
8 Sundeen G. Processed meats. *Meat Probe* 1987;4(2).

GILBERT A. LEVEILLE

Dietary Guidelines: Steps for the Food Industry

I have spent some time in both camps but I have spent more time being an academician than I have being on the industry side, so I can take some liberty and say a lot of things that some of my industrial colleagues might not be able to say!

Let me start out by making a few observations that I think are relevant. I am going to try to keep my comments very brief. First, it is important to realize that the food industry is not a single industry. Everyone talks about the food industry's role related to the implementation of dietary guidelines, of providing products to facilitate the implementation of dietary guidelines. But remember that you are talking about an aggregate of companies that have very different goals and very different objectives, selling very different products, whose profitability is influenced in a whole array of ways. You may make changes that benefit one segment of the industry but wreak considerable harm on the rest of the industry.

Secondly, it is important to recognize that as a consumer product industry, food processing companies respond to consumer wants. Whatever the consumer purchases in the market place determines what we manufacture. I'll give you some specific examples. We are often accused of using questionable marketing strategies to foist upon consumers products that they do not want, and our marketing people wish that were true, that we knew how to do that. Let me assure you that we do not. We do respond to consumer needs. We try to anticipate things that will sell, obviously, and more often than not we fail. We don't make the right judgment. One needs only to look at the number of products entering the market place and the very small proportion, fewer than 10%, that succeed in the long term.

Finally, it is important for you to keep in mind that the food industry is a capitalistic industry for a capitalistic society. Stockholder equity drives what we do to a large extent. We have to be concerned about profitability, and to produce products that cost more is certainly possible, but that cost is clearly going to be passed on to the consumer. It is not going to be absorbed by the manufacturer. I think it is important to recognize that the industry can only respond to the direction that is provided by the scientific and the health community. That direction needs to be clear. If there is ambiguity in the messages, if there is confusion, if there are various points of view, then all that has been done is to open the total market place to potental exploitation, because manufacturers will select that particular bit of advice, those particular opinions, which suit their particular marketing strategy. So it is very important that there be a single message that the food industry can respond to and work from. The important point, it seems to me, is not so much expecting the industry to be pro-active in producing products and trying to convince consumers to purchase those products. The important point is an education program which generates a level of awareness in a consuming public to a point where they are willing to purchase and in fact are demanding new products.

Let me give a case in point. We have seen the proliferation of a whole array of new calcium-fortified food products entering the market place, driven not by any new scientific evidence (we really have not had anything dramatically new in the last decade in the area of calcium metabolism), but driven by a markedly increased level of consumer awareness among women about the ravages of osteoporosis and a potential relationship to calcium intake. Now I am not going to try to defend the kinds of products that are marketed, how valid they are, or how much of a role they play. The point is that the products were introduced into the market by virtue of a high level of consumer awareness. Most of the products have failed, because in the rush to get them out poor ones were often produced. No matter what consumers' perceptions are of health and well-being, they simply will not purchase and consume food products that do not taste good. Therefore, that becomes a very top and primary objective.

The point of education in the generation of consumer awareness is an important one, and frankly I do not feel that responsibility should fall upon the food industry. As a consumer, I do not want to see it there. Industry does have a role in terms of providing products that are useful, for which there is a demand, and which consumers will accept. Let me give you one more example of that. Sodium and hypertension is a topic that has received enough attention to generate a high level of awareness. In a recent *Good Housekeeping* survey women were asked what foods or ingredients in a diet contributed to hypertension. Over two-thirds recognized that salt/sodium were associated. This high level of recognition has resulted in the success of a number of reduced-sodium products. Not all reduced-sodium products have been successful. Those that were able to match their traditional counterparts in terms of taste were accepted. On the other hand, there have been a number of failures, where the reduction in sodium significantly reduces the sensory attributes of the products. But sodium is a case which demonstrates that if the scientific and health care community can develop a high level of awareness that something is important, the food processing industry will provide products that meet the need that has been created.

Let me touch on one area of particular concern in the United States (I am not sure what its status is in Canada), and that is the area of health claims. What you will hear from manufacturers is that if indeed they are going to try to meet this need, they have to be allowed to tout the attributes of their products. Let me warn you that this opens a Pandora's box. On the one hand, no one objects to honest and truthful claims, but it is important to recognize that it is virtually impossible to establish a regulatory environment, allowing such claims, without opening opportunities for the faddists and quacks to make an array of claims regarding their products. This is an area that requires attention from the standpoint of public health policy.

Let me end by saying that I think the needs beyond what I have mentioned are for ways of bringing the academic community, government agencies, and industry together to discuss the issues and how they can best be resolved, and how each segment of our society can contribute in a meaningful way to their resolution. I think if there is a challenge for us, it really is that. How do you bring about meaningful, productive dialogue which can contribute to a final resolution?

HEATHER NIELSEN

Dietary Guidelines: Steps for Dietitians/Public Health Nutritionists

Dietary guidelines are the focal point for policies and programs undertaken by the majority of dietitians and public health nutritionists around the world. Consequently, you are actively involved in implementing the dietary guidelines whether they are simple statements of carbohydrate and fat requirements, the more complex guidelines for general health, those for specific disease states, or for specific age groups such as the Nutrition in Pregnancy: National Guidelines recently released in Canada.

The steps that are taken emanate from activities in the work environment, in professional associations, and in individual actions. Dr. Beare-Rogers will be describing the process that we are entering into in the review of the Canadian dietary guidelines – Nutrition Recommendations for Canadians. Dietitians and public health nutritionists are and will be actively involved in the consultation process collectively through national groups such as the Federal-Provincial Subcommittee on Nutrition and the Canadian Dietetic Association. They are also involved through representation on major health-related groups such as the Canadian Cancer Society and the Canadian Diabetes Association. From past experience, I know that you will also be involved as individuals.

Most of you are in a unique position to (a) lead and participate in the formulation of dietary guidelines; (b) promote an understanding of the scientific evidence and rationale underlying dietary guidelines; (c) interpret the dietary guidelines for policy formulation; and (d) implement the dietary guidelines through multifaceted, integrated strategies.

The role of the dietitian/public health nutritionist is to bring about change as required in individual behaviour as well as to build a supportive environment for change. To accomplish this, it is necessary that the steps be global in nature and, at the same time, respond to the practical everyday concerns of the consumer.

One major step for your involvement in implementing dietary guidelines is setting goals and objectives and getting commitment to action on the goals. In general terms, a desirable objective could be: informed food choices for healthy eating in a safe food supply.

Setting specific goals for targeted populations, such as increasing fish consumption from *x* variety of fish considering *y* sources, e.g. sea, fresh water, and potential problems of toxicity for northern adult males represents much more of a practical challenge.

Another major step is the selection of a framework in which appropriate strategies for implementing dietary guidelines can be undertaken. This will be an important consideration for the Communications/Implementation Committee.

A broad framework can be used to illustrate the scope of work which is feasible for participation of dietitians/public health nutritionists. *Achieving Health for All: A Framework for Health Promotion* (1), released in November 1986 at the International Conference of Health Promotion, represents such a framework.

Dietary guidelines are an integral part of health promotion and disease prevention. They are needed to meet current health challenges, such as reducing health inequities, increasing prevention efforts, and enhancing the individual's ability to cope. The mechanisms which can be used to meet the challenges include self and mutual aid and building a supportive environment.

Five major strategies form the basis of actions for dietitians and public health nutritionists. The strategies are essential at a time when demand for nutrition is ever increasing and services are often being pushed to their limits.

Healthy Public Policy

Depending on the state of policy development, contributions to creation, modification, and/or coordination of nutrition policies in healthy public policy must be made. At all levels, actions to coordinate policies and programs which address health, social, economic, and environmental issues are needed. Key steps include:

• *intersectoral coordination* – initiating collaborative actions among agencies, government groups, professional associations to bring about change in food consumption patterns;
• *economic measures* – analyzing the impact and recommending those measures such as taxes and subsidies which would support positive changes in food selection, i.e. supporting incentives such as health insurance plans which include nutrition counselling;
• *regulations and standards* – developing and implementing those which would ensure the availability of foods in food delivery systems consistent with the dietary guidelines.

Community Services

Dietitians and public health nutritionists participate in the delivery of nutrition within the framework community services, particularly community health services, so as to implement dietary guidelines. The steps that are now needed may involve reorientation of services, strengthening of existing services, or increasing the availability of services to implement the guidelines successfully. Key steps include:

• *increasing access to services* – ensuring access to nutrition counselling when required for individual behaviour change (this necessitates support for preventive as well as therapeutic treatment);
• *professional development* – organizing and presenting programs related to the interpretation of dietary guidelines to health professionals in both training programs and in continuing education programs.

Public Participation

The dietitian/public health nutritionist must take steps to increase and strengthen citizen actions. Increased involvement of individuals and communities in the decision-making process will impact favourably on acceptance of dietary guidelines. For many, the role assumed by dietitians and public health nutritionists will shift from deliverer to facilitator. Key steps include:

• *strengthening voluntary groups* – providing professional or expert advice initiated by self-help groups such as weight control groups;

• *facilitating communication among groups* – initiating and supporting interdisciplinary, intergroup activities such as a network for information sharing on specific issues within dietary guidelines.

Public Information and Education

Information and education programs have traditionally been seen as steps taken to implement dietary guidelines and they will continue to play an important role in the context of other strategies. For dietitians and public health nutritionists, ensuring consistency in messages for the general public is a key concern. Moving from the general statement of "reduce fat intake" to the specific individual request for "how much" and "what do I reduce" does necessitate direct actions and judgment calls. Key steps include:

• *availability of timely information* – ensuring that the information given is both relevant and up to date, while responding to changing information within dietary guidelines;
• *application of appropriate education models* – assessing existing models from all areas and incorporating into the broad picture;
• *development of personal skills* – supporting programs in the workplace which encourage opportunities to develop and practise skills in food selection and preparation. (There is a return to practical activities such as cookbooks with specific directions to reduce fat intake.)

Research and Knowledge Development

Dietitians and public health nutritionists play an important role in implementing dietary guidelines through active participation in the identification of research priorities. The questions that arise as a result of developing and evaluating programs provide useful input into setting research priorities. For example, we need to study changing values and attitudes towards weight as a basis for advocating change in stereotyping among media or the need for new products.

Conclusion

Participating in both academic and community-based research builds a solid foundation for action.

The five strategies represent the breadth of knowledge, skills, and abilities which are needed for dietitians and public health nutritionists to take the steps to implement dietary guidelines.

REFERENCE

1 Epp J. *Achieving health for all: a framework for health promotion*. Ottawa: Health and Welfare Canada, 1986.

JOAN DYE GUSSOW

Dietary Guidelines: Steps for Nutrition Educators

As the third to last speaker on the last day of a two-and-a-half-day conference, I feel blessed, as I am sure you do, by the fact that I have been asked to speak for only ten minutes. I don't want to listen to anyone – including myself – for even that long this morning. Nevertheless, I am here, representing nutrition educators, and I am supposed to tell you what we educators might do to help implement the dietary guidelines.

Ideally, we might do a lot. In the interest of time, I would like to ignore the question of whether nutrition education works, asserting simply that we have evidence that under the right circumstances nutrition education can and does work. I will also not deal with the question of which are the best devices or motivational tricks or experiences we can make use of to induce consumers to change their behaviour on the basis of appropriate information. I can assure you, however, that we know increasing amounts about how to make nutrition education work to produce behavioural change – given the right circumstances. What I want to focus on today are the *actual* circumstances under which nutrition education professionals are now trying to work. What is the environment in which we try to reach the public with relevant, complete, accurate – and motivating – information about diet and health?

To begin with, the environment is one in which publicly funded nutrition education efforts are scattered and inconsistent in quality, so most children never receive a thorough grounding in ways of thinking rationally about food and their own well-being. Corporate wellness programs reach some adults who are part of corporations large enough to afford them, but many such programs pay nominal attention to teaching people how to make sense of the changing food supply. So most people's exposure to wit and wisdom on food and nutrition comes not from organized efforts at promoting nutrition literacy, but from the global buzz; the environment in which nutrition educators try to work is one in which the noise to signal ratio is very high.

You have only to look around you to realize that consumers – of both food and information – are being exposed to a lot of data these days about eating in relation to well-being. Twenty years ago, even fifteen years ago, you could not have interested a newspaper editor or a food manufacturer in using "nutrition" to promote her or his products. Nutrition was, by definition, boring. Today newspaper people who know varying amounts about either food or science comb the pages of the *New England Journal of Medicine* for their everyday story ideas; most newspapers have "science" and "food" sections which regularly report the latest nutrition discovery; and national newsmagazines schedule cover stories on subjects like "The Diet Wars" in which foods are consigned to the "bad" column or dragged back into the "good" column based on a single report from the latest issue of *Science*.

Just to give you a feeling for what this means, I have collected, quite casually, a few of the *major* stories that have appeared in the *New York Times* in the last two months – stories that appeared in much less careful detail elsewhere throughout the media of both our countries. On April 19, Jane Brody, writing under the headline "New Index Finds Some Cancer Dangers Are Overrated and Others Ignored," describes Bruce Ames' new ranking system for carcinogens in which the daily consumption of one peanut butter sandwich is described as producing ten times the risk of eating 3½ oz. of cooked bacon a day. (Since that 3½ oz. is eight (8) slices, the equivalent of more than half a pound of raw bacon a day, one must assume that Dr Ames was thinking only of the nitrosamine hazard, and not of bacon's fat or salt content, which might lead some of us to discourage the consumption of four pounds of bacon a week!) Brody's follow-up "Personal Health" column on the Human Exposure Dose/Rodent Potency Index clearly shows tap water to be more dangerous than PCBS, EDBS, and DDT. (Personally, I find it hard to believe that Ames called it a HERP index without tongue in cheek, but with scientists, one never knows.)

On May 7 women got the bad news that they had to avoid any alcohol at all. The carry-over story in the *Times* was headed "Drinkers Warned on Breast Cancer," but "drinkers" turned out to include even

Aunt Minnie, who only sipped the wine at mass, since NIH researchers were said to have found that "any amount of alcohol, even the equivalent of less than one drink weekly, raises the breast cancer risk by at least 40%." So the choice clearly is to drink DDT, since water, alcohol, and coffee have been proved harmful, but pesticides are safer than you think.

But even that reassurance might not have calmed the consumers who read on May 13 and May 21 about successive NAS reports indicating that 1) chemical and microbial contamination of poultry was widespread in the U.S. and 2) pesticide regulation was spotty at best. The riskiest foods, according to the pesticide report, were tomatoes, potatoes, and beef, oranges, lettuce, apples, peaches, pork, wheat, soybeans, beans, carrots, chicken (again), corn, and grapes. Obviously a daunting list to those of us attempting to convince consumers to eat more fruits, vegetables, grains, and poultry. Consumers could learn from the story that 8.75 of 10,000 of those who ate tomatoes over a theoretical 70-year lifetime "will develop cancer from pesticide residues."

I well remember a professor I once had who, when a student came up and asked him about a study that was reported in the paper, replied contemptuously, "I don't do my science reading in the newspapers." Well, scientists may not, but the public does. So when one group of researchers comes to the conclusion, based on a relatively short-term study of the diets of a relatively restricted age group of women, that the women (in their group) with the highest fat intake do not differ in cancer risk from those with the lowest fat intake, the press coverage headline "Fat Not Implicated in Breast Cancer" may convince the female public that does not have a private nutritionist to consult that they may as well eat that four pounds of safe bacon a week.

Moreover, the confusion produced by the presumably well-meaning is compounded by the confusion sowed – not always unintentionally – by the entirely profit-minded. At a time when the public is suddenly fascinated by "healthy foods" or what marketers describe as "foods that *appear* to be healthy," everyone is selling the appearance of health. And in a deregulated marketplace, the fall-out can be remarkably confusing. In the good old days, 16 or so years ago, I was trying to help devise ways of regulating the advertising of foods so that it would help rather than baffle the consumer. At that time many of us came to understand 1) that consumers needed information that was "relevant, complete, and accurate" and 2) that those terms were going to prove hard to define. Unfortunately, today no one is even *trying* to define them. In the U.S. the present administration – as is well known – has very different views on how to achieve market efficiency. The free-play of the marketplace – the invisible hand of self-interest – will, they believe, ultimately serve the consumer best.

And how *has* the consumer's interest in learning how to select healthful foods been served by information in the public marketplace? A quick glance through some of the recent campaigns featuring "nutrition" is sobering. Admittedly, the manufacturers of bran cereals have told you that the National Cancer Institute recommends fibre to prevent bowel cancer. What they have not told you is that the evidence on fibre is very confusing, that it is not at all clear that the fibre of bran is as important as the fibre in fruits and vegetables, and so on. As a former advertising man, Richard Manoff, wrote in a recent issue of *Advertising Age*, "It is always possible to tell *a* whole truth without telling *the* whole truth. Advertising, by definition, is prejudiced in behalf of product." This means, of course, that no advertiser can ever tell you to eat *less* of *his* product, however beneficial cutting down might be in terms of your reduced risk of disease.

A perfect example of this is visible in recent advertisements for beef, and in the recent plague of "facts about food" articles (planted on the front pages of local newspapers' food sections) informing you that meat is healthful, low in fat, and so on. There is nothing intrinsically wrong with beef, and there is nothing wrong with consuming amounts of it that are by current standards small. What the advertisements (especially those from a well-known hamburger purveyor) do not tell you is that the portion of meat consumed by most Americans is – like the standard burger ordered at the fast food establishments that most ardently promote their good nutrition – much higher in fat and salt, and served with a meal much lower in certain other nutrients than is considered healthful by any nutritional standards. Of course you can "dilute" those limitations by eating only fruits and vegetables, unbuttered whole-grain breads, and other low-fat, low-salt foods for the remainder of the day. But the advertisers do not tell you that either.

Even more disquieting is the way in which brand new products are being invented and promoted as "healthy" before the scientific community has come to agreement about their virtues. The current mania for "health promotions" (as opposed to "health promotion") seems to have begun with bran and reached a climax (at least this year's climax) with calcium. Nutrition educators of necessity view the calcium fad with real alarm.

The facts about how calcium *qua* "calcium" affects osteoporosis are far from clear cut, and in their present uncertain state should not be influencing food *marketing* at all. (This is also true of the omega-3 fatty acids, whose costliness as an ingredient may be the only thing saving us from a spate of fatty acid-enriched products.) Just to give you a feeling for where the marketers' and consumers' interests most clearly diverge, let me quote from a story that ran in *Advertising Age* in August of last year. The story was headed "Calcium Market Shrugs Off Study." "The booming market in calcium supplements," the story begins, "seems fit as a fiddle despite a new study suggesting that added calcium may not prevent osteoporosis." The story went on to say that although *unpublished research* reported at a medical meeting the previous month showed women's bone calcium levels unaffected by dietary calcium, "the impact has not been felt on the calcium supplement and additive market which was built on earlier studies that linked calcium deficiency to osteoporosis."

Now, frankly, I do not want food marketers prescribing calcium for the public by dumping the mineral into every medium that will hold it, from breakfast cereals to soft drinks. Nor do I want them planting fibre in my breakfast cereals or omega-3 fatty acids in my butter. We are having enough trouble sorting out the truth without having to explain each new tentative finding to consumers who have gotten their information from food marketers.

The reality is that we are in the midst of a diet and health *fad* in which everyone with a product, a newspaper, or a magazine to sell has something to say about diet and health. Not all of it is true, all of it is partial, much of it is not helpful, and very little of it is set appropriately within the overall context of diet and disease. And what this means for nutrition educators – not a powerful or high status group to begin with – is that we are shouting into the wind.

What can be done about this? Fortunately, my time is short, since I can better describe the problem than suggest realistic remedies. We *could* regulate health claims in food advertising, but I am not optimistic about that possibility in the U.S. given the present anti-regulatory climate in Washington. We *could* put a 1% tax on the marketing budget of the largest industry in the U.S., the food industry, to provide a fund for public media education. The marketing budgets of just 13 major companies (reported in *Advertising Age*) came to over $5 billion last year. One percent of that is about $53 million, which would provide $1.00 for every school child in the U.S. – twice as much as was provided by the only mandatory (and short-lived) nutrition education program our country ever had. But I am not optimistic about this coming true either.

As for the well-meaning, what can we ask of them? We could ask the press not to cover the *New England Journal of Medicine*. We could ask scientists to inform reporters forcefully of the modesty of their own results, to remind reporters that one swallow does not a summer make, and that results from one epidemiologic study should not be the basis for widespread dietary change. We could pay teachers and fund education to produce a public that can *reason*, that can sort through the masses of trivia that flood the media to pick out what is essential in creating reliable pictures of the world. Since we do not have a public that can make sense of fields much more essential than nutrition, I am not optimistic about producing critical consumers of nutrition education – even though I have written a book aimed at doing just that.

Despite this admittedly gloomy picture, I believe we have some evidence that people are improving their diets. I would be interested in hearing from the audience and my fellow panelists during the discussion that follows 1) whether you believe that to be the case, and 2) what combination of intentional and unintentional "nutrition education" has brought it about.

RICHARD B. GOLDBLOOM

Nutrition, Diet, and Health: The Physician's Role

The topic of this symposium relates to preventive medicine in the broadest sense – as it applies not only to physicians, but to other health professionals and public health authorities. Implementing some of the solutions proposed poses several major problems. Those problems can be quite variable, depending on whether they apply to the individual patient sitting in the doctor's office or to community public health policies.

Let me confess a personal bias at the outset. I was brought up in the school of nutritional philosophy typified by the American writer Jack Douglas, who uttered the immortal statement: "If I had my life to live over, I'd live over a delicatessen." Admittedly, those temples of salt, nitrite, and saturated fat have had a rough time of it at this gathering.

For the past decade, I have been involved with Canada's Task Force on the Periodic Health Examination and more recently with the analogous U.S. Task Force on Preventive Services. These two bodies are charged with reviewing the quality of evidence for preventability of various harmful conditions and making recommendations for preventive interventions based on such critical assessments. It is interesting to observe how relatively cautious the views of such independent assessment bodies are on preventive strategies when compared to those of equally sincere groups committed to dealing with a particular disease, such as cancer, heart disease, or diabetes. This difference was exemplified by yesterday's discussions in which NIH recommendations concerning diabetic diet were contrasted with those of the American Diabetic Association.

In preparing to discuss implementation issues for physicians, I sought solace as well as hard data from the scientific literature. I wanted to review the evidence for how much doctors really know about diet, nutrition, and health; about how much they need to know; and about how much of such advice their patients not only absorb but actually translate into altered behaviour with the final desired improvement in health. (The final part of the question is the one that really counts.)

The literature review reveals some harsh realities. First, it is clear that most doctors are trained to diagnose and treat disease and injury rather than prevent them. This fact is often cited as a basic educational evil, but I think we should carefully consider why this is so. In the first place, most patients are more concerned with care of present problems than with prevention of future ones. Second, there are problems with the knowledge base. Physicians are poorly informed on many issues of nutrition, diet, and disease. Besides, it has been shown that physicians' personal habits determine to a considerable degree what they counsel their patients. Nutritionists should not take any special satisfaction from this observation because, as Dr Philip James pointed out, a study in the U.K. showed that nutritionists' dietary habits were no different from those of the general public. Then there is the issue of our faith in health promotion activities. My concern here extends not only to the promotion of good nutrition but also to other health issues such as accident prevention. Those who review the evidence will be forced to admit that the track record for health promotion is rather poor, and the scientific knowledge base to validate the efficacy of health promotion is not large. Despite this, health promotion in North America has become a major cottage industry. But I suggest to you that there is remarkably little evidence that all the brochures, handouts, and other means of public communication have a major impact on changing preventive behaviour.

Finally, there is the expectation, right or wrong, of low compliance. Many doctors believe that patients are unlikely to follow recommended diets, so that counselling may be largely a waste of time. Those who read the literature critically are also concerned that there may be instances of assigning guilt by statistical association, resulting in associated phenomena being designated "risk-factors." Guilt by association and proof of *causality* are two very different things.

Just how appalling is the physician's knowledge of nutrition and diet? One study, conducted in 1982, showed that among some 49 physicians, knowledge of the sodium content of food turned out to be at the same level as that of the general public. As I mentioned earlier, there is a limited amount of information which suggests that doctors preach what they practise.

In 1978, Elizabeth Johnson and Nancy Schwartz studied physicians' nutritional knowledge and practices. They found that the physician was the individual whom the public relied on most for information about nutrition as it related to disease. However, as noted previously, doctors were not particularly expert in that aspect of their profession. Not surprisingly, pediatricians attended post-graduate courses with nutrition content much more often than did other types of physicians.

Deficiencies in nutrition knowledge do not constitute the only problem in medical practice. There is also a problem of misapplication of nutrition knowledge. One may cite the continuing extensive use of vitamin supplements for children over two years of age who are consuming perfectly good diets. Or the continuing extensive use of vitamin and mineral supplements for pregnant women whose nutritional intake is also entirely satisfactory.

How are these identified problems to be rectified? There is remarkably little information in the medical literature to answer this question. In one investigation conducted at the University of Minnesota, physicians attending an update program were provided with lunches for a five-day period which conformed with a type of "prudent" diet. A separate group of physicians was tested prior to the introduction of the trial and 29% of them rated the diet as palatable. However, among those who unknowingly consumed the diet for the five-day period, 64% rated the diet as palatable and, one year later, 55% stated that they had increased the amount of nutrition counselling in their daily practices. However, this type of study must be interpreted with some caution because of the unreliability of self-reported behaviours.

There are other factors that place limits on implementation of preventive behaviours. One is that in North American health care systems, there is frequently no remuneration for preventive services, including counselling. Such counselling requires a considerable amount of time in clinical practices where there is often a great deal of pressure for therapeutic services. For some issues in preventive nutrition, communication between doctors, governments, and the food industry is vitally important. I recall that, during my years as a practising pediatrician in Montreal, we were still seeing about 100 children a year with vitamin D deficiency rickets, at a time when the condition had disappeared from most other provinces. The problem disappeared immediately when the provincial government was finally persuaded to legislate the supplementation of milk with vitamin D. Thus, in some situations, strategies and solutions that deal with the population as a whole rather than the individual patient in the doctor's office can be far more effective.

It is tempting to believe that problems like atherosclerosis, obesity, and hypertension are preventable by nutritional modifications. The truth is that for many of our patients the best solution would be to trade in their genes for a better set. But since this is not easily accomplished, my final plea would be that until we have sufficient knowledge to be sure of our ground in nutritional approaches to the prevention of disease, we should practise patience and restraint. Medical history is littered with examples of today's dogma becoming tomorrow's malpractice. Let me recall Dr Roncari's beautiful presentation of new information about the problem of obesity. His findings suggest that some of the advice on caloric restriction we have traditionally given to obese patients may be not only unhelpful, but possibly harmful. Recognition of our own ignorance should not be misinterpreted as apathy. I am reminded of the woman who answered her doorbell to be confronted by a gentleman who announced that he was conducting a national survey. "Madam," he said, "we want to know which you consider to be the biggest problem affecting Canadians – apathy or ignorance?" to which she replied, "I don't know and I don't care!"

In a collection of essays entitled *The Medusa and the Snail*, Dr Lewis Thomas takes as his theme the seven healthy life habits which have been widely promoted by the Blue Cross in the United States, and which have to do with proper diet, exercise, and all the virtuous aspects of lifestyle. Let me quote his final paragraph:

> Nobody can say an unfriendly word against the sheer goodness of keeping fit, but we should go carefully with the promises. There is also a bifurcated ideological appeal contained in the seven life habits doctrine, quite apart from the subliminal notion of good luck in the numbers involved – 7 come 11. Both ends of the political spectrum can find congenial items. At the further right, it is attractive to hear that the individual, the good old free-standing, free-enterprising American citizen is responsible for his own health. When things go wrong it is is his own damn fault for smoking, drinking and living wrong and he can jolly well pay for it. On the other hand, at the left, it is nice to be told that all our health problems including dying are caused by failure of the community to bring up its members to live properly, and if you really want to improve the health of the people, research is not the answer.

You should upheave the present society and invent a better one. At either end you can't lose. In between, the skeptics in medicine have a hard time with it. It is much more difficult to be convincing about ignorance concerning disease mechanisms than it is to make claims for full comprehension, especially when the comprehension leads, logically or not, to some sort of action. When it comes to serious illness, the public tends understandably to be more skeptical about the skeptics, more willing to believe the true believers. It is medicine's oldest dilemma, not to be settled by candor or by any kind of rhetoric. What is needs is a lot of time and patience, waiting for science to come in, as it has in the past, with the solid facts.

JOYCE L. BEARE-ROGERS

Dietary Guidelines: Steps by Government Agencies

Nutrition Recommendations came to Canada in 1977. They arose, somewhat mellowed, from the Report of the Committee on Diet and Cardiovascular Disease, popularly known as the Mustard Report, and became the foundation for educational programs and regulatory actions relating to nutrition.

These early recommendations gained the support of other federal government departments concerned with food, and with provincial governments, professional organizations, as well as food producers and consumers. Dr T.K. Murray, then Director of the Bureau of Nutritional Sciences, spearheaded their development and acceptance. They were generally seen as moderate and sensible guidelines based upon the strongest scientific evidence available at that time.

Subsequent reviews of the scientific literature provided assurance that the guidelines were still valid. The Nutrition Recommendations for Canadians, as stated, appeared to be serving their purpose, but posed some difficulty in practical application, particularly in reducing the level of fat to 35% of dietary energy. Ways for decreasing fat intake a consumer could understand and methods for quantitating the fat intake needed improvement. Ten years after the introduction of Nutrition Recommendations for Canadians, the scientific basis and the implementation of recommendations require updating and revision.

Provision of dietary advice has proliferated in North America and touched upon fears of developing specific diseases. Individuals may be forgiven their confusion about which disease they are trying to prevent. For example, a food that is high in both calcium and saturated fat may be promoted to prevent osteoporosis but condemned for increasing the risk of cardiovascular disease. The Canadian diet should be one that maintains nutritional health, which also implies a decrease in the risk of a degenerative disease. Those trying to prevent specific problems would benefit from a common base for good nutritional practices. Well-founded nutrition guidelines must be applicable to the general population and understandable to the users.

The National Institute of Nutrition played a valuable role in bringing together organizations generating or using dietary advice with a view to discerning the need for nutrition guidelines. As a result the Department of National Health and Welfare made a commitment to revise the Nutrition Recommendations for Canadians. Federal leadership seemed imperative for broadly-based, national recommendations.

In mid-March of 1988, Mr Jake Epp, Minister of National Health and Welfare, approved the formation of two committees to report jointly to the Health Services and Promotion Branch and the Health Protection Branch. One committee will be responsible for scientific review and assessment of strength of evidence and the other committee will be responsible for the communication and implementation aspects of the revised nutrition recommendations.

A consultative process is underway with interested parties who are proposing names of persons who might make a contribution. It is anticipated that specific task groups will report to the appropriate committee.

Further educational and regulatory programs will be formulated in the environment engineered by revised nutrition recommendations. They will be given renewed impetus by the knowledge that not only can they depend on and refer to the best available assessment of the scientific evidence, but that a great deal of fresh thought has been given to overcoming difficulties in communication and implementation.

We expect that government agencies with different mandates and constitutional responsibilities will come together to implement dietary guidelines in a harmonized and harmonious way. This will aid in the promotion and protection of the health of Canadians and be a cornerstone of federal and provincial accords in public health. Naturally, we shall seek cooperation with academia, with industry, with communities, and with the many voluntary organizations who have so much to offer.

Implementation over the years will surely require more population monitoring, research and demonstration projects, appropriate regulatory changes, periodic reviews, and greater exchange of information. This meeting is a prelude to what we hope will be something of a renaissance in Canadian nutrition.

Public Health and Mortality

JOHN CAIRNS

The History of Mortality

One of the major human accomplishments in the last 200 years has been the prevention of premature death. Readers of this article should realize that, if they had been born at any time before the middle of the eighteenth century, a quarter of them would have died before even learning how to read.

As we shall see, throughout the history of Homo sapiens, until about 1750, the balance of life and death hardly changed at all. Populations survived because each woman of reproductive age produced on average five or six children; of the two or three that were female, one survived to become her mother's successor. Today, in most nations, childhood mortality is so low that the size of the population will be maintained if women have slightly more than two children each; indeed, the population of the world as a whole now has an average life expectancy that is higher than the highest achieved by any nation before the twentieth century. In each country, the change in mortality came several generations before the change in birth-rate, and that is why there has been an explosive increase in population.

The causes for these demographic changes have been the subject of much argument among economists and social and medical historians. One way of approaching the problem is to concentrate on a single parameter, the obvious choice being mortality. Unlike health or happiness, it is a precisely measurable variable. Furthermore, there are reasonably accurate ways of estimating the force of mortality at different times in human history.

Measurement of Life Expectancy: Life Tables

Collection of vital statistics has been a preoccupation of rulers and governments since the beginnings of recorded history, because the size of a population determines how large an army it can mobilize and how much it can produce in taxes. The number of adult males in the tribes of Israel, for example, was counted by Moses and King David as a prelude to their attacking the neighbouring tribes; the Romans needed regular censuses so that they could tax their colonies; the Normans recorded in minutest detail the population of conquered England in the Domesday Book, because even the humblest peasant was considered part of the taxable assets of each rural estate. Interestingly, none of these early surveys was concerned with the longevity, suffering, and mortality of the population being surveyed. Even the first United States census of 1790, which was carried out for the democratic purpose of ensuring that each state should have the right number of representatives in Congress, went no further than to subdivide the white male population into those under or over the age of 16.

Despite the absence of any information on life expectancy, governments found themselves having to enact laws about life insurance and annuities, and the way they did this shows us how unsophisticated were their thoughts about the force of mortality. Roman law, for example, accepted the simple rule that anyone under the age of 20 could expect to live for another 30 years, and anyone over 20 could expect to live to the age of 60. Similarly, in seventeenth-century England, the official table for calculating annuities (certified by Newton himself) assumed that each person, irrespective of age, would survive on average for an additional ten years. Some populations do show this kind of exponential decline in numbers, where the force of senescence is not detectable and the probability of dying is constant for each time interval: radioactive atoms are constrained to behave in this manner by the Principle of Uncertainty; for some birds the hazards of their normal environment are so great that almost none of them live into old age, and the decline of each cohort is effectively exponential; and there have been human populations, such as the inhabitants of ancient Rome (see below) and certain groups of fighter pilots in World War II that were similarly overwhelmed by their circumstances. But it seems extraordinary to us today that a government in what, after all, was to be the beginning of the Age of Enlightenment should have been so fatalistic as to accept exponential decay as a fitting description of human mortality. (By chance, at just about this time, Leibnitz, the co-inventor of calculus, was urging that there should be some effort to determine what were the actual statistics of mortality.)

The formula for calculating life-expectancy in seventeenth-century England was so unrealistic that annuities became much too good an investment for foreign capital. This led to a desperate search for some source of information that would show the exact relationship between age and death-rate. The answer was eventually found by the English astronomer Edmund Halley, who learnt that the town of Breslau had, for some years, been keeping a record of age at time of death for every death within the city. He obtained a copy of the register covering a period of five years, and with this and a record of the number of births in the city he was able to construct the first *life table* (1). The method for preparing such tables can be illustrated using his example.

The Breslau registry of births reported that, on average, 1238 children were born each year. The register of deaths showed that each year, on average, 348 children died before their first birthday; if we assume that there had been no net immigration or emigration of infants during this period, it follows by subtraction that each year, on average, 890 children survived at least to celebrate their first birthday. Each year, 69 children died who were between one and two years old; this implies that each year only 821 of those 890 children would survive to their second birthday. The same calculation can then be made for every subsequent year of life using the average number of deaths observed in each one-year age group. The final result shows us how many of the 1238 children born in any one year would on average live to celebrate any particular birthday (see Table 1). Halley realized that this procedure would be valid only if there had been no movement of people in or out of the city and no change in the force of mortality; for example, the calculation assumes that when the children born in 1690 reach 50 years of age they will be subject to the precise annual mortality that was being suffered by those who had reached 50 in 1690 (i.e., were born in 1640). Also, because he only had records for five years, he could not exclude errors due to migration or to changes either in birth-rate or in mortality, although he pointed out that during this period the annual birth-rate roughly equalled the annual death-rate, as it should in steady-state conditions (actually, he observed that there were on average 64 fewer deaths than births each year, but he attributed this to some deaths having occurred in foreign wars and therefore not being counted, and

Table 1
The Life Table for Seventeenth-Century Breslau*

Age	*Number*	*%*	*Age*	*Number*	*%*	*Age*	*Number*	*%*	*Age*	*Number*	*%*
0	1238	100	21	586	47	42	422	34	63	207	17
1	890	72	22	581	47	43	412	33	64	197	16
2	821	66	23	576	47	44	402	32	65	187	15
3	776	63	24	570	46	45	392	32	66	177	14
4	744	60	25	564	46	46	382	31	67	167	13
5	716	58	26	558	45	47	372	30	68	157	13
6	692	56	27	551	45	48	362	29	69	147	12
7	665	54	28	542	44	49	352	28	70	137	11
8	654	53	29	534	43	50	342	28	71	126	10
9	643	52	30	527	43	51	331	27	72	115	9
10	637	51	31	519	42	52	320	26	73	104	8
11	630	51	32	511	41	53	309	25	74	93	8
12	624	50	33	503	41	54	298	24	75	83	7
13	619	50	34	494	40	55	287	23	76	73	6
14	615	50	35	485	39	56	277	22	77	63	5
15	613	50	36	476	38	57	267	22	78	53	4
16	610	49	37	467	38	58	257	21	79	44	4
17	607	49	38	458	37	59	247	20	80	36	3
18	603	49	39	449	36	60	237	19	81	29	2
19	598	48	40	440	36	61	227	18	82	23	2
20	592	48	41	431	35	62	217	18	83	18	1

*The first complete life table, prepared for the city of Breslau at the end of the seventeenth century, by the astronomer Edmund Halley. On average, 1238 children were born in the city each year, and the table shows how many of this annual crop of children would still be alive at each subsequent birthday up to the age of 83 (1).

The table published by Halley is somewhat different from the version given here because his object was to calculate the number of people alive at any moment. For example, the number of children who were in their first year of life on any arbitrarily chosen day would be somewhere between 1238 (the annual birth-rate) and 890 (the number surviving a whole year). Thus the first entry in his table was 1000; subsequent entries were roughly halfway between the adjacent numbers shown here (855 in the second year of life, 798 in the third, etc.).

so he surreptitiously made up the difference by adding a few extra deaths to the older age groups). Halley realized that he could have checked some of his assumptions if a census of the population had been taken, because the table can also be read as an estimate of the age distribution of the population at any given moment, and therefore the total of about 34,000 for all the numbers in the table should equal the total population of Breslau.

For many purposes, it is convenient to summarize such a table by calculating the average number of years lived by each person in the population – in this case, the total number of years lived by the cohort of 1238 people whose fate is described in the table, divided by 1238. The calculation proceeds as follows. We can assume that the 348 who died in their first year died half-way through the year and so contributed 174 person-years to the total; the 69 who died in their second year contributed 1.5 years each, or 103.5 person-years; and so on. From the total of all those person-years (lived by the cohort born in any given year) divided by 1238, we get an estimate of average *life expectancy* at age zero. For Breslau in 1690 it was 26.4 years; in modern Wroclaw, life expectancy will be over 70 (unless, of course, there is war).

Halley's method for estimating the force of mortality can be used whenever we have records of age at time of death, provided we have reason to think that the total size of the population is not changing. For example, we can estimate the life expectancy of prehistoric man, because we can determine the age of the skeletons in Palaeolithic burial sites; the Roman obsession with astrology made them record on each tombstone the exact date of birth and death, and this gives us the age at death for at least those people who were important enough to deserve a gravestone; and of course the births and deaths in the ruling families of Europe are part of recorded history. From such records we can therefore estimate what life expectancy was for certain groups of people in the distant or not so distant past.

For the more recent past, however, Halley's procedure is not adequate. When the size of a population is steadily increasing (as it was in most industrial nations from about 1750 onwards), the number of births each year exceeds the number of deaths. Since the deaths are occurring among cohorts that were born many years earlier when the annual birth-rate was lower by some unknown amount, we have no way of deducing the original size of each birth cohort nor how many of them are still alive, and so we cannot translate total numbers of deaths in each group into age-specific death-rates. If we want to measure life expectancy in an unstable population, we therefore have to have a census that shows the number of people in each age group.

Fortunately, early in the nineteenth century it became the custom in many nations to conduct regular censuses that recorded each person's age. Indeed, many of the reforms in public health that came later in the century were stimulated by these surveys, which showed for the first time just how appalling were the conditions in cities like

Paris and London. Before dealing with these more modern statistics we should, however, go back to the beginnings of mankind. Homo sapiens has spent at least ten times longer being a hunter-gatherer than an agriculturalist, and the city dweller is a still more recent invention. We should therefore expect to find that much of our biochemistry and our pattern of reproduction was selected to be suitable for what we would now think of as an alien lifestyle, and so we may find that some of our present diseases can be traced to our departure from the habits and lifestyle to which we were adapted. To give just one example, breast cancer is now the commonest cancer for women in the Western world, but there are good reasons to think that it would become one of the rarer cancers if we all were to go back to the diet and breeding habits of hunter-gatherers.

The History of Mortality to 1700 A.D.

One of the most extensive and best documented Palaeolithic burial grounds was found in a cave at Taforalt in Morocco (2). Forty thousand years ago this was the site of a small community. They have left us 186 skeletons, and these give us a distribution of age at time of death, which can then be translated into a life table. (Halley's calculations were based on the observed birth-rate in Breslau, and he added a few extra deaths so that births and deaths were equal; we know nothing about the birth-rate in Taforalt, and so we have to assume that the number of births in any given period of time – in this instance, the functioning life of the cemetery – roughly equalled the number of deaths.) Figure 1 shows graphically this life table for Palaeolithic Man compared with a similarly constructed life table for a Neolithic settlement of early agriculturalists living in Hungary around 3000 B.C. (2), and the life table for a contemporary tribe of hunter-gatherers living in the Kalahari desert of Africa (3).

Considering the changes that are to come later, these three curves are remarkably similar; indeed, their similarity suggests that they are fairly accurate. The !Kung are doing slightly better than our distant ancestors (which is to be expected since they have survived so well that they have elected to resist all the temptations of civilization), but it seems likely that the pattern of birth, life, and death was probably much the same for the three groups. The !Kung have been carefully studied over many years, and the dynamics of their population are well documented (3). On average, each breeding woman produces 4.5 children, spaced about four years apart. Of these, 2.2 are girls,

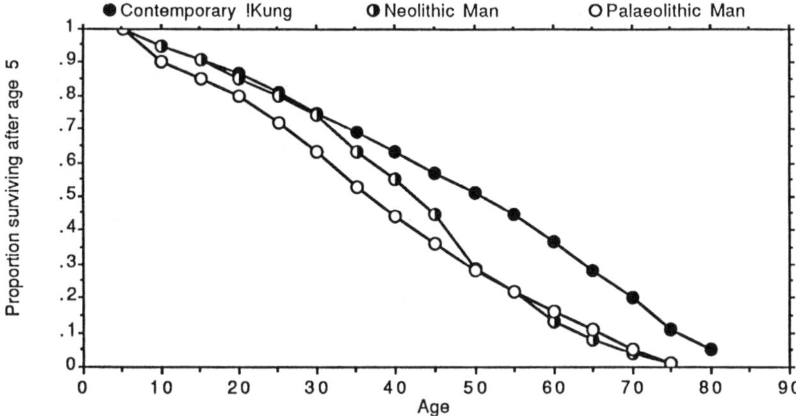

Figure 1. Life tables for Palaeolithic man (40,000 B.C.) and Neolithic man (10,000 B.C.), based on the excavation of burial grounds in Morocco and Hungary (2), and for the contemporary !Kung tribe of hunter-gatherers in the Kalahari desert (3). Because infant death would probably be underestimated, deaths under the age of five are excluded.

and of them one survives to be the replacement for her mother. In this way, births balance deaths, and the population tends to maintain itself at a constant level from one generation to the next. Much has been written about the four-year interval between successive births. It is probably essential for tribes such as these; for the mother in a nomadic family carries some of the baggage and also has to carry the youngest child, so she cannot easily carry another child (4). Part of the long interval between births is due to prolonged lactation, which is believed to inhibit ovulation (the diet of nomads is difficult to eat if you have no teeth, and so the mother has to breast feed each child for about three years (5)). However, the tribe undoubtedly has some unexploited capacity for increase that is kept in check by abortion, infanticide, and restrictive rules governing matrimony. For the ancient non-nomadic communities shown in Figure 1, mortality was somewhat higher and so each breeding woman must have had to produce more children to maintain the population.

The invention of agriculture, around 10,000 years ago, vastly increased the capacity of land to support human populations (6). Palaeolithic communities seldom achieved densities higher than 0.1 per square kilometer, whereas early Neolithic agriculturalists reached one person per square kilometer, and by the time of the Roman Empire several countries had reached 15 persons per square kilometer. Presumably the increased productivity of the countryside, brought about by agriculture, improved the nutrition of its inhabitants and this then led both to an increase in their fertility and to a decrease in their mortality. The invention of agriculture, however, brought other changes that were much more important than the mere increase in population. It has regularly been observed that the inhabitants of agricultural communities have to work much harder than hunter-gatherers (7). In this sense, agriculture can be seen as the invention that allows people to generate more food by working harder – in particular, more food than they themselves can consume. So it brings into existence societies in which some people not only produce food for themselves but are forced to produce food for others – a development that has been called "macroparasitism" (8). Such societies are the very essence of civilization. But with their arrival the human race acquired rulers and armies, and these had to be supported by yet more work, which in turn created the demand for more births to add to the working population – an idea that is explicit in the Roman choice of the word "proletarius" to describe the segment of the population who were not landowners and whose prime function was to produce offspring ("proles").

It may never be possible to disentangle the many interactions between the inventions of agriculture and the birth-rate and death-rate of these early populations; and the same problem will return when we come to consider the demographic changes that occurred at the time of the Industrial Revolution. However, one consequence of the invention of agriculture was of enormous importance for the evolution of human diseases, and that was the development of cities. Once large numbers of people are in close contact with each other, infectious agents can survive from one year to the next even if they produce life-long immunity in their host, because there will now always be a high enough concentration of susceptible children waiting to be infected (9). So we see new human diseases arising that had probably never existed before, such as measles and smallpox. Even diseases that had existed since earlier times achieved a prevalence they probably never had among scattered, isolated communities. As a result, cities came to be called the graveyards of mankind. We see this clearly from the records of Roman cemeteries (10). The life table for the inhabitants of the Roman colonies in North Africa in 0–400 A.D. shows life expectancy to have been very like that of the !Kung. In contrast, Rome itself, even for those rich enough to deserve gravestones, must have been an extraordinarily hostile environment. As Figure 2 shows,

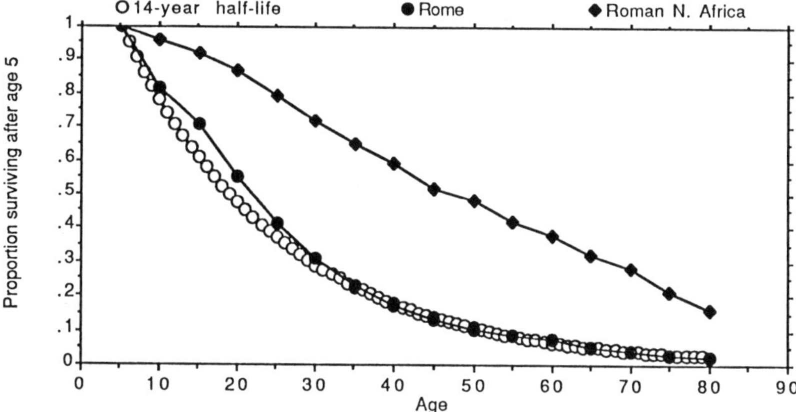

Figure 2. Life tables for urban and rural populations in the Roman Empire between 0 and 200 A.D., based on the age distribution at death determined from the inscriptions on gravestones (10). The survival of people living in the city of Rome is seen to be close to the survival expected for objects with a half-life of 14 years. As in the previous figure, survival is followed after the age of five.

the force of mortality there was so overwhelming that senescence ceased to be very important; in any year, you had roughly a one-in-twenty chance of dying irrespective of your age (namely, a half-life of about 14 years). Such a population cannot sustain itself without infusion from outside, and so the surrounding countryside had continually to provide Rome not only with the tribute of food and taxes but also with young recruits for its workforce. (Incidentally, this example allows us to see how great a change has recently taken place in our ideas of what constitutes the best of all possible worlds; just two hundred years ago the historian Edward Gibbon declared that "If a man were called to fix the period of the world during which the condition of the human race was most happy and prosperous, he would, without hesitation, name that which elapsed from the death of Domitian (96 A.D.) to the accession of Commodus (180 A.D.).")

Ancient Rome may have been an extreme case, but it was not until the twentieth century that any city became able to sustain itself without continual influx of people from outside. Indeed, it was the contrast in the statistics of life and death in the towns and country districts of eighteenth- and nineteenth-century Europe that first stimulated sanitary reform and gave rise to the science of public health. As we shall see, the way these reforms came about is interesting, because it shows how much can be achieved on the basis of empirical evidence even when your underlying beliefs as to mechanism are completely fallacious.

The Seventeenth and Eighteenth Centuries

In 1662 John Graunt published a study of the weekly record of mortality for London (11). He showed that the city regularly recorded more deaths than births and was being maintained by immigrants from the country, and he ascribed its unhealthiness rather vaguely to pressures of population and to the ever-increasing smoke as the nation turned to coal for its source of heat. Even though he discussed the rise and fall of various diseases, he seems to have been uninterested in their causes. Indeed, he ends his book discreetly by saying, "whether the knowledge [of births and deaths, migration and disease] be necessary for many, or fit for others than our sovereign and his chief ministers, I leave to (the) consideration (of others)."

People's attitude to disease seems to have been a strange mixture of activism and passivity. Everyone knew that plague was a contagious disease which could be escaped by avoiding any contact with victims. That was why Boccaccio's talkative ladies and gentlemen were sequestered in the country in 1348 (the very word "quarantine" comes from the practice, in fourteenth-century French and Italian ports, of holding ships at anchor off-shore for 40 days if they had come from countries suffering plague). But the general force of mortality, as it weighed upon the populace from one year to the next, was treated as if it were something ordained by God, immutable and not to be meddled with. Thus in 1741, when Johann Süssmilch wrote what is generally considered to be the first treatise on population, he carefully entitled it "Die Göttliche Ordnung in den Veränderungen des menschlichen Geschlechts, aus der Geburt, dem Tode, und der Fortplanzung desselben erwissen" (The God-given order to the changes in male and female births and deaths, from one generation to the next).

Times were changing, however. Within one generation, Johann Peter Frank produced the first of a series of books describing how the cities could be kept clean and free of disease, and how the German authorities should encourage the population to produce children who then would be properly looked after, educated, and protected from accident. His "System einer vollständigen medicinischen Polizey" (A system for the policing and control of medical hygiene) appeared in six volumes between 1779 and 1817, and may perhaps be counted as the first statement of the concept of public health. Unfortunately, like many really original suggestions, this one seems to have had little impact. (A similar scheme was proposed, at about the same time, to the revolutionary Constituent Assembly of France by Dr Guillotin, but it too was not acted upon, and his lasting fame rests upon a very different invention.)

For some years, Sweden had been keeping a complete record of births and deaths. After comparing the records for urban and rural Sweden and England, Richard Price, the English theologian and revolutionary, wrote:

> From this comparison it appears with how much truth great cities have been called the graves of mankind. [The comparison] must also convince all that ... it is by no means strictly proper to consider our diseases as the original intention of nature. They are, without doubt, in general, our own creation. Were there a country where the inhabitants led lives entirely natural and virtuous, few of them would die without measuring out the whole period of the present existence allotted them; and death would come upon them like a sleep, in consequence of no other cause than gradual and unavoidable decay. Let us, then, instead of charging our Maker with our miseries, learn more to accuse and reproach ourselves. (Essay on the population of England, sent as a letter to Benjamin Franklin in 1769.)

Price then goes on to lay the blame firstly on the luxury and debaucheries of town life, and secondly on the general filth of all cities; so his stance is still slightly tainted with the moralism of an earlier age. He was, however, one of the founders of the first life assurance company, and it seems likely that his influence can be detected in the wording of the U.S. Declaration of Independence.

The end of the eighteenth century was above all a time of high ideals and revolution. That was when people started to collect statistics on mortality, and it seems to have been about then that governments and rulers started to adjust to the idea that one of the most important responsibilities of the state is to provide a happy longevity for its citizens – that is, for all its citizens, rather than just the rich and the powerful. It had seemed perfectly reasonable that Frederick the Great, when pursuing his family squabbles on the largest of scales, should urge on his troops with the cry, "You rascals, do you want to live forever?" Yet, less than twenty years later, Thomas Jefferson was writing a draft of the U.S. Declaration of Independence and asserting that we all have a right to "the preservation of life, liberty, and the pursuit of happiness." And, significantly, it was about then, at the end of the eighteenth century or early in the nineteenth, that life expectancy started to climb. For those lucky enough not to be in large cities, life expectancy had been roughly 40 for hundreds or even thousands of years (except, of course, in times of famine and pestilence). Over the next 150 years, however, the industrial nations of the world were to see average life expectancy move up to 75 and beyond.

We would obviously like to know what actually were the technical, social, and political changes that produced such a sudden improvement in the human condition. How many of the changes were meant to improve public health and how many were fortuitous? How often did the reforms confer such obvious benefits that they were instantly accepted by everyone, and how often did they have to be forced on the population by some paternalistic authority? It is also worth considering what, at the time, were believed to be the causes of premature mortality; as we shall see, the arguments that raged then over the causes of what we now call the infectious diseases were extraordinarily like some of the present arguments about the causes of cancer. By looking at this period, we may learn some important lessons about the practice of public health and preventive medicine.

We should start with the crude facts. The exact historical records of life and death in the ruling families of Europe show that, for the rich, life expectancy started to go up somewhere between 1650 and 1750 (12,13). The uncertainty stems from the fact that the seventeenth century may have been a period of unusually high mortality, and so the first part of the increase in life expectancy could be considered as the natural rebound rather than part of a long-term trend; after 1750, however, there is no doubt about the trend. The common people had to wait another 100 years before their lot improved (14), although the rise in their life expectancy, when it finally came, was steeper than it had been for the rich (Figure 3). (Even to this day, the rich tend to live longer than the poor: in most Western nations, apart from Sweden, life expectancy is still about ten years greater for the highest social classes than for the lowest (15); in the United States, for example, the richest ethnic group is the Japanese and the poorest is the blacks, and the life expectancies for Japanese, Caucasian, and black women in 1960 were 80, 75, and 67 respectively (16).)

Surprisingly, the prime causes of the increase in life expectancy are still somewhat obscure. If the only information at our disposal were the statistics for the total population of a nation such as England, we would be forced to conclude that nothing happened to life expectancy

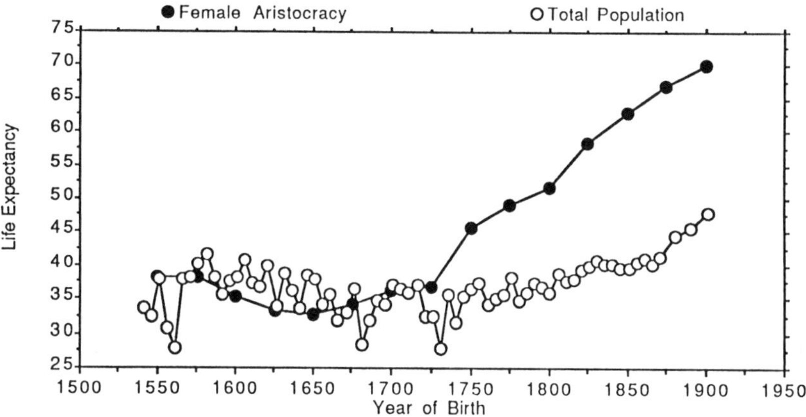

Figure 3. Change in life expectancy in England since 1540. The values for female members of the aristocracy come from family records (12). The values for the general population come from a reconstruction of parish records (14). Note that it is not yet possible to determine the average life expectancy for cohorts born after 1900 because so many of these people are still alive; for an estimate of the likely change in life expectancy in the twentieth century, see Figure 10.

until the middle of the nineteenth century, especially since we know that this was the time of great sanitary reform. But mortality had started to change much earlier for the rich, and so before we give all the credit to the reformers of the nineteenth century we should look at what was happening a hundred years earlier.

The eighteenth century saw one conspicuous innovation in public health – the introduction of immunization against smallpox – and this may have had a significant effect on overall mortality. In Sweden, for example, smallpox was responsible for more than 10% of all deaths in the middle of the century, but the figure had dropped to about 1% a hundred years later (17). (In England the effect would have been masked (save perhaps among the rich) because industrialization was drawing people into cities; in the eighteenth century, London's share of England's population went from 5% to 12%, and this would have tended to raise mortality.)

Other important changes were taking place. Increasing trade with the new world was bringing in new crops, plus the great wealth engendered by such trade. Agriculture was becoming vastly more sophisticated and efficient, so that many people probably had access to at least a more varied diet (18). Wool (which shrinks when washed) began to be replaced by cotton, so that it became practical to wash your clothes repeatedly and therefore worthwhile to wash yourself at the same time, and people at last started to be fairly clean, which must have diminished the spread of many contagious diseases (19). Lastly, there seems to have been a great change in attitude. Books on health became best-sellers. In France, a book entitled "Avis au peuple sur sa santé" (Advice to the population on its health) (Tissot, 1762) went through ten editions in six years, and a German equivalent, "Gesundheitkatechismus" (A catechism for health) (Faust, 1794), sold 150,000 copies.

The emphasis of the times, at least among the reading public, seems to have been on cleanliness. Unfortunately, this could be extended to the general public only in those situations where there was some centralized authority – as in certain hospitals, army camps, and ships of the navy. For the poor, whether they lived in the city or the country, the struggle for survival allowed little time for inventiveness, and so they were not involved in these changes nor initially did they benefit from them. Nevertheless, we should date the beginnings of public health to at least as far back as the eighteenth century. Frank, who was mentioned earlier in connection with his treatise on public health published between 1779 and 1817, studied the state of medicine in northern Italy and concluded that most disease could be traced to the abject poverty imposed on the population by the nobility and clergy, who owned all the land. In this, he was far ahead of his time, and in consequence his attempts at reform were fruitless even though he had the backing of the Emperor Joseph II. In a famous graduation day address at the University of Pavia in 1790 (entitled "De populorum miseria: morborum genitrice" [The suffering of the people: the genesis of disease]), he pointed out a paradox that, to some extent, remains unresolved to this day. "Why is it," he asked, "that a vast amount of illness originates in the very society that men of old inaugurated in order to enjoy a safer life?"

Although most of the well-known heroes of public health are nineteenth-century figures, my own feeling is that the change can be traced back to the philosophers of the Age of Enlightenment, who persuaded the world that the human condition is not the subject of Divine Will but is essentially a matter of choice. That, I think, was the foundation of what was to happen in the next 100 years.

The Nineteenth Century

The population of Europe has suffered at least two periods of great decline – during the Dark Ages which followed the fall of the Roman

Empire, and during the fourteenth century when there was a succession of epidemics of plague, the worst of which killed one out of every three people. But apart from these major setbacks the number of people living in Europe (and in the world as a whole) had been growing fairly steadily at the rate of about 7% per generation (i.e., was doubling every 300 years or so). In the nineteenth century, this was suddenly to change. Europe's population doubled in 100 years and would almost double again before reaching its present relatively stationary state; indeed, England went further, doubling between 1800 and 1850, and again between 1850 and 1900, which amounts to a 50% increase in each generation.

The exact process underlying this period of growth is still the subject of debate (14,18,19,20). Obviously, for a population to increase, births must exceed deaths; and if the increase is to be more than just temporary, the growth must apply to the breeding population – that is, must come in the form of either an increase in birth-rate or a decrease in childhood mortality. Since the force of mortality did not change in England for the nation as a whole until after 1850 (Fig. 3), the explosion in population that occurred in the nineteenth century must initially have been due to an increase in birth-rate. As mentioned earlier, the circumstances of a !Kung tribeswoman determine that she has rather little unexploited capacity for producing children. In contrast, the modern European woman was plainly able to produce enough children to increase the population by more than 50% per generation, and nineteenth-century England was so organized (in terms of marriage and reproduction) that she did exactly that. Historical demographers have therefore had to decide whether there was a sudden change in marriage customs (proportion of women who married, how young they were, etc.) or in the fertility of married women, and how much the change was a physiological one – due, perhaps, to improvements in nutrition – and how much was the result of a conscious effort to have more children. (Incidentally, any explanation has to accommodate the awkward fact that a similar acceleration was occurring at the same time in India, China, and Japan (21).)

Whatever the underlying cause, the increase in Europe's population was accompanied by a migration into the cities in pursuit of the wealth that was being generated by the Industrial Revolution. Over the course of 100 years, the populations of London and Paris increased about five-fold, while Berlin increased ten-fold. By 1900, London contained over six million people and the other two cities each contained two to three million. As this growth occurred at a time when there were few if any restrictions on the design and occupancy of buildings,

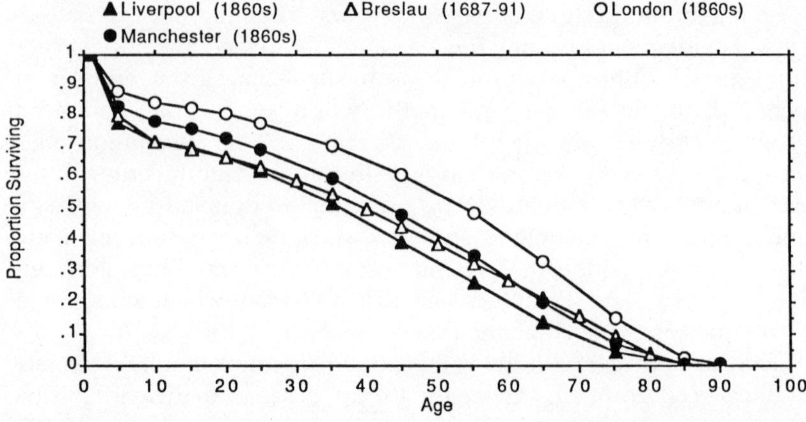

Figure 4. Halley's life table for seventeenth-century Breslau compared with the life tables for London, Liverpool, and Manchester at the height of the Industrial Revolution. In this and the next figure, deaths under the age of one are excluded.

or minimum standards to be met by landlords, the major cities of the Western world maintained a squalor and level of mortality almost matching that of ancient Rome.

The conventional view of the Industrial Revolution is that it worsened the lot of the masses. Yet the statistics on mortality do not support this idea. I would have guessed that life in seventeenth-century Breslau was much like Wagner's idyllic portrait of life in sixteenth-century Nurenberg. In fact, Halley's life table shows that the conditions in Breslau were as bad as those of the worst of English cities (Liverpool) at what must have been about the worst time in the Industrial Revolution (Figure 4). As for life in the country, the rural districts of England in the 1860s were subject to roughly the same level of mortality as the agrarian community in Roman North Africa nearly 2000 years earlier (Figure 5) (22). What had changed, however, were people's thoughts about disease and death. The world was now ready for reform.

The earliest actual numerical studies of mortality among the poor were carried out in France (23). In 1829, in the first issue of *Annales d'hygiène publique et de médecine légale,* Villermé reported that most paupers' prisons in France were imposing on the wretched prisoners an average annual mortality of about 25%; the cause had to be the indifference of the authorities to the fate of the poor, rather than any calculated severity, because mortality was much lower in maximum

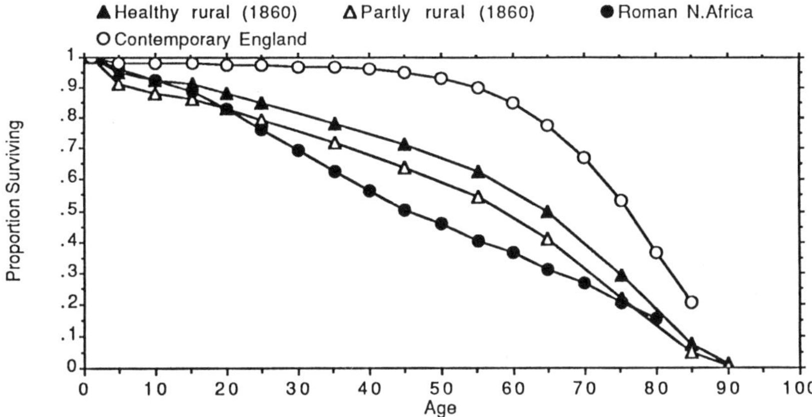

Figure 5. The life table for Roman North Africa in 0–200 A.D. compared with that of 53 sparsely populated ("healthy rural") and 137 more densely populated rural ("partly rural") districts of England during the Industrial Revolution, and with that of present-day England.

security prisons where there was forced labour. From prisoners, Villermé then turned his attention to the citizens of Paris. Figures were available for mortality, and the affluence of various districts could be assessed indirectly by determining the proportion of people who paid rents that were high enough to be taxed. Using these statistics, he showed that mortality was about 50% higher in the poorest districts than in the richest. From there he went on to look at mortality for different occupational groups and produced a table giving life expectancy at several ages for sixteen occupations. The differences were very great: for example, at age ten the children of manufacturers and merchants could expect to live for another 42 years; for factory workers the figure was only 28 years.

Villermé's second report, "Tableau de l'état physique et moral des ouvriers" (A tabulation showing the physical and moral condition of workers), came out in 1840 and was followed, two years later, by Chadwick's "Report on the Sanitary Conditions of the Labouring Population of Great Britain." The conclusion was all too clear. The businessman who built a factory and created jobs was bringing wealth to some but he was certainly not bringing health to the workers in the factory. For example, one of England's major sources of wealth was the manufacture of cotton fabrics (by the 1830s about 1% of the entire population was engaged in the cotton industry). The southern states of the U.S. were becoming the main suppliers of raw cotton, and this was made possible by the triangular trade – slaves from West Africa to the U.S., cotton from the U.S. to England, and cotton (and other) goods from England to Africa (and elsewhere). For people who were rich, cotton fabrics made it much easier to be comfortable and clean, and as mentioned earlier this cleanliness may have contributed to their increasing life expectancy; for both the West African slaves (24) and the English cotton-spinners, life expectancy at birth seems to have been about 20 years.

The Industrial Revolution brought another very unwelcome result. In 1831, trade with India introduced cholera to Europe for the first time, and by the following year it had spread to the United States. Like plague, cholera is a readily identifiable disease and typically produces sudden violent outbreaks with a high mortality. For example, the 1892 outbreak in Hamburg (which at the time had a population of about half a million) produced a thousand new cases a day of whom half were to die, and one nineteenth-century epidemic in Cairo killed 13% of the inhabitants. Europe had been free of such cataclysmic epidemics for several generations; the last outbreak of plague had been in Marseilles in 1720, and smallpox could by now be fairly well contained thanks to vaccination. So the sudden appearance of a new epidemic disease precipitated a prolonged and historically very important controversy about the causes of mortality. It also stimulated the collection and use of proper statistics. Just as the plague of 1592 had been the stimulus for the collection and publication of the weekly London Bills of Mortality, so it was that the arrival of cholera in the 1830s made the British Parliament create, in 1848, a central Board of Health with the power to enforce the sanitary reforms that were being advocated by those who knew the statistics. The first half of the nineteenth century was therefore a time for assembling statistics, arguing about causes and preparing for a reform in public health.

The main causes of death were certain infectious diseases that we have now almost completely eradicated. Indeed, the most important of these (tuberculosis, diphtheria, cholera, dysentery, typhoid, and typhus) are caused by micro-organisms that most people in the Western world should now never meet unless they travel. Some of these diseases are airborne, spreading directly from person to person; others are carried in food or water. None of this, however, was known at the start of the nineteenth century. Smallpox had been shown to be contagious; indeed, the practice of inoculation was based on that idea. Plague and leprosy had for centuries been regarded as infectious. But the other diseases, that we now know to be infectious, were often not well distinguished one from another, and for the most part their incidence did not vary greatly from one year to the next. So there was ample excuse for not realizing that they were infectious diseases. Furthermore, with the French and American revolutions fresh in everyone's mind, it was very much part of the spirit of the times to look for political, rather than technological solutions for the ills of humankind. Villermé and Chadwick had shown that the greatest cities had the greatest mortality and that the poor lived less long than the rich. Since mortality went hand in hand with density of population and the general filth of cities, it was natural to propose that diseases were caused simply by the miasma (smell) of people and the filth and squalor that accompanies extreme poverty. So there arose, early in the century, a strong anti-contagionist school which believed that diseses were, with a few exceptions, not due to infective agents transmitted from one person to another, but could arise spontaneously wherever the miasma of poverty existed. (The issue has fascinating similarities to the controversy, in the 1940s, about the origin of mutations; interestingly, the arguments were resolved in opposite directions, but each controversy lies at the heart of a scientific discipline – respectively, clinical microbiology and classical genetics.)

The anti-contagionists included some strange bedfellows (25,26). Many scientists felt that the arguments of the contagionists were very weak, and this rather negative reason made them, illogically, into anti-contagionists; they did, however, remain experimentalists at heart and would fearlessly use themselves to prove that one or another disease was not contagious, the most famous instance occurring in 1892 when von Pettenkofer swallowed a culture of the newly isolated *Vibrio cholerae* in the hope of proving that it was not a cause of disease. The social reformers, with even less logic, tended to be anti-contagionists because they believed that social reform was all that was needed to resolve the problem of disease; for example, the great German pathologist, Rudolf Virchow, was a staunch believer in the social causes of diseases (e.g., that social conditions decided whether your disease appeared as typhus or typhoid); it was thanks largely to his efforts that Berlin was transformed into one of the healthiest cities in Europe, and Pettenkofer was to do the same for Munich (indeed, Virchow went further than most people and declared that medicine is essentially a social science and politics is nothing more than medicine on a large scale). Many priests were *laissez faire* anti-contagionists because they wanted to believe that disease was a sign of sinfulness. Big business was anti-contagionist because it did not want any form of quarantine to interrupt international trade and it also did not want any social reform; its position was therefore at least internally consistent (unlike, for example, the present-day American tobacco industry which asks that the growers be subsidized and the marketers be left free to advertise their lethal product). Lastly, even the medical establishment was occasionally driven by self-interest to take an anti-contagionist stance; for example, in 1897 the New York Academy of Medicine opposed legislation that would make tuberculosis a notifiable disease, because this would diminish the power and independence of the doctors (27).

Certain unfortunate experiments greatly strengthened the anti-contagionist cause. Most of the people like Pettenkofer, who deliberately employed themselves as experimental animals, escaped unscathed, for many human pathogens are of rather limited virulence and tend to become attenuated on culture. In the 1820s, the French conducted a series of very careful studies of several outbreaks of yellow fever, in the New World and the Old, and showed beyond doubt that the disease could arise in people who had not come into contact with other cases; yellow fever was, however, an unfortunate choice, because it is transmitted by mosquitoes, and consecutive cases can therefore arise far apart from each other. As a result of these studies, the French Academy of Medicine produced a strongly anti-contagionist report in 1828, and this led to a similar position being taken on many other diseases (including cholera) and to the widespread abolition of quarantine. (We should not blame them too much for this; the contagiousness of diseases such as plague and smallpox had been a more obvious and acceptable idea in earlier centuries when most people lived in small towns or villages, travel was slow and difficult, and a belief in contagion had rather few economic consequences.)

It is easy to list the sequence of discoveries that should have been the decisive events in establishing, once and for all, that most mortality at that time was due to pathogenic micro-organisms; hindsight makes wise men of us all. What actually happened seems to have been much less tidy. In 1840, a young German pathologist, Jacob Henle, produced a masterly review of the literature, "Von den Miasmen und Kontagien" (On miasmas and contagions), in which he outlined all the reasons for thinking that many of the common epidemic diseases were caused by micro-organisms. His argument was partly by analogy: fermentation and putrefaction had recently been shown, experimentally, to be the result of contamination with living creatures, such as yeasts and fungi, that do not arise spontaneously; like the process of fermentation, the development of a disease such as measles, scarlet fever, or smallpox takes time (i.e., each disease has a characteristic incubation period); during this time the causative agent must be increasing in quantity because we know, from direct observation, that in a disease such as smallpox a single pustule contains enough of the agent to infect many people each of whom will, in due course, bear many pustules; and it is this ability of the causative agents of smallpox and the other epidemic diseases to multiply which shows that they must be alive, since living creatures are the only things that can multiply in number.

Unfortunately, Henle's elegant reasoning seems to have had little influence on his contemporaries, and anti-contagionism remained the dogma of the day. Curiously enough, part of the problem came from Darwin's recently published account of evolution and the origin of species. If species emerge spontaneously, one from another, under the pressure of changes in their environment, then it follows (so the argument went) that there must have been a primary act of spontaneous generation that gave rise to the first species; and if such an event *can* occur, then who is to say that it is not occurring the whole time? (Interestingly, a similar controversy raged in the 1930s over the nature of the viruses of bacteria (bacteriophages), and once again the wrong side was temporarily victorious; Burnet, in Australia, believed that the bacteriophages were viruses and should be classified as living because they exhibited, as he put it, "genetic continuity" from one generation to the next (28); unfortunately, Northrop and others, who were biochemists and therefore somewhat unreliable on matters of biology, argued that the bacteriophages were inanimate toxic enzymes which could induce a bacterium to make more such enzyme molecules but were not alive and could not multiply. Their view prevailed for several years – perhaps because Northrop had won a Nobel Prize and Burnet, at that time, had not.)

In 1854, a third epidemic of cholera hit Europe, and it gave rise to two reports that, at least in retrospect, should have settled once and for all what was the immediate cause of the disease and how it was spread. John Snow's report, published in 1855 ("On the Mode of Communication of Cholera"), showed, beyond all reasonable doubt, that that particular outbreak of cholera was spread chiefly by contamination of water supplies, and that some 600 cases could be traced to one particular water pump in London. Furthermore, this local epidemic provided him with several significant "controls," for he noted that the people occupying a nearby brewery and workhouse (each of which had its own independent water supply) were spared, whereas those who collected their water at the pump had a high risk of cholera even if they happened to live far away. His book, which describes the outbreak around the Broad Street pump in the district of Soho and a rather similar episode south of the river Thames in the suburb of Lambeth, is a *tour de force*. Indeed, it marks the beginning of investigative epidemiology. As it happened, another report was published at about the same time by Filippo Pacini describing and naming the unusual bacterium that is present in almost pure culture in the intestines of people dying of cholera ("Osservazioni microscopiche e deduzione patalogiche sul colera asiatico," 1854). It is sad that neither of these reports seems to have made any lasting impression on the governments of the time. In England, the compiler of the Registrar General's Annual Reports, William Farr, persuaded himself as the result of further epidemiological studies that Snow was right, and it seems that many doctors were equally persuaded and, by their efforts, cut short many outbreaks of cholera. But central authorities were not persuaded; indeed, in an orgy of *laissez faire* capitalism the Parliament in London shortly after this abolished Chadwick's Board of Health, which until then had been responsible for sanitary reforms in the cities of England. The issue seems to have been the familiar one of power politics, the lobbying of certain vested interests, and the gullibility of those who read newspapers. The London *Times* rejoiced in the decision by saying that "we prefer to take our chance of cholera and the rest than be bullied into health." Chadwick retired. Snow died at the age of 45. And although Pacini survived until 1883 he too died a disappointed man, unaware that his discovery was just about to be confirmed.

From the vantage point of the twentieth century, we can see that the central, scientific issue was the question of spontaneous generation. If some disease is caused by a miasma and can appear in a totally isolated community whenever the right physical conditions are present, then the causative agent must be capable of arising by spontaneous generation (i.e., is not like the living creatures we see around us, that can only increase by producing replicas of themselves); conversely, if the disease spreads solely by direct contact (contagion), that must be because the causative agent is a living creature and cannot arise *de novo*. Although experiments had already been performed that seemed to exclude the possibility of spontaneous gen-

Table 2
Death Rates (per Million) in England and Wales, Classified by Causative Agent.[1]

Conditions attributable to micro-organisms	*1848-54*	*1971*
Airborne		
Tuberculosis	2901	13
Bronchitis, pneumonia, influenza	2239	603
Scarlet fever, diphtheria	1016	0
Whooping cough	423	1
Measles	342	0
Smallpox	263	0
Upper respiratory tract infections	75	2
Carried in food and water		
Cholera, dysentery	1819	33
Typhoid (and typhus2)	990	0
Non-respiratory tuberculosis	753	2
Transmitted in other ways		
Infections in infants	1322	0
Appendicitis, peritonitis	75	7
Puerperal fever	62	1
Syphilis	50	0
Other infections	635	52
Total attributable to micro-organisms	12965	714
Conditions not attributable to micro-organisms	8891	4670

Source: After Thomas McKeown, "The Role of Medicine: Dream, Mirage, or Nemesis" published by the Nuffield Provincial Hospitals Trust London, 1976.

Notes
[1]Rates have been standardized to the distribution of age and sex in the population in 1901.
[2]Typhus is transmitted by lice, but in the early nineteenth century it was still not properly distinguished from typhoid fever.

eration of the invisible causes of disease, the issue remained in doubt until the 1860s, when Pasteur showed conclusively that any material or culture medium that had been properly sterilized by heat would remain sterile indefinitely provided it was protected against microbial contamination from outside. His proof required the concept that substances can be sterilized by heat. This may seem a trivial notion, but it is the foundation of the sophisticated technology that he and others were developing for the study of bacteria. Once developed, these techniques made it possible to identify all the major pathogenic bacteria (i.e., the immediate causes of most of the diseases listed in Table 2). Appropriately, the dominant figure at this time was a pupil of Henle's, Robert Koch. In 1882, Koch isolated the bacterium that is the cause of tuberculosis, and in the following year he went to Cairo to investigate an outbreak of cholera and quickly identified the bacterium that was responsible. On his return to Germany he was accorded a hero's reception, perhaps in part because the Egyptian exercise had been a joint (but competitive) venture by Germany and France, and so Koch's success could be given nationalistic overtones.

Some doubters remained, however, even among the scientific community. The doctors could not have liked seeing so many of their cherished beliefs cast aside. The bacteriologists must have seemed to them like arrogant intruders, for this was really the first time that laboratory science had invaded the practice of medicine. As the president of the New York Academy of Medicine said, in 1885, "Have we not had enough yet of the monthly instalments of new bacilli which are the invariably correct and positive sources of disease ... ?"

Any residual doubts about the cause of cholera were settled by Koch's study of the 1892 epidemic in Hamburg, in which he showed that the hardest hit parts of the city were those that had the oldest water supply. Interestingly, his epidemiological evidence was less elegant and clear-cut than John Snow's, a generation earlier. But now the world was ready for the discovery and, more to the point, ready for all its implications. Over the previous 30 or 40 years there had been a revolution in people's attitude to public health, and it was now widely accepted that health and disease were proper subjects for legislation. Boards of Health had been created in most major cities and the process of cleaning up the environment was already well underway. (As Virchow had put it, "Medicine is a social science ... Politics is nothing but medicine on a large scale." Cicero had said rather the same thing almost 2000 years earlier – "Salus populi suprema est lex" – although he probably meant that the prime consideration of the law should be the welfare of the populace, rather than their freedom from disease, which he would not have thought of as a controllable variable.)

With the knowledge that cholera is caused by a bacterium, it became much easier to police the laws about water supply and sewage disposal and to enforce rules of quarantine during epidemics; for example, in the great outbreak of 1892 six infected ships visited the port of New York, but the local Board of Health was able to stop the disease from entering the city. Henceforth, any population could in principle be shown how to halt an epidemic of cholera by instituting a few simple precautions. It is important to note here that although the discovery of the bacterium *Vibrio cholerae* required some fairly high technology (good microscopes and all the other paraphernalia of bacteriologists), the end result was a solution to the problem that was within the reach of even the humblest peasant. Incidentally, this seems to have been true for many of the important biological discoveries; in biology, as in other fields of human endeavour, "knowledge itself is power" (Francis Bacon).

The conquest of cholera is a particularly useful example because it illustrates so clearly the interplay between epidemiology and laboratory science – the kind of interplay, incidentally, that is becoming characteristic of much of present-day cancer research. But the final years of the nineteenth century were filled with other similar discoveries of enormous importance for the health of the human race. The transmission of malaria and yellow fever by mosquitoes, the role of symptomless carriers in the spread of diseases such as typhoid and diphtheria, the discovery of the immune system – the list seems endless. It was obviously one of those moments when a fresh cast of mind is sufficient to achieve a scientific revolution. For the full impact of these discoveries upon the health of the world, we must, however, look at the twentieth century.

The Twentieth Century

Once they had identified the most important bacterial causes of human disease, the early bacteriologists moved on to study the mechanisms underlying acquired immunity to those diseases. The history of this period can be illustrated by considering the example of diphtheria. This is a disease, usually of the upper respiratory tract, that is dangerous because the bacterium *Corynebacterium diphtheriae* secretes a very potent toxin. In 1890, workers in Koch's laboratory showed that the blood of guinea pigs who had survived infection contained antibodies which would inactivate the toxin. Their discovery quickly led to two important developments – the mass production of antitoxin (in horses) for the treatment of human cases of diphtheria, and the production of toxin (suitably modified to diminish its toxicity) for the preventive immunization of human populations. This was the first time science offered not only a specific treatment (passive immunity against the bacterial toxin) but also a way of preventing an infectious disease (active immunization). These procedures (plus the antibiotics that came in the 1940s) are still, to this day, the weapons used to control diphtheria, and so the history of diphtheria records what amounted to a competition between those who treat and those who

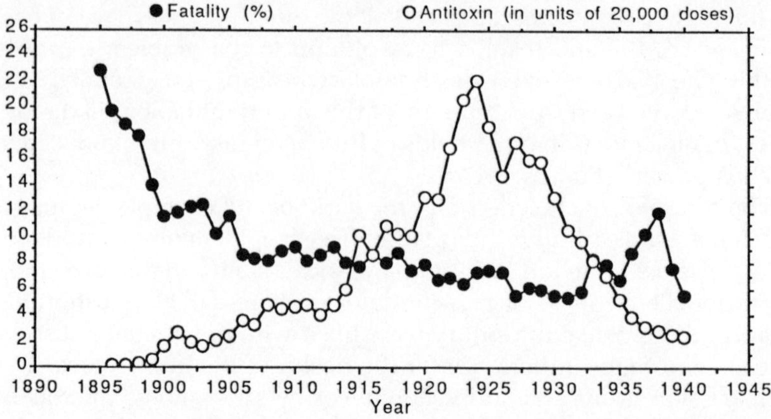

Figure 6. The change in the fatality of diphtheria in the state of Massachusetts (percent of cases that were fatal) in relation to the production of diphtheria antitoxin (number of doses distributed in Massachusetts each year).

seek to prevent. For our study of the history of diphtheria, any good source of statistics will serve. For example, since the 1890s the state of Massachusetts has kept a record of the number of cases of diphtheria occurring each year, what proportion of the cases were fatal, how much diphtheria antitoxin was distributed and later (when immunization became practicable), how much modified toxin was distributed. The statistics are shown in Figures 6 and 7. The first thing we see (Fig. 6) is that the fatality of the disease had dropped steeply in the 1890s (before antitoxin became available) and has remained between 5% and 10% from then on. To judge from these overall numbers, therefore, treatment with antitoxin seems to have been of rather little avail (even with today's antibiotics, the fatality of cases is still about 10%). There does, however, seem to have been some control over the incidence of diphtheria, because no major epidemics occurred after about 1907 (Fig. 7). This was the year the state installed Inspectors of Health whose job it was to see that every case of a dangerous infectious disease was reported. Although these inspectors had very limited powers, they would advise about quarantine and could arrange for bacteriological tests to determine who were chronic carriers of diphtheria, and it seems not unreasonable therefore to assume that the drop in incidence of diphtheria was at least partly due to their efforts. Finally, with the introduction of active immunization in the 1920s diphtheria ceased to be an important cause of

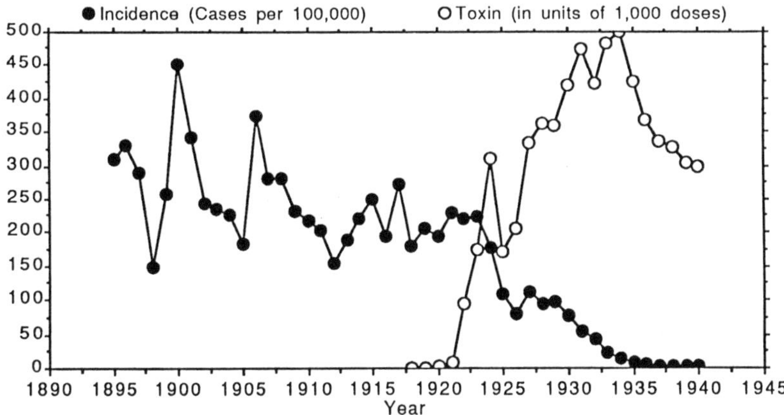

Figure 7. The change in the incidence of diphtheria in Massachusetts (cases per 100,000 people per year) in relation to the production of diphtheria toxin for immunization (number of doses distributed each year).

death. If therefore we look back over the history of this one disease, we would have to say that it was largely conquered by prevention – first as part of the general reduction in mortality from many diseases that came at the end of the nineteenth century (perhaps because of improvements in nutrition), and somewhat later as the result of direct efforts to restrict the spread of the disease, and finally as the result of a specific program of immunizaton. Advances in the treatment of diphtheria, in particular the discovery of antibiotics, have had only a minor effect on mortality.

When technical measures are introduced that involve interference with specific mechanisms of disease, it is easy to accept their efficacy and think of their discovery as having been a turning point in human affairs. For this reason, the obvious impact of active immunization upon the incidence of infections like diphtheria tends to blind us to the effects of other less specific ways of controlling the spread of infectious diseases. But we should remember that more than half of the reduction in mortality from diphtheria had already been achieved before the technological solution was available. Therefore we should now look specifically at the history of some infectious disease for which no technological solution was available.

The pre-eminent example is tuberculosis. As a cause of death this was far more important than diphtheria; in Massachusetts, for example, one in 1000 people died of diphtheria each year, but four times as many died of tuberculosis. No really effective treatment for tuberculosis became available until the 1950s, and immunization was never adopted in the United States on a large scale. Yet the mortality went steadily downwards during the nineteenth century. It is not clear when this trend started; rates of 500 per 100,000 were not uncommon at the beginning of the nineteenth century, and so the decline was probably well underway by the time that the statistics were collected that are shown in Figure 8. The change could hardly have been due to any deliberate attempt at prevention, because the disease had been thought to be hereditary. Although Villemin showed, in France in 1865, that tuberculosis was transmittable to rabbits, his experiments seem not to have been believed, and it was only when Koch isolated the bacterium, in 1882, that the contagiousness of tuberculosis became widely known. By then the death rate had already dropped by a third or more.

Tuberculosis is a relentless indicator of social conditions. We can see this in the way the privations caused by World Wars I and II temporarily raised the mortality of the civilian population; in each war about 15,000 more people died from tuberculosis in Britain than would have been expected from the rates in the years either side of the two wars; and Vienna and Budapest, during World War I, again achieved annual death rates of about 600 per 100,000. So we should be looking for possible social explanations for the drop in mortality in the nineteenth century. Various ideas have been proposed – for example, an increase in resistance of the population (as the gradual epidemic of tuberculosis, brought about by urbanization, gained momentum and then receded) (29), or an improvement in nutrition (due to new crops and to advances in agriculture) (18), or an increase in real wages (due to the Industrial Revolution) (14,30), or the efforts to improve people's living conditions (brought about by publication of the very statistics we are discussing). Apart from the first strictly biological explanation (which is largely supposition), these various underlying changes are known to have taken place and each of them was in some sense, directly or indirectly, a product of the philosophical and technological revolutions of the eighteenth and nineteenth centuries.

If statistics on mortality are a fair index of the human condition, it seems that the fortunes of the masses were steadily improving in the second half of the nineteenth century, rather than going continuously downhill in the way Karl Marx predicted. (Engels first visited England in1842 and, stimulated by what he saw in the factories of Manchester,

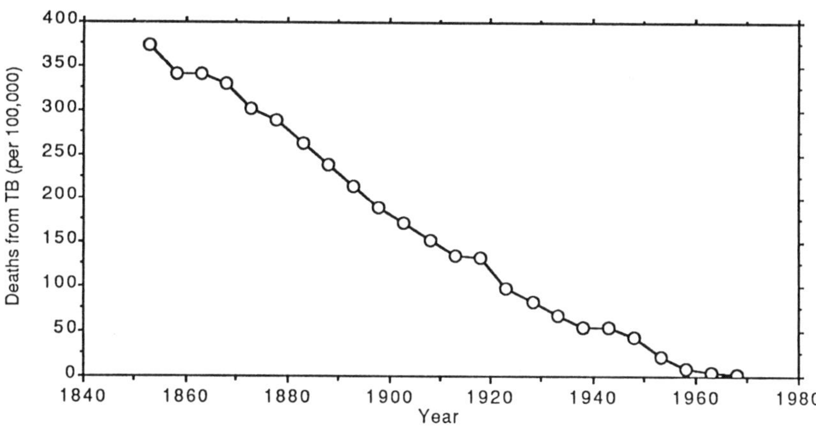

Figure 8. The change in the number of deaths each year from tuberculosis in England and Wales since 1853 (the death rates have been standardized to the age/sex distribution of the population in 1950).

wrote his famous book, *Die Lage der arbeitenden Klasse in England* (The condition of the working class in England), published in 1845. The material for the book was derived, for the most part, from the many official studies on the social conditions in England and Scotland that had been published in the previous fifteen years. But neither he nor Marx (who was strongly influenced by Engels' book) seemed to have realized that this sudden flood of reports was itself a sign that the capitalist world was about to embark on a gradual social revolution.)

Looking at the smooth decline in mortality from tuberculosis shown in Figure 8, it is tempting to say (as others have done) that the discoveries of the 1880s and 1890s had absolutely no impact on events. Yet when we read the annual reports of local authorities such as the Boards of Health of Massachusetts and New York, it is hard to believe that science was not making a contribution. Within one year of Koch's discovery of *Mycobacterium tuberculosis*, the Massachusetts Board had started on its campaign to eradicate bovine tuberculosis, and New York had made consumption a notifiable disease (though it was not compulsorily notifiable until three years later). Interestingly, in some cities the medical profession resisted the idea that tuberculosis was contagious, because they felt that the principle of notifiability was an infringement of the delicately lucrative relationship between physicians and their patients; thus they complained that the New York Board was "not only, by means of alarming bacteriological edicts, directly interfering with the physician in the diagnosis of the patient, but in the end, by the creation of a public suspicion of his ignorance, possibly depriving him of one of the means of legitimate livelihood."

In many ways, the campaign against tuberculosis was like the present drive against cancer. For it involved a nation-wide attempt to achieve earlier diagnosis (by chest x-rays, and testing for hypersensitivity to tuberculin) plus an expensive outlay for special hospitals (sanatoria) where patients could undergo prolonged treatment. Even in retrospect, the results are just as difficult to judge as the results of the war against cancer. Part of the difficulty is that we can view any medical advance or social reform in several different ways, depending on where we ourselves stand with respect to the change. For the average citizen, the drop in tuberculosis death rate from 350 to 250 per 100,000 in England between 1860 and 1885 conferred exactly the same absolute benefit as the drop from 250 to 150 that occurred over the next 25 years; each of them lowered the probability of dying in any one year by exactly 0.001. For those who have invented or implemented a new way of curing or preventing some disease, part of the measure of success should be the factor by which their discovery has lowered incidence or mortality, rather than the absolute number of people saved from sickness or death; thus rival claims for success in the war against tuberculosis (or cancer or heart disease) might best be judged by looking at changes in morbidity or mortality on a logarithmic scale. Last but not least, for those who know that they have a potentially fatal disease, the important statistic is simply the current fatality of their disease; this is a single point on a curve and so its value is not coloured by choice of scales.

The modern period in the campaign against tuberculosis in the U.S. started in 1930, when annual deaths were running at 70% of the rate of diagnosis of new cases (i.e., about two-thirds of all patients were eventually dying of their disease). This was the time when mass screening by chest x-ray came increasingly into play, and that was presumably why the recorded incidence of new cases now started to go up, rather than steadily down. These extra cases were apparently not contributing to mortality, because the death rate continued on its gradual decline until some time in the late 1940s, at which point it dropped away more steeply as antibiotics became available for the treatment of tuberculosis. Before this time, however, the annual mortality had already dropped from 400 to 30 per 100,000. Thus the invention of an effective treatment did not arrive until more than 90% of the mortality had already been avoided by other means.

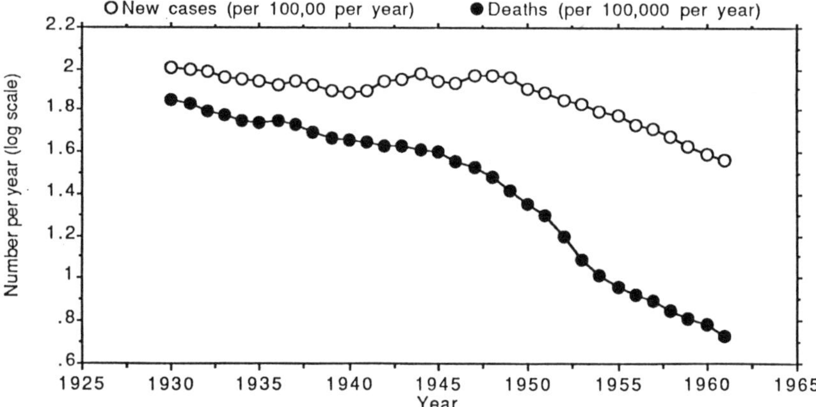

Figure 9. The relation between the rate of notification of new cases of tuberculosis and the death rate from tuberculosis in the United States during the period when treatment with antibiotics became available (streptomycin was first introduced in 1947 and isoniazid in 1952).

Although tuberculosis and cancer may seem at first sight to have little in common, the sequence of events shown in Figure 9 may have been a foretaste of what is now happening for certain cancers. In North America the mortality from cervical cancer has been going steadily downwards for 50 years (over much of this time at a rate, like tuberculosis, of about 5% per year), whereas the apparent incidence of pre-cancerous conditions of the cervix has gone up in the last 20 years as more and more women are screened by cervical smears; for much the same reason, the incidence of conditions that are thought to be early stages in the development of breast cancer gives the appearance of having increased, whereas the mortality from breast cancer is staying level or may even have started downwards. Actually, the similarity extends also to changes in age distribution. As the mortality from tuberculosis went down and a generation came along who had grown up in an environment that was essentially free of tubercle bacilli, the disease changed from being mainly a disease of adolescents to being commonest in old age (i.e., among those who dated back to the previous era). This same change is now being seen in the overall mortality from non-respiratory cancers (we have to put to one side all respiratory cancers because these depend chiefly on the energy and effectiveness of the cigarette companies). For the non-respiratory cancers, mortality has stayed approximately constant for the oldest age groups, but it is going down significantly in middle

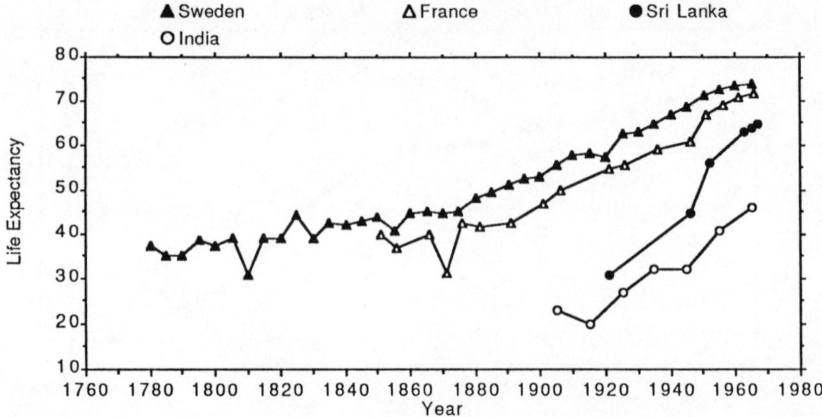

Figure 10. The recent change in life expectancy in Sweden, France, Sri Lanka, and India.

age and quite rapidly for people under 40. This analogy is very encouraging; perhaps the steady improvement in living conditions, diet, and environment that has occurred in the industrialized nations of the world during the past 200 years has not only protected us from the more lethal infectious diseases but will eventually extend to protecting us from many forms of cancer.

The revolution in mortality that started among the wealthiest inhabitants of the wealthiest countries some 250 years ago (Fig. 3), has not been confined to industrialized nations. To see what has happened on a world-wide level, we should look at both the highly developed and the less developed nations. Sweden was the first country to collect proper statistics and, perhaps for this reason, it was some ten years ahead of the other European countries in raising life expectancy. But now the process has spread throughout the world and the pace has accelerated. Sri Lanka and India, for example, have achieved more in one generation than Sweden achieved in 100 years (Figure 10).

The Future

The history of human disease has to be based almost entirely on what we know about the changes in mortality and life expectancy: illness and suffering do not lend themselves to hard statistics, whereas births and deaths can be counted. To learn about the way diseases have been conquered in the past we have, therefore, to look at mortality. From this study we see that the major lethal diseases were conquered not so much by discovering how to treat them as by prevention. For example, although we rightly admire the discoverers of the antibiotics, we should not forget that pencillin was discovered at about the time that life expectancy in Western nations had already reached the biblical limit of three score years and ten.

The attack on mortality began at the start of the nineteenth century, at a time of revolution and reform, and greatly accelerated when the causes of many diseases were discovered at the end of the century. Even in the twentieth century, the greatest improvements are still being achieved by prevention rather than treatment. Part of our difficulty in accepting this conclusion lies in our attitudes and beliefs about the practice of medicine. We tend to think that the typical patient is someone whose life is being saved, whereas this is actually the exception rather than the rule; most patients, even those in hospitals, are receiving what might be called minor repairs. Most treatments are concerned with curtailing illness rather than holding back death, and that is perhaps why the force of mortality in the developed nations of the world bears no strong relation to the number of doctors in each country or their salaries (indeed, infant mortality actually tends to go up rather than down as the density of doctors increases (31,32)). The great achievement is that the streets of most great cities are no longer filled with the maimed and the halt and the blind. We now consider it our right to live into old age, free from the misery of chronic illness.

In this discussion of mortality I have left out one of the most important sources of premature death, namely war. But it seems proper, in the twentieth century, to discuss war as if it were just another problem in public health. For this purpose, we can take the statistics for almost any European country. Figure 11 compares (a) the calculated survival of the children born in France in 1895, assuming that no further improvements in life expectancy occurred after that year, and (b) the actual survival of these children (33). We see that life expectancy has been increasing, because the female children have lived much longer than expected. The males, however, have survived much less well than expected, because one-third of them were killed in World War I. For this group of males, all the advances in medicine and public health of the twentieth century were not sufficient to compensate them for the losses they suffered in the war.

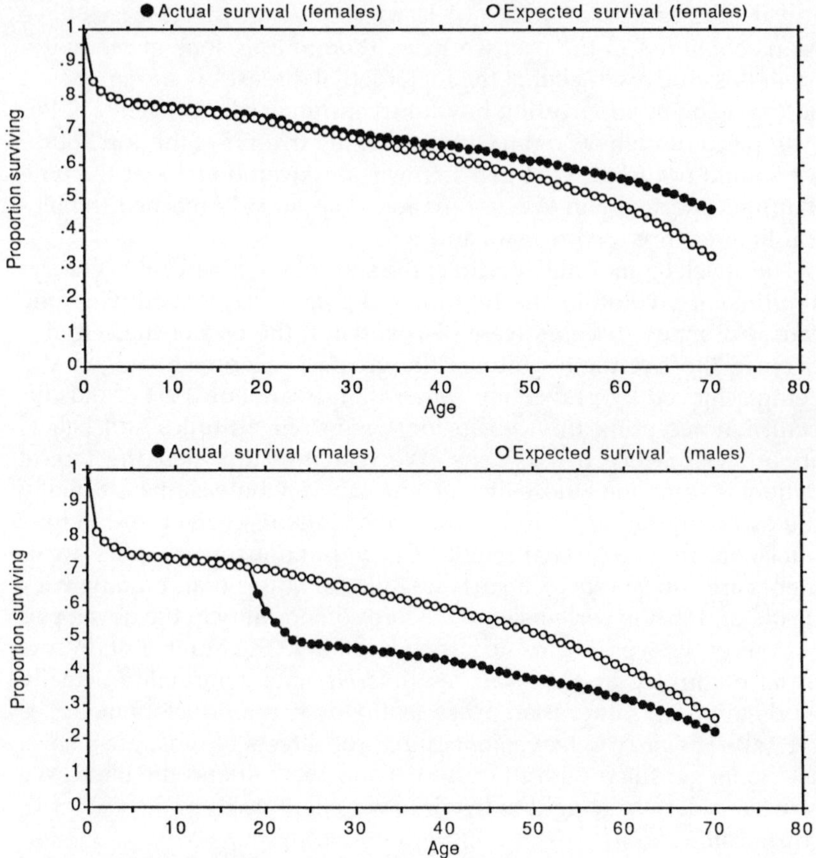

Figure 11. The *actual survival* of the cohort of (a) female and (b) male infants born in France at the very end of the nineteenth century, compared with the *expected survival* that might have been predicted for them, knowing the age-specific mortality rates obtaining in France at the time of their birth.

Early in the history of public health, in the 1860s, the newly formed New York Board of Health wrote the following words in its second annual report: "The health department of a great commercial district which encounters no obstacles and meets with no opposition, may safely be declared unworthy of public confidence; for no sanitary measures, however simple, can be enforced without compelling individuals to yield something to the general welfare" (34).

These words were written about the politics of health, but surely apply just as well to the politics of peace.

REFERENCES

This article was first published in German in *Mannheimer Forum* 85/86.

1 Halley E. An estimate of the degrees of the mortality of mankind, drawn from curious tables of the births and funerals at the city of Breslau; with an attempt to ascertain the price of annuities upon lives. Phil Trans 1693;17:596–610. Rpt in: Smith D, Keyfitz N, eds. *Mathematical demography: selected papers*. Berlin: Springer-Verlag, 1977.

2 Acsadi GY, Nemeskeri J. *History of human life span and mortality*. Budapest: Akadémiai Kiadó, 1970.

3 Howell N. *Demography of the Dobe !Kung*. New York: Academic Press, 1979.

4 Dumond ED. The limitation of human population: a natural history. *Science* 1975;187:713–721.

5 Frisch RE. Population, food intake, and fertility. *Science* 1978;199:22–30.

6 McEvedy C, Jones R. *Atlas of world population history*. London: Penguin Books, 1978.

7 Boserup E. *Population and technological change: a study of long-term trends*. Chicago: University of Chicago Press, 1981.

8 McNeill WH. *Plagues and peoples*. Garden City, NY: Anchor Press/Doubleday, 1976.

9 Black FL. Measles endemicity in insular populations: critical community size and its evolutionary implication. *J Theoret Biol* 1966;11:207–211.

10 MacDonell WR. On the expectation of life in ancient Rome, and in the provinces of Hispania and Lusitania, and Africa. *Biometrika* 1913;9:366–380.

11 Graunt J. *Natural and political observations mentioned in a following index, and made upon the Bills of Mortality. With reference to the government, religion, trade, growth, ayre, diseases, and the several changes of the said city.* 1662; rpt. New York: Arno Press, 1975.

12 Hollingsworth TH. The demography of the British peerage. *Popul Studies Suppl* 1965;18(2).

13 Peller S. Births and deaths among Europe's ruling families since 1500. In: Glass DV, Eversley DEC, eds. *Population in history*. Chicago: Aldine Publishing, 1965.

14 Wrigley EA, Schofield RS. *The population history of England, 1541–1871: a reconstruction*. Cambridge, MA: Harvard University Press, 1981.

15 Black D, Morris JN, Smith C, Townsend P. *Inequalities in health*. London: Penguin Books, 1982.

16 Kitagawa EM, Hauser PM. *Differential mortality in the United States: a study in socioeconomic epidemiology*. Cambridge, MA: Harvard University Press, 1973.

17 Razell PE. Edward Jenner: the history of a medical myth. *Med Hist* 1965;9:216–229.
18 McKeown T, Brown RG, Record RG. An interpretation of the modern rise of population in Europe. *Popul Stud* 1972;26:345–382.
19 Razzell PE. "An interpretation of the modern rise of population in Europe" – a critique. *Popul Stud* 1974;28:5–17.
20 Braudel F. *Capitalism and material life, 1400–1800*. New York: Harper and Row, 1974.
21 Durand JD. Historical estimates of world population: an evaluation. *Popul and Devel Rev* 1977;3:253–296.
22 Farr W. *Vital statistics: a memorial volume of selections from the reports and writings of William Farr*. The History of Medicine Series, no. 46. Metuchen, NJ: Scarecrow Press, 1975.
23 Coleman W. *Death is a social disease: public health and political economy in early industrial France*. Madison, WI: University of Wisconsin Press, 1982.
24 Roberts GW. A life table for a West Indian slave population. *Popul Stud* 1952; 5:238–243.
25 Ackernecht EH. Anticontagionism between 1821 and 1867. *Bull Hist Med* 1948;22:562–593.
26 Tesh S. Political ideology and public health in the nineteenth century. *Intl J Health Serv* 1982;12:321–342.
27 Shrady GF, ed. The Health Board and Compulsory Reports – editorial. *Medical Record* 27 Feb 1897:305–306.
28 Burnet FM. Bacteriophage and cognate phenomena. In: *A system of bacteriology in relation to medicine*, Vol. 7. London: HMSO, 1930:463–509.
29 Burnet FM. The natural history of tuberculosis. *Med J Austral* 1948;1:57–63.
30 Hollingsworth TH. Book review of Wrigley EA, Schofield RS, The population history of England, 1541–1871: a reconstruction, London: Edward Arnold, 1981. In: *Popul Stud* 1982;36:495–499.
31 Keyfitz N, Flieger W. *World population: an analysis of vital data*. Chicago: University of Chicago Press, 1968.
32 *World population year*. Committee for International Cooperation in National Research in Demography (CICRED) Series. World Health Organization, 1974.
33 Vallin J. *La mortalité par génération en France, depuis 1899*. Paris: Presses Universitaires de France, 1973.
34 Duffy J. *A history of public health in New York City, 1866–1966*. New York: Russell Sage Foundation, 1974.

Index

Adipocytes, 121–124
Aging: economic and social changes, 157; osteoporosis, 191; physiological changes, 156; psychological changes, 156–157. *See also* Elderly
Agriculture, implications of dietary guidelines for, 268–282
Alcohol, 50–51, 176–186; and hypertension, 99
Alcoholics, treatment of, 185
American Health Foundation, food plan, 151
Ames test, 209
Amines, heterocyclic, in cooked food, 207–221
Amino acids: and kidney function, 132–133; metabolism, 130–131
Apolipoprotein E, 26–27
Aspartame, in diabetic diet, 114
Atherosclerosis, 73–75

Bioenergetics, and obesity, 124–125
Blood Pressure. *See* Hypertension
Bone loss. *See* Osteoporosis
Bone mass, 195–197
Breast cancer, 147, 243–247

Caffeine, and hypertension, 99
Calcium: and hypertension, 97–98; fortified food products, 285; requirements by the elderly, 161; requirements in osteoporosis, 193–197; urinary excretion, 199
Calories, 50; and cancer, 250–254; and hypertension, 93–95; in the elderly, 158–160
Cancer, 207–254; breast, 147, 243–247; calories and, 250–254; case-control studies, 245–246; cohort studies, 246–247; dietary fat and, 145–148, 252; micronutrients, 148; mortality from, 230–233, 238–241, 339; prevention, 221–222; risk factors, 234; stomach, 229–241
Carbohydrate, dietary, 47–49, 111–112
Carcinogens, formed during cooking, 207–221
Cardiovascular disease, 19–82. *See also* Heart disease
Case-control studies of cancer, 245–246
Children, blood cholesterol levels, 149
Cholera, 326–333
Cholesterol: blood, 149–150; dietary, 36–40, 57; lipoprotein, 20–29, 39–45, 95; mass screening for, 150; plasma, 37–46, 74–81; serum, 22, 87, 143–144
Cholesterol-saturated fat index, 53–56
Chylomicrons, 21–22
Cohort studies of cancer, 246–247
Colon cancer, 243–247
Committee on Medical Aspects of Food Policy (COMA), 8–9
Cooked foods, carcinogens in, 209, 219

Coronary heart disease: epidemiological studies, 20–21; genetic disorders, 25–27; intervention studies, 27–28; population and individual approaches to, 28–30; prevention and treatment by diet, 33–66; prevention trials, 73–82, 85–88; risk factors, 33–34

Diabetes, 103–117
Diet: low-fat, high-carbohydrate, 48, 54–65; Mediterranean, 42–43; palaeolithic, 97, 141
Dietary goals, 262–263
Dietary guidelines: European policy, 3–15; financial consequences of, 275–279; implications for agriculture, 268–282; steps by government agencies, 303–305; steps for dietitians/public health nutritionists, 287–290; steps for nutrition educators, 292–297; steps for the food industry, 284–286; for whole populations versus high risk populations, 259–266
Dietary recommendations: application of, 148–151; for diabetes, 105–106; for hypertensives, 100–101
Dietitians, and dietary guidelines, 287–290
Diphtheria, 333–335
Drugs, cholesterol lowering, 76–81

Elderly, nutritional assessment, 157–167. *See also* Aging
Endocrine factors affecting osteoporosis, 191–192
Energy. *See* Calories
Exercise: and osteoporosis, 192; as therapy for diabetes, 115–116

Familial hypercholesterolemia, 25–26, 38, 52–53
Fat, dietary: and cancer, 145–148, 244–247, 250–253; effects on plasma lipids and lipoproteins, 40–46; reduction, 86–87; reduction by hypertensives, 95; saturated, index, 53–56; sources of, 57; and thrombosis, 46–47
Fat-modified menus, 271–279
Fatty acids: medium-chain, 41; monounsaturated, 42–43; polyunsaturated omega-3, 43–47, 115; polyunsaturated omega-6, 43–47; saturated, 41–42, 46
Fibre, dietary, 49; deleterious effects of, 110; effects on cancer, 245–247; in diabetes, 107–109
Fibre modified menus, 271–279
Fish Oil, 44–45
Food policy: in Britain, 4–10; in Europe, 10–15
Food industry, and dietary guidelines, 284–286
Fructose, in diabetic diet, 113–114

Genetic disorders of plasma lipoproteins, 25–27
Glucose, blood, 107–108
Glycaemic index, 111–112

Health: education programs, 148–149; maintenance, 141–152
Heart disease, 143–145. *See also* Cardiovascular disease
Hypercholesterolemia, familial, 25–26, 38, 52–53
Hypertension, 87, 93–101, 235, 237, 286; dietary recommendations, 100–101

Industrial revolution, 324–326
Insulin, 93, 95, 103–104, 125–126
Intervention trials, 27–28. *See also* Prevention trials
Intestinal malabsorption, related to alcohol, 179–180
Iron, status of elderly, 161–164

Joint Advisory Committee on Nutrition Education (JACNE) 9

Keto acid therapy of uremia, 132–134
Kidney disease, 130–136

LDL receptors, 23–27
Lecithin, 52
Life expectancy, 321, 340; measurement of, 310–314
Life tables, 310–315, 317, 324, 325
Lipid metabolic pathways, 76–77
Lipids, plasma, effects of dietary fats on, 40–46
Lipoprotein lipase, 22–23, 122–123
Lipoproteins, 20–30, 33, 75–77; effects of dietary cholesterol on, 36–40; effects of dietary fat on, 40–46; genetic disorders of, 25–27; high density, 20–21; low density, 20–28; very low density, 21–28

Meal pattern, effects on obesity, 121–122

Menu modification, 271–279
Minerals, 52
Mortality: history of, 309–342; stomach cancer, 230–233, 238–241; stroke, 230–233, 238–240
Mutagens, formed during cooking, 207–221

National Advisory Committee on Nutrition Education (NACNE) 6–8
Nutrient goals, European, 14
Nutrition, in the elderly, 158–168
Nutrition educators, and dietary guidelines, 292–297
Nutritionists, public health, and dietary guidelines, 287–290

Obesity, 121–127
Osteoporosis, 188–201; factors affecting, 191–192

P/S value, 46
Paleolithic man, diet of, 97, 141
Phosphate, dietary, and osteoporosis, 199–200
Physicians, role in nutrition, diet, and health, 298–302
Potassium, and hypertension, 97
Preadipocytes, 123–124
Protein, dietary: and cardiovascular disease, 49–50; and diabetes, 114–115; and kidney disease, 131–132; and osteoporosis, 199–200; in the elderly, 160
Public health and mortality, 307–342
Public health policy, 260–262

Renal: function, 114; insufficiency, 134–136. *See also* Kidney disease

Salt, 229–241
Seventh-Day Adventists, 142, 245–246
Sodium, and hypertension, 95–96, 286
Stomach cancer, 229–241; etiology of, 237; risk factors for, 234
Stroke, 229–241; risk factors for, 234
Sucrose, 48–49
Sweetners, in diabetic diet, 112–114

Tarahumara Indians, 142–143
Thermogenesis, diet-induced, 125–126
Thrombosis, and dietary fat, 46–47
Thyroid hormone, 125
Triglycerides, 21, 126; medium-chain, 41
Tuberculosis, 335–339
Tumours, 250–251. *See also* Cancer

Uremia, keto acid therapy, 132–134

Vitamin D, and osteoporosis, 197–199
Vitamin E, as antioxident, 165
Vitamins, 52; effects of alcohol in, 180–185; in the elderly, 164–167

Watanabe rabbits, 25–26
World Health Organization (WHO), 11–12

RA
784
.D43

1989